THE RATIONAL USE OF ADVANCED MEDICAL TECHNOLOGY WITH THE ELDERLY

Freddy Homburger, MD, is Research Professor of Pathology at the Boston University School of Medicine. He was one of the early cancer chemotherapists at Memorial Hospital in New York City and for 10 years founded and directed the Cancer Research Unit of the Tufts University School of Medicine. He became a toxicologist and directed the Bio-Research Institute in Cambridge, Massachusetts from 1957 to 1984.

Dr. Homburger's book, *Medical Care of the Aged and Chronically Ill*, had three editions. He edited 33 volumes of a series, *Progress in Experimental Tumor Research*, for S. Kager SA of Basel, Switzerland.

THE RATIONAL USE OF ADVANCED MEDICAL TECHNOLOGY WITH THE ELDERLY

Freddy Homburger, MD

Editor

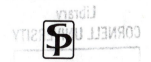

Springer Publishing Company
New York

Springer Publishing Company, Inc.
536 Broadway
New York, NY 10012

94 95 96 97 98 / 5 4 3 2 1

Library of Congress Cataloging-in-Publication Data

The rational use of advanced medical technology with the elderly /
  Freddy Homburger, editor.
     p. cm.
  Includes bibliographical references and index.
  ISBN 0–8261–8410–3
  1. Geriatrics—Technological innovations. I. Homburger, Freddy.
  [DNLM: 1. Health Services for the Aged. 2. Technology, Medical.
WT 30 R236 1994]
RC952.5.R27 1994
618.97—dc20
DNLM/DLC
for Library of Congress   94–1496
                                                 CIP

Printed in the United States of America

Chapter 6 is adapted from the article, "Decision-Making Regarding
the Initiation of Tube Feedings in the Severely Demented Elderly: A
Review" by R.M. Meyers and M.A. Grodin, originally published in the
Journal of the American Geriatrics Society, volume 39, number 5,
pages 526–531, © 1991 Williams & Wilkins.

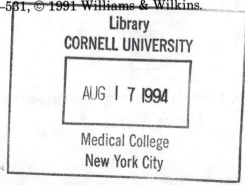

Contents

Contributors   *vii*

Foreword by Knight Steel, M.D.   *xi*

Introduction   *xv*

Chapter 1   Assessment of Geriatric Patients   1
                P. P. Barry, MD

Chapter 2   Uses and Misuses of Laboratory Tests in the
                Aged   10
                L. D. Berman, MD

Chapter 3   Prophylactic (Preventive) Therapies in Old
                Age   44
                L. J. Kerzner, MD, and S. Van B. Wilking,
                MD

Chapter 4   Defensive Medicine in Geriatric Practice   67
                M. B. Kapp, MD, JD, MPH

Chapter 5   The Role of the Physician in Decisions to
                Use or Forgo Life-Sustaining Technologies   75
                L. O'Donnell, EdD, and
                M. Z. Solomon, EdD

Chapter 6   The Rational Use of Tube Feeding in
                 Elderly Long-Term Patients   96
                 R. M. Meyers, MD, MPH, and
                 M. A. Grodin, MD

Chapter 7   Advanced Diagnostic Technology in
                 Cardiovascular Disease of the Aged   111
                 K. E. Fleischmann, MD, and R. T. Lee, MD

Chapter 8   Cardiovascular Surgery in the Elderly   132
                 S. F. Aranki, MD

Chapter 9   Diagnostic Tests in the Elderly with
                 Neurological Disorders   146
                 P. A. Cyrus, MD, J. Jankowiak, MD, and
                 R. G. Feldman, MD

Chapter 10   Dialysis in the Geriatric Population   168
                 T. I. Steinman, MD

Chapter 11   Joint Replacement in the Aged   187
                 I. G. Yablon, MD, and D. J. Covall, MD

Chapter 12   Laparoscopic Surgery in the Aged   205
                 D. Birkett, MD

Chapter 13   Problems and Opportunities for the
                 Diagnosis and Treatment of Prostatic
                 Cancer   214
                 M. Grégoire, MD, M. A. O'Donnell, MD, and
                 W. C. DeWolf, MD

Chapter 14   Advanced Cancer Treatment of the Elderly   236
                 W. L. Akerley, III, MD, and P. Calabresi, MD

Chapter 15   The Progress and Promise of Effectiveness
                 Research in Aged Patients   250
                 C. W. Maklan, MPH, PhD

Index   271

Contributors

Wallace L. Akerley, III, MD
Department of Medical
   Oncology
Rhode Island Hospital
Providence, RI 02903

Sary F. Aranki, MD
Division of Cardiac Surgery
Brigham and Women's
   Hospital
Boston, MA 02115

Patricia P. Barry, MD
Geriatrics Section
Boston University School of
   Medicine
Boston, MA 02118

Leonard D. Berman, MD
Jewish Memorial Hospital
Boston, MA 02119

Desmond Birkett, MD
Department of Surgery
University Hospital
Boston, MA 02118

Paul Calabresi, MD
Department of Medicine
Rhode Island Hospital
Providence, RI 02903

David J. Covall, MD
Department of Orthopaedic
   Surgery
Boston University Medical
   Center
Boston, MA 02118

Pamela A. Cyrus, MD
Department of Neurology
Boston University School of
   Medicine
Boston, MA 02118

William C. DeWolf, MD
Urologist-in-Chief
Beth Israel Hospital
Boston, MA 02115

Robert G. Feldman, MD
Department of Neurology
Boston University School of
  Medicine
Boston, MA 02118

Kirsten E. Fleischmann, MD
Brigham and Women's
  Hospital
Boston, MA 02115

Mireille Grégoire, MD
Service d'urologie
Hôtel-Dieu de Québec
Québec, Canada G1R 2J6

Michael A. Grodin, MD
Health Law Department
School of Public Health
Boston University
Boston, MA 02118

Janet Jankowiak, MD
Department of Neurology
Boston University School of
  Medicine
Boston, MA 02118

**Marshall B. Kapp, MD, JD,
  MPH**
Professor, Department of
  Community Health
Director, Office of Geriatric
  Medicine and Gerontology
Wright State University School
  of Medicine
Dayton, OH 45401

Lawrence J. Kerzner, MD
The Jewish Memorial Hospital
  and Rehabilitation Center
Boston, MA 02119

Richard T. Lee, MD
Noninvasive Cardiac
  Laboratory
Cardiovascular Division
Brigham and Women's
  Hospital
Boston, MA 02115

**Claire W. Maklan, MPH,
  PhD**
Agency for Health Care Policy
  and Research
Rockville, MD 20852

**Roberta M. Meyers, MD,
  MPH**
Department of Medicine
Division of Geriatric Medicine
Minneapolis, MN 55415

Lydia O'Donnell, EdD
Education Development Center
Newton, MA 02160

Michael A. O'Donnell, MD
Department of Urology
Beth Israel Hospital
Boston, MA 02215

Mildred Z. Solomon, EdD
Education Development Center
Newton, MA 02160

Knight Steel, MD
World Organization for Care in
  the Home and Hospital
Washington, DC 20002

Theodore I. Steinman, MD
Director, Dialysis Unit
Beth Israel Hospital
Boston, MA 02115

Spencer Van B. Wilking, MD
Geriatrics Section
Boston University School of
  Medicine
Boston, MA 02118

Isadore G. Yablon, MD
Department of Orthopaedic
  Surgery
Boston University Medical
  Center
Boston, MA 02118

Foreword

The single greatest achievement of humankind has been the extraordinary increase in longevity that has taken place in the 20th century. From the dawn of man until the year 1900 the average life expectancy has increased by about 25 years. A person born in the United States in 1900 had a life expectancy of 47 years. In the years since then—less than 100 years—an additional 30 years has been added to that life expectancy. In the United States and throughout the Western world this has been brought about mostly by improvements in public health and the control of infectious diseases. This phenomenon has taken place in all developed countries, and is occurring in most developing countries as well. For example, in China, it is estimated that there will be 300 million Chinese aged 60 years and over by the year 2025.

A result of this increased life expectancy is that the characteristics of the population that medicine is serving are strikingly different today when compared with those of 20 or 30 years ago. Age tends to limit, in various degrees, the reserve of most physiological systems. In addition, the majority of persons now enter old age with a host of chronic conditions. These conditions, which are accumulated throughout life, frequently diminish functional capabilities. This elderly segment of the population, representing about 12 percent of the total, accounts for as many as half of all hospital-bed-occupancy days in some hospitals.

Each patient, whether in the hospital or the outpatient setting, rep-

---

The opinions expressed in this article are those of the author and do not necessarily reflect those of the World Health Organization.

resents a unique diagnostic and management problem. Superimposed on the patient's present illnesses or crises are the debilitating changes brought about by aging and chronic disease. Over the past 15 or 20 years a wide array of sophisticated technology has been invented both for diagnostic and therapeutic purposes. An increasing amount of skill is required from both the specialist and the primary-care physician to determine the most appropriate time and under what circumstances to apply this technology. Not only clinicians, but health-care planners and the elderly themselves are very concerned about which diagnostic and therapeutic instruments to use and when to do so. Too often decisions may be made without all available scientific knowledge and, on occasion, are arrived at in response to unsound or irrelevant considerations.

The need for this book emanated from this state of affairs. It seems to be not only timely but essential to try to provide doctors with the scientific information that would help them choose most appropriately just when to employ a certain high-tech procedure. No volume could address all clinical situations; however, this book presents the benefits and risks of many commonly used procedures used in the care of the elderly. Special attention should be given to the chapter by Dr. Patricia Barry on the assessment of geriatric patients, for this—to a great measure—is how the information unique to the patient is gathered. Without these data the proper decisions certainly cannot be made. I would also highlight the chapter by Dr. Lawrence Kerzner on the prophylactic and preventive therapies, for the institution of such measures will surely limit the need for high-tech interventions at a later time. And although I would advise the reader that this volume does *not* substitute for clinical judgment (the distinction between the care of the individual and group studies must always be clear, Diamond & Denton, 1993), nonetheless, I earnestly believe this book makes it possible for that judgment to be improved.

All of us, as we age, wish to have a knowledgeable, thoughtful, and caring doctor—one who can assess our very specific needs and then utilize the vast array of technological services now available to address them in the most effective and human manner possible.

KNIGHT STEEL, MD
Chief, Health of the Elderly Program
World Health Organization

REFERENCE

Diamond, G. A., & Denton, T. A. (1993). Alternative perspectives on the biased foundations of medical technology assessment. *Ann Int Med, 118,* 455–464.

Introduction

Before leaving his Professorship in Geriatrics at Boston University to become Chief, Health of the Elderly Program of the World Health Organization in Geneva, Switzerland, Knight Steel shared with us his idea of the need of developing a manual of guidelines on the rational use of advanced diagnostic and therapeutic medical technology with the elderly. Only a short time ago decisions as to what measures to apply in any given case of disease were quite straightforward, regardless of the age of the patient. The diagnostic and therapeutic tools available were relatively safe and unlikely to be harmful, just as their effectiveness often was limited. Now the diagnostic and therapeutic armamentarium is replete with two-edged swords that are potentially as effective as they are dangerous and costly.

Physicians often find themselves in ethical and scientific quandaries. Should technology that prolongs life be used? Does the risk of a procedure outweigh its potential benefit? Is an expensive diagnostic test likely to yield data to benefit the patient? Is it worth taking the risk of an invasive procedure?—of highly toxic chemotherapy? Given the rapid multiplication of highly sophisticated tests and therapies, teaching has not kept up with developments. This volume intends to narrow this gap and to provide a survey of actual knowledge on the effectiveness and drawbacks of advanced diagnostic and therapeutic technologies, with special emphasis on their use in aged patients. Our goal is to follow as closely as possible the "weighing of the relevant options resulting from the objective assessment of benefits, risks and costs of diagnostic tests, drugs and other therapeutic approaches," as recently and succinctly stated by J. P. Kassirer (1991):

> Benefits are assessed in terms of the accuracy of tests and the efficacy of treatments, and risks in terms of morbidity and mortality. When one choice yields benefits that clearly outweigh the risks we embrace it, and when the reverse obtains we reject it. When the comparison of benefits and risks fails to yield an unambiguous choice, we develop either a formal or an informal benchmark, or threshold, based on the benefits and risks, that defines how a procedure or treatment should be used. We would use the procedure of treatment when out suspicion of a certain disease exceeds this threshold, and we would avoid it when it falls short of the threshold.

In addition, close attention will be paid to the evaluation of the patient to whom procedures may or may not be applied, based on age and medical condition, what is the likely life expectancy, what kind of quality of life may be expected with or without the contemplated procedure, what are the patient's capabilities to understand the options, and what are the patient's wishes or those of health-care proxies? The task we have set ourselves is a complex and difficult one and may raise some questions to which there are as yet no answers. No single person can adequately cover this subject; this volume is therefore a multiauthor endeavor. It is intended to facilitate some decisions and to answer some questions—but above all, to stimulate interest and concern in a crucial area of medicine: to find a way through the maze of technical innovation to do what is best for the patient.

F.H.

REFERENCE

Kassirer, J. P. (1991). Editorial. *New England Journal of Medicine*, 325(23), 1647–1649.

Chapter One

Assessment of Geriatric Patients

Patricia P. Barry

Although the majority of elderly persons are in good health, a significant number suffer from multiple illnesses and disabilities. Since physical, mental, and social aspects of illness are closely interrelated, the diagnosis-oriented approach has significant limitations and may not correlate well with overall health and functional status. To evaluate and plan appropriately for the long-term health care of such frail persons, information must be obtained and organized regarding five basic domains: performance of activities of daily living (ADLs), physical health, mental health, socioeconomic resources, and the environment. Since the interrelationship among these factors is especially important, a coordinated multidimensional, multidisciplinary approach, referred to as geriatric assessment, has evolved in order to collect such information systematically. In addition, specific instruments for geriatric assessment have been developed for use in administration, policy-making, education, research, and patient care. The focus in this chapter will be on the use of geriatric assessment in the clinical setting.

GERIATRIC MULTIDIMENSIONAL ASSESSMENT

In 1988, the National Institutes of Health sponsored the Consensus Development Conference (1988) on Geriatric Assessment Methods for Clinical Decision-making. The Consensus Statement issued by the conference noted that the goals of assessment, as listed in Table 1.1, are often interdependent so that diagnostic accuracy leads to appropriate interventions and better use of available services, re-

TABLE 1.1   Goals of Assessment

1. Improve diagnostic accuracy
2. Guide selection of interventions to restore or preserve health
3. Recommend optimal environment
4. Predict outcomes
5. Monitor clinical change

sulting in improved level of function and optimal placement. As noted in Table 1.2, geriatric assessment can (and should) be performed in many different clinical settings, both institutional and community.

The Consensus Statement points out that two aspects of geriatric assessment are particularly important. First is the need to *target assessment to those persons most likely to benefit*, especially those who are "frail" but not terminally ill; those at critical transition points, such as consideration of nursing home placement; and those at times of decline, both in health and in function (Table 1.2). Second is the need to *link assessment with care management and follow-up services* in order to implement the recommendations resulting from assessment. Geriatric assessment is thus a *process* (Table 1.3) involving referral, collection of information; and assessment, development, and implementation of a care plan, with periodic reassessment and modification of that plan.

Geriatric assessment often involves several health care professionals, including a physician, nurse, and social worker. Goals of

TABLE 1.2   Structure of Assessment

Locations
Institutional settings: hospitals (medical, psychiatric, rehabilitation), nursing
    homes
Ambulatory settings: office, clinic home
Occasions
Critical transition points:
    Actual or potential decline in health or function
    Change in living situation
    Stress
Elements
Physical health
Mental health
Social and economic status
Functional status
Environmental characteristics

TABLE 1.3 Process of Assessment

Referral: relatives, community service agencies, physicians
Assessment and development of care plan: patient, family, team (physician, nurse, social worker)
Implementation of care plan: case management
Periodic reassessment and modification of care plan

assessment should be clearly defined and instruments selected that are most likely to achieve them. Decisions regarding the choice of instruments need to consider the purpose, population, clinical setting, and method of administration. The use of valid and reliable existing instruments offers several advantages: they are more likely to be comprehensive, to allow for comparisons over time, and to enable better communication among care providers. Instruments should be objective, rather than subjective, and should have been adequately evaluated for validity (accurately reflecting the characteristic being assessed) and reliability (obtaining the same result with different measures in the absence of real change). They should be of length and complexity acceptable to both staff and frail elderly patients. The method of measurement should be clinically useful, and the instrument should be both sensitive (minimizing false negatives) and specific (minimizing false positives) for the clinical factor under consideration. Attributes being measured should be amenable to intervention and clinically important.

Although lengthy multidimensional assessment instruments may be useful for research and needs assessment for policy decisions, combinations of individual instruments targeting such important domains as mental status or ADLs may be better suited to the needs of individual patients and more appropriate to the clinical setting. In addition, numerical scores and scales, although useful in the research setting, are often less appropriate in the clinical setting than the specific characteristics of the patient's performance, such as identification of the need for evaluation of urinary incontinence or ambulatory difficulty.

Existing assessment instruments can be used for several purposes in the clinical setting. Screening instruments may be used to determine the need for more thorough evaluation of identified problems. Diagnostic instruments may reveal unsuspected illness and lead to planned interventions. Monitoring instruments may be used to assess the effectiveness of treatment or follow the progress of disease. Some instruments may even be useful in predicting outcomes. Instruments are available that are useful in the clinical setting, especially in the domains of mental and functional status.

Geriatric assessment has been utilized in inpatient units, outpatient programs, and long-term care facilities. Multidisciplinary teams are usually involved, providing examinations, identifying problems, and suggesting solutions. A case-management system should be available for follow-up care. Special programs may address specific problems, such as cognitive disorders or rehabilitation. Well-designed studies have demonstrated the value of assessment in improving diagnostic and therapeutic outcomes in settings such as geriatric inpatient and outpatient units, involving assessment by multidisciplinary teams, usually with follow up case management. Although several studies have demonstrated that geriatric assessment in the office and hospital practice of the individual physician can identify previously unsuspected problems, the impact on outcome depends on targeting appropriate patients and the ability to identify resources and services necessary for follow up care.

PHYSICAL HEALTH

The standard medical history and physical examination probably provide the most useful clinical evaluation of physical health, although they do not allow for overall measures of health status, indicators of severity, or the patient's perceptions of illness. In the elderly, extra time may be required, and the information may need to be collected over several visits. It is important to speak clearly and distinctly and to allow the patient time for a complete response. The "chief complaint" may not be a classic symptom of a specific disease but rather a vague or nonspecific problem such as fatigue or confusion. Special attention should be directed to the past medical history, which may be complex and detailed. Medications (prescription and nonprescription) are especially important in the elderly, and patients should be instructed to bring all medications with them at their appointment. Not infrequently, elderly persons may also take medication prescribed for someone else. A personal history of present and/or past use of tobacco, alcohol, or other substances should be obtained, in addition to the patient's previous employment, marital history, and living situation. During the review of systems, specific questions regarding nutrition, exercise, vision and hearing, ambulation, sexual function, sleep pattern, falls, incontinence, and immunizations should be asked.

The examiner should be familiar with the physical manifestations of normal aging. For example, obvious manifestations of aging include gray hair, wrinkles, and thinning hair. The examiner should also be aware of the shortening of stature and thinning of skin, mild kyphosis, and redistribution of fat to the abdomen and hips occur with normal aging. Presbycusis (high-frequency hearing loss) and presbyopia ("far-sightedness") are normal aging changes. Loss of vibratory sensation in the lower extremities and decreased ankle jerks are frequently found in normal elderly.

Laboratory studies should be obtained as indicated. Normal values are essentially unchanged with age, except for nonspecific elevations of the sedimentation rate and slight elevations in serum glucose (see Chapter 2).

In general, a focus on recent changes and the identification of illness that is treatable and affects function is especially useful in the evaluation of the elderly patient. In addition, the patient's values and advance directives regarding end-of-life decisions should be elicited and documented by the physician as part of the comprehensive assessment.

FUNCTION

Good medical care is an essential component of geriatric management. However, diagnosis and treatment of diseases is only the first step in helping the elderly person to achieve maximum independence and quality of life. Attention to the patient's functional status and ability to provide self-care is essential. In order to evaluate function, measurement of ADLs is necessary, including critical items of self-care: bathing, toileting, feeding, dressing, and ambulating. In community-residing elderly, assessment of instrumental activities of daily living (IADLs), which require a higher level of function, may identify impairment at an earlier stage. IADLs usually include the following: managing finances, managing medication, preparing meals, housekeeping, shopping, using a telephone, and arranging transportation. It should be noted, however, that IADLs are "biased" toward activities performed by women and thus may overestimate deficiencies in men who cannot perform meal planning, shopping, or housekeeping due to lack of familiarity with such tasks.

Although the most accurate evaluations of function probably come from direct observation, it is also possible to obtain useful information self-reported by the patient or described by the family. To determine which services are needed for assistance, it is useful to grade performance of ADLs and IADLs into three levels: (1)independent, (2) need for some assistance, and (3) unable to perform (even with assistance). Persons who need mechanical aids but do not require caregiver assistance may be considered independent.

MENTAL STATUS

Mental status tests may be used to assess both cognition and affect; some patients may require further psychiatric, neurological, or neuropsychological evaluation. Cognition includes orientation, memory, perception, judgment, and intelligence, as well as psychomotor skills. Measures of cognition are used in the clinical setting to identify cognitive impairment, such as that caused by delirium or dementia. Short tests, such as Folstein's Mini-mental State (Table 1.4) have been widely used and validated.

Affective measures usually attempt to identify depression, which is common, treatable, and an important cause of dysfunction in the elderly. Although evaluation by a skilled psychiatrist remains the "gold standard" for this diagnosis, routine use of one of several instruments is justified in patients at risk of this disorder. The Zung Self-Rating Depression Scale, the Beck Depression Inventory, and the Geriatric Depression Scale (GDS) have all been found useful in the clinical setting. Behavioral problems such as wandering, agitation, or sleep disturbance, may be an important indication for intervention.

SOCIOECONOMIC STATUS

Social measures have been developed to assess both well-being and social resources. The former has proved to be relatively difficult to assess, since concepts are not easily defined and are heavily influenced by cultural factors and individual value systems. Identification of social resources is especially important for appropriate clinical care, specifically those caregivers available to provide help and their willingness and ability to do so, the strength of interpersonal

TABLE 1.4 "Mini-mental State"

I. *ORIENTATION (Maximum Score 10)*
"What is the _____?"

	Date (1)
	Month (1)
	Day (1)
	Season (1)
	Year (1)
"What is the name of this hospital?"	Hospital (1)
"What floor are we on?"	Floor (1)
"What town (or city) are we in?"	Town/City (1)
"What county are we in?"	County (1)
"What state are we in?"	State (1)

II. *Registration (Maximum score 3)*
Say "ball," "flag," "tree" clearly and slowly, about one second for each. After you have said all 3 words, ask patient to repeat them. This determines the score (1-3). Keep repeating them (up to 6 trials) until the patient can repeat all 3 words. If all three are not learned, recall cannot be meaningfully tested.

Ball (1)
Flag (1)
Tree (1)

III. *Attention & Calculation (Maximum score 5)*
Ask the patient to begin at 100 and count backwards by 7, stopping after 5 subtractions. Score one point for each. *Or,* if the patient cannot or will not perform this task, ask him/her to spell the word "world" backwards (D,L,R,O,W). The score is one point for each correctly placed letter.

"93" (1)
"86" (1)
"79" (1)
"72" (1)
"65" (1)

_____ (5)
D L R O W

IV. *Recall (Maximum score 3)*
Ask the patient to recall the three words you previously asked him/her to remember:

"ball" (1)
"flag" (1)
"tree" (1)

V. *Language (Maximum score 9)*
Naming: Show the subject a wrist watch and a pencil and ask "What is this?" Score one point for each item.

"watch" (1)
"pencil" (1)

Repetition: Ask the patient to repeat, "No ifs, ands, or buts." Score one point if correct.

Repetition (1)

3-Stage Command: Give the subject a piece of blank paper and say, "Take the paper in your right hand, fold it in half and put it on the floor," Score one point for each action performed correctly.

Takes in rt hand (1)
Folds in half (1)
Puts on floor (1)

Reading: On a blank piece of paper, print the sentence "Close your eyes." in large letters. Ask the patient to read it and do what it says. Score if (s)he actually closes his/her eyes.

Closes eyes (1)

(continued)

TABLE 1.4 *(Continued)*

Writing: Give the patient a blank piece of paper and ask him/her to write a sentence. It must contain a subject and verb and make sense. Ignore grammar, spelling and punctuation.	Writes sentence (1)
Copying: On a clean piece of paper, draw intersecting pentagons, each side about 1 inch, and ask patient to copy it exactly as it is. All 10 angles must be present and two must intersect to score 1 point.	Draws pentagons (1)
	TOTAL SCORE (30)

relationships, and the sources of stress and support of the caregiver.

Community resources available may include services such as day care, respite care, home health care, and homemakers. Information about financial resources is necessary to determine eligibility for programs such as Medicaid and to assess the ability to pay for needed services not otherwise able to be provided.

ENVIRONMENT

Descriptions of the environment are an important part of the elderly person's assessment and include such factors as convenience, safety, and availability of services and social supports. A home visit by the physician or other health care professional may provide essential information to determine the need for specific interventions. These may include physical equipment (ramps, grab bars), special services (homemakers, meals), and increased social activity (visitors, day care). Obviously, the need for environmental intervention is largely determined by the elderly person's functional status and requirements for assistance.

CONCLUSION

The routine use of comprehensive functional assessment has been recommended in the evaluation of frail elderly patients, including all of those over 75. An efficient, short-form procedure that could be used in the office or hospital to screen for indications for more detailed investigation of functional deficits would indeed be useful, but no adequately evaluated instrument currently exists for this purpose. Clinicians should select from among existing instruments, appropriately target frail elderly, and routinely incorporate multidimensional assessment into the evaluations of such persons, with special attention to implementation of their recommendations by means of appropriate referrals and care management.

References

Applegate, W. B. Use of assessment instruments in clinical settings. *J Am Geriatr Soc, 35*: 45–50. 1987.

Applegate, W. B., Blass, J. B., & Williams, T. F. Instruments for the functional assessment of older patients. N Engl J Med, *322*: 1207–14.

Barry, P. P., & Ibarra M. Multidimensional assessment of the elderly. *Hospital Practice, 15*: 117–128. April 1990.

Consensus Development Panel (Solomon, D., Chairman), National Institutes of Health Consensus Development Conference Statement: Geriatric assessment methods for clinical decision-making. *J Am Geriatr Soc, 36*: 3422–347. 1988.

Folstein, M. F., Folstein, M. E., & McHugh, P. R. Mini-mental State: A practical method for grading the cognitive state of patients for the clinician. *J Psychiatr Res, 12*: 189–98. 1975.

Health and Public Policy Committee, American College of Physicians: Comprehensive functional assessment for elderly persons. *Ann Intern Med, 109*: 70–72. 1988.

Kane, R. A., & Kane, R. L. *Assessing the Elderly: A practical guide to measurement.* Lexington, MA: Lexington Books. 1981.

Rubenstein, L. The clinical effectiveness of multidimensional geriatric assessment. *J Am Geriatr Soc, 31*: 758–765. 1983.

Rubenstein, L. Z., Campbell, L. J., & Kane, R. L., Eds. Geriatric Assessment. *Clin Geriatr Med,* Vol 3. 1987.

Yesavage, J. A., Brink, T. L., & Rose, T. L., et al.: Development and validation of a geriatric depression scale: A preliminary report. *J Psychiatr Res, 17*: 37–49. 1982.

Chapter Two

Uses and Misuses of Laboratory Tests in the Aged

Leonard D. Berman

Over the past several decades advances in clinical laboratory medicine have occurred in the four major areas listed below.

1. The development of new tests to identify or assess the pathophysiology of disease states, those newly recognized as well as those that have preoccupied clinical medicine for quite some time.

2. The development of more advanced (usually more automated) technology to improve speed and accuracy and reduce specimen sample size. This has involved the streamlining of existing technology or, in many cases, the development of entirely new technology. In most instances this also involves reductions in expense; however, occasionally the reverse has been true.

3. Changes in the rationale and strategy for use of laboratory tests. Whereas, in the past, laboratory testing was primarily used to diagnose patients with symptomatic disease, today's clinicians largely use laboratory tests to monitor patients as to whether their disease has progressed, remained stable, or improved under therapy. They also use the laboratory to screen asymptomatic individuals in order to detect early phases of treatable disease.

4. The development of quality control of analytical processes to ensure the utmost accuracy of laboratory results. Quality control measures have included statistical evaluation techniques and

the initiation of proficiency surveys in which prepared samples are distributed to large numbers of laboratories. Results are compared, and individual laboratory performance is evaluated.

In assessing the effect of these advances on the practice of geriatric medicine, three areas will be focused upon.

1. The improvements in technology, statistical analysis, and quality control programs have all contributed to a refinement in analytical precision previously unattainable. This has resulted in a more precise definition of normal reference ranges. It has also enabled investigation as to whether reference ranges in the elderly differ from those in the general population.

2. Advances in technology have had other effects on geriatric medical practice, in addition to the improvement in test accuracy noted above, with both positive and negative aspects. Factors to be considered include expense, timeliness, specimen size, and the effect of the modern multitest analyzers.

3. The availability of new tests and the evolution of laboratory usage in medical practice have raised questions concerning the usefulness, effectiveness, and appropriateness of laboratory testing, which will also be discussed in this chapter.

NORMAL VALUES

Since chronic diseases are quite prevalent in the elderly, it becomes crucial to be able to distinguish an abnormal laboratory value associated with disease from one associated purely with the aging process. It is therefore essential that any discussion of the appropriateness of laboratory testing in the elderly must be preceded by awareness of possible differences in the normal reference ranges as a result of the aging process per se, in the absence of subclinical or clinically apparent disease.

Any discussion of normal values in the elderly must also be prefaced by consideration of the variability of that population. The elderly are a dynamically heterogeneous population, with two subgroups, and most people fall somewhere in between. The "healthy elderly" are those who function independently in society, are ambulatory, and have not lost appreciable muscle mass because they attain a level of physical activity sufficient to retard significant losses. They may suffer from some chronic diseases, but the severity of their condition is not sufficient to retard their physical activity. On the other extreme are the "frail elderly." These are mainly occupants of nursing homes or other chronic care facilities. They perform little, if any, physical activity, are frequently bedridden, and have lost appreciable muscle mass. They suffer from overt chronic diseases (frequently chronic obstructive pulmonary disease or cardiac or renal failure) that preclude many, if not most, physical activities. However, the elderly population is dynamic and, except for those who die suddenly (or after a short illness), most of the elderly will eventually progress from the healthy to the frail group as the sum total of the effects of chronic disease take their toll.

The relevance of this discussion to the subject of normal laboratory values is that laboratory values can be quite different in the two groups. The healthy elderly usually have laboratory values closer to the universally accepted normal reference ranges, the reverse being true in the frail elderly. It is therefore questionable as to whether studies of "normal" laboratory values are at all appropriate in the frail elderly, a population characterized by multiple organ system failure and inanition. Furthermore, even the healthy elderly are frequently affected with a number of chronic conditions, many of them nondisabling or subclinical, which may also have an effect on studies of normal values. These changes can convey the false impression that certain laboratory values tend to change as a result of "normal aging." In these cases, it is the high incidence of disease, rather than the normal aging process, that is responsible for the age-related changes of laboratory values in the elderly. That is not to say that changes due to normal aging do not occur. The confusion of true normal, age-related changes with those due to underlying disease has been the source of much controversy. In some cases these issues have not been completely resolved.

These factors also impinge on the selection of populations to use for reference range studies. If age-related changes in the value of an analyte are the result of the normal aging process, then reference ranges for the elderly should be based on values obtained from the healthy elderly, because those values will reflect the age-related change. Care should be taken, however, to exclude those with clinically apparent diseases, as well as those on medications that might have some effect on laboratory tests. If, however, age-related changes in laboratory values are not the result of the normal aging process, then reference ranges should remain based on the traditional groups of healthy adult subjects.

Other population variables that may affect age-related changes are obesity and race. The former has been shown to affect metabolic tests such as glucose tolerance. The latter has not been thoroughly investigated, although there is one such report on hematology reference ranges in black Americans (Castro, Haddy, & Rana, 1987).

SPECIFIC TESTS

A summary of the following section, including the effect of age and whether changes are probably age- or disease-related, is given in Table 2.1. It will be noted that age-related changes apparently do occur with a number of analytes. In some cases, these changes fall within the generally accepted reference ranges. In other cases, more overt changes will frequently go beyond reference range thresholds.

Hematology Tests

The effect of age on the hemoglobin/hematocrit has been a controversial subject. Although most studies have shown a decline in the elderly (Hale, Stewart, & Marks, 1983, Htoo, Kofkoff, Freedman, 1979; Nilsson-Ehle, Jagenburg, Landahl, Svanborg, Westin, 1988; Salive et al., 1992; Timiras & Brownstein, 1987), other reports have failed to demonstrate this trend (Caird, 1973; Mattila, Knusela, & Palliniemi, 1986; Myers, Saunders, & Chalmers, 1968; Zauber & Zauber, 1987). The differences are probably related to the particular patient population studied. However, even among those who found an increasing incidence of anemia in the elderly, in three of these studies this was attributed to pathologic causes rather than to normal aging (Htoo et al., 1979; Nilsson-Ehle et al., 1988; Salive et al., 1992). Where anemias were worked up, causation was attributed to a combination of iron deficiency and the anemia of chronic disease (Nilsson-Ehle et al., 1988, Salive et al., 1992). Some cases of anemia, especially mild anemia, showed no obvious cause. These frequently reverted to normal upon retesting (Nilsson-Ehle et al., 1988). Although macrocytosis was occasionally found, vitamin B^{12} and folate deficiency were uncommon. Anemia was also associated with smoking, alcohol abuse, cancer, renal insufficiency, and hypoalbuminemia (Gambert, Csuka, Duthie, Tiegs, 1982; Salive et al., 1992; Zauber & Zauber, 1987).

Although some reports showed a decrease in white count with

TABLE 2.1 Laboratory tests in the elderly as compared to generally accepted values in the overall adult population.

Analyte	General Elderly	Healthy Elderly	Frail Elderly	AR/DR
Hemoglobin/hematocrit	↓–	↓↓	–/+	
WBC	(↓)–			–/+
Platelets	(↑)–			
ESR	↑	–	↑↑	–/+
Fibrinogen	↑	↑		?
Clotting tests	–			
Glucose	↑	(↑)		+/+
Glucose Tolerance Test	↑↑	↑↑	↑↑	+/+
Albumin	↓	(↓)	↓↓	+/+
Cholesterol	Plateaus at age 55–65		↓	–/+
Electrolytes (Na, K, Cl, CO_2)	–			
Calcium, Phosphorus (generally)	(↓)			
Urea, Creatinine	(↑)		↑	+/+
Uric acid, creatinine clearance	↓	↓	↓↓	+/+
Alkaline phosphatase	↑			+/+
Bilirubin & other liver enzymes	(↑)–			+/+
Magnesium	(↓)			
Thyroid function				
T_3	↓	(↓)	↓	+/+
T_4	–			
TSH	↑	(↑)	↑	(–)/+
Vitamin B_{12}	↓		↓	–/+
Folate	–			
Iron	↓	–		–/+
Arterial blood gas				
pH	–			
pO_2	↓	↓	↓	+/+
pCO_2	(↑)			?/+
Rheumatoid factor/ANA	↑	↑		–/+
Asymptomatic bacteriuria	↑	(↑)	↑↑	?
Tuberculin sensitivity	↓			?

() = Changes which are mild or controversial
AR = Normal age related change
DR = Disease related change

age (Caird, 1973; Gambert et al., 1992; Salive et al., 1992; Zauber & Zauber, 1987), this was not confirmed by most other studies (Dybkaer, Lauritzen, Krakauer, 1981; Jernigan, Gudat, Blake, Bowen, & Lezotte, 1980; Lehtonen, Eskola, Vainio, Lehtonen, 1990; Salive et al., 1992; Zaubert & Zauber, 1987). As in the case of hemoglobin, the abnormals were probably explained by pathophysiology in the form of drug reactions, latent infections, or other conditions. One study found elevated platelet counts with advancing age, presumably on the basis of intercurrent disease (Nilsson-Ehle et al., 1988). Other studies, however, showed no such platelet abnormalities (Cavalieri, Chopra, & Bryman, 1992; Salive et al., 1992).

The relationship of the erythrocyte sedimentation rate (ESR) to the aging process has also been controversial. Most studies have found elevated percentages of accelerated ESR in the geriatric population (Caird, 1983; Dybkaer et al., 1981; Gambert, et al., 1982; Griffiths et al., 1984; Shearn & Kang, 1986; Sparrow, Row, Silbert, 1982) and attributed these findings variously to disease or "normal aging." Griffiths et al. (1984) questioned whether normal aging was a factor and attributed all elevations to disease. Crawford et al. (Crawford, Eye-Boland, Harvey, & Cohen, 1987) found that age per se had no influence on the ESR in their study population of 111 ambulatory elderly. The abnormalities detected could be attributed to such factors as anemia or hypoalbuminemia, which are known to nonspecifically affect the ESR. Serum albumin acts to decrease the ESR by inhibiting rouleaux formation. The main serum factors tending to elevate the ESR are fibrinogen, globulin, and acute phase reactants, substances frequently elevated in the elderly (Gambert et al., 1982; Hamilton, Dawson, Ogston, & Douglas, 1974; Meade, Chahrabarti, Haines, North, & Sterling, 1979). Again, it is not clear whether this elevation is associated with "normal aging" or pathophysiology. Coagulation tests were unaffected by age. (Cavalieri et al., 1992).

Chemistry Tests

Glucose, albumin, and cholesterol have been the most thoroughly studied analytes in the elderly because of their association with three of the most important geriatric degenerative conditions: diabetes mellitus, nutritional status, and atherosclerosis, with its complications of ischemic heart disease and stroke.

Although most studies have shown rises in fasting glucose with age (Caird, 1973; Cavalieri et al., 1992; Dybkaer et al., 1981; Jernigan et al., 1980), this effect is frequently minimal or even occasionally absent (Blunt, Barrett-Connor, & Wingard, 1991). The glucose tolerance test (or 2-hour postprandial glucose) is a much more sensitive indicator of derangements in carbohydrate metabolism. All studies have found it to be significantly elevated in advancing age (Blunt et al., 1991; Shimokata et al., 1991; Broughton & Taylor, 1991; Busby et al., 1992; Cavalieri et al., 1991; Dybkaer et al.,

1991). Although most of these reports consider the elevation to be related to age per se, variables such as level of physical activity, waist-to-hip (fat) ratio, and body mass index were also found to be factors (Broughton et al., 1991; Busby et al., 1992; Shimokata et al., 1991). Insulin resistance, combined perhaps with delays in monosacharride absorption, is the probable underlying mechanism (Broughton et al., 1991). These factors, even as a result of normal aging, contribute to the predilection of the elderly to develop non-insulin-dependent diabetes mellitus.

Many reports have cited an age-related decline in serum albumin levels (Campion, de Labry, Glynn, 1988; Cavalieri, et al., 1992; Cooper & Gardner, 1989; Dybkaer et al., 1981; Greenblatt, 1979; Keating, Jones, Elveback, Randall, 1969; Leto, Kiergst, Barrows, 1970; Munro et al., 1987; Orwoll, Weigel, Oviatt, Meier, & McClung, 1987). In some of these studies there was indication that the changes were directly age-related (Munro et al., 1987; Shibata et al., 1991), whereas in others, using an ambulatory population, the decline was attributed to the presence of disease (Campion, et al., 1988; Cooper & Gardner, 1989). However, in the latter studies there was a small decrease of serum albumin in the "elderly elderly" that was attributed to normal aging. Although albumin levels are related to nutritional state and are depressed in chronic heart, liver, and renal disease and in cancer, there is also evidence that albumin synthesis may be impaired in the elderly, a factor unrelated to nutritional state, protein intake, or, necessarily to disease (Gersovitz, Munroe, Eldall, & Young, 1980). The diminution of albumin in the elderly would also affect the activity of therapeutic drugs, many of which are ordinarily complexed by albumin in the circulation.

In regard to cholesterol, most population studies have shown elevations in total cholesterol to ages 50–65, followed by a plateauing or slight decline thereafter (Caird, 1973; Cavalieri, et al., 1992; Coodley, 1989; Dybkaer et al., 1981; Kashyap, 1987; Rock, 1984), until in the very old (>81 years), the levels decline more markedly (Fritzsche, Tracy, Speirs, & Glueck, 1990). The implications of these data are that, in the middle-aged and healthy elderly, cholesterol increase is a reflection of dietary habits and other similar epidemiologic factors, as in the younger adult population. The decrease in the very old and in the frail elderly probably represents the effect of chronic disease and malnutrition. Indeed, cholesterol levels have been cited as a prognostic factor in these populations (Fagard et al., 1991; Noel, Smith, & Ettinger, 1991).

The other chemistry analytes have not been as thoroughly studied because progressive age-related changes do not have as much obvious direct clinical significance.

Electrolytes show no age-related change (Caird, 1973; Cavalieri, et al., 1992; Coodley, 1989; Dybkaer et al., 1981; Rock, 1984). Calcium and phosphorus in general also show little if any change; however, one study showed a slight general diminution with age (Sorva, Valvanne, & Tilvis, 1992). One a diminution in males only (Keating et al., 1969) and one an elevation in elderly females only (Caird, 1973). Another report showed a low phosphorus in the elderly (Jernigan et al., 1980). Although one might expect the calcium to follow the downward trend of protein and albumin, this is not apparently the case. Phosphorus is typically labile, being affected by such ubiquitous factors as exercise, eating, and sleeping. Urea (BUN), creatinine, and uric acid tend to undergo some variable age related elevation in a number of different reports (Caird, 1973; Cavalieri et al., 1992; Coodley, 1989; Dybkaer et al., 1981; Keating et al., 1969; Rock, 1984). One would suspect that this effect was probably disease- rather than age-related, considering the prevalence of some degree of chronic renal insufficiency in the elderly. The fact that creatinine is not more definitely elevated in the elderly might have to do with the fact that the depressing effect of diminished muscle mass somewhat offsets the elevating effect of chronic renal failure. Creatinine clearance, however, does show a distinct age-related diminution and is a much more sensitive indicator of impaired renal function (Cavalieri et al., 1992). This effect is due to decreased renal blood flow, a diminished number of glomeruli, and a decline in glomerular filtration rate, all of which are age-related (Gambert et al., 1982; Jernigan et al., 1980).

In regard to enzymes and liver function tests, there is a clear consensus that alkaline phosphatase shows an age-related increase in the elderly (Caird, 1973; Cavalieri, et al., 1992; Coodley, 1989; Dybkaer et al., 1981; Kampmann, Sinding, & Moller-Jergenson, 1975; Keating, et al., 1969; Morgan, 1983; Rock, 1984), possibly associated with extrahepatic conditions such as bone disease, malabsorption, or renal insufficiency (Gambert et al., 1982). However, the possibility of a true age-related change cannot be excluded. Results of lactate dehydrogenase, alanine aminotransferase, and aspartate aminotransferase are variable, with some studies reporting a slight age-related elevation, sometimes in only one sex (Coodley, 1989; Dybkaer et al., 1981; Rock, 1984; Tietz et al., 1984), and other studies reporting no change (Cavalieri et al., 1992; Kampmann et al., 1975). Creatinine kinase (CK) and bilirubin showed no general age-related change. However, in the case of CK, although the upper limits of the elderly range were higher than those of the regular normal reference range, the mean was not elevated and was perhaps even somewhat lower (Tietz et al., 1984). This, again, may be explained by the loss in muscle mass in the elderly, countering an otherwise age-related tendency toward elevation. Studies of magnesium levels were variable. Two studies showed low amylase activity in the elderly (Jernigan et al., 1980; Mayer & Necheler, 1940), a finding attributed to possible decreased enzyme catalytic activity or inactive enzyme in that age group.

Thyroid function testing in the elderly has received much attention due to the high incidence of hypothyroidism in this population. Although the literature is full of conflicting claims, some facts do stand out: (1) the elderly have an increased incidence of thyroid test abnormalities, manifest in a diminished triiodothyroxin (T3) and elevated thyrotropic hormone (TSH) levels (Cavalieri et al, 1992; Coodley, 1989; Drinka, Nolten, Vocks, & Langer, 1991; Dybkaer et al., 1981; Herrmann, Heinen, Kroll, Rudorff, Kruskemper, 1981; Rock, 1984, 1985; Runnels, Garry, Hunt, & Standefer, 1991; Sundbeck, Lundberg, Lindstedt, Jagenburg, & Eden, 1991); (2) these abnormalities most often are manifest before the age of 60 (Kampmann et al., 1975; Tietz et al., 1984); (3) elevated TSH frequently occurs in the presence of normal T3 and thyroxine (T4) (Drinka et al., 1991; Runnels et al., 1991). In some cases, the mildly elevated TSH subsequently reverts to normal (Drinka et al., 1991), indicating that these changes may be an effect of intraindividual (within subject) variability or due to the presence of nonthyroid disease (cardiovascular, hepatic, and renal), altered states of binding proteins, or concomitant medication (Coodley, 1989). Some of the TSH may also be nonfunctional (Gersovitz et al., 1980). A minority of patients with isolated elevated TSH go on to develop more overt hypothyroidism (Drinka et al., 1991), especially when TSH levels are more markedly elevated and other manifestations of thyroid disease, such as positive antithyroglobulin or microsomal antibody titres, coexist (Drinka, et al., 1991). Unless there is overt disease, T4 levels usually remain normal, due perhaps to decreased hormonal degradation counteracting decreased secretion (Rock, 1985). The implication of the above findings is that the thyroid function test abnormalities in the elderly are probably the result of a combination of intraindividual variation and subclinical disease (Nilsson-Ehle et al., 1988). Age-related increased parathyroid hormone levels in the elderly have been reported (Jernigan et al., 1980; Wiske, 1979).

Among the vitamins, folate and cobalamine (B^{12}) are the most frequently clinically assayed and studied. B^{12} is commonly diminished in the elderly, folate much less so (Caird, 1973; Cape & Shinton, 1961; Cavalieri et al., 1992; Coodley, 1989; Drinka & Goodwin, 1991; Dybkaer et al., 1981; Hanger, Sainsbury, Gilchrist, Beard, & Duncan, 1991; Nilsson-Ehle et al., 1988; Rock, 1984). Although the reason is far from clear, the concensus appears not to favor normal aging, even though the changes do not appear to be directly related to diet and nutritional state. Lower levels of other vitamins have also been observed in the elderly and have been attributed, at least in some cases, to nutritional or environmental factors (Coodley, 1989; Drinka et al., 1991; Morgan, 1983). Results of serum iron studies have been variable, due perhaps to the particular population studied (Coodley, 1989; Dybkaer et al., 1981; Nilsson-Ehle, et al., 1988; Rock, 1984; Zauber & Zauber, 1987). However most reports have shown a slight age-associated drop, probably related to disease. The possibility that there is some physiological age-related decline in iron absorption cannot be excluded (Gambert et al., 1981). If true, however, this would have only a minor effect.

In regard to arterial blood gases, there is a definite consensus that PO_2 decreases with age, a change related to reduced lung function and vital capacity due to diminished lung elasticity, decreased alveolar surface area, and increased chest wall stiffness as well as decreased cardiac output (Cavalieri et al., 1992; Dybkaer et al., 1981; Rock, 1984). Whether this is normal aging or related to chronic obstructive pulmonary disease is a moot point, since the two blend together in a continuum, the latter being the overtly clinical manifestation of the former, a widespread ubiquitous finding in the elderly. PCO_2 was found to show a slight age-related rise in some studies (Dybkaer et al., 1981) and to remain stable in others (Cavalieri et al., 1992). This divergence may be related to differences in the populations studied, since the elevated PCO_2 may be a further extension of the processes manifested by the decreased PO_2. All reports show no essential change in pH.

In regard to immunologic tests, there is one report of elevated IgM, IgA, and alpha-1–antitrypsin in the elderly (Jernigan et al., 1980). Antinuclear antibody (ANA) and rheumatoid factor (RF) changes are discussed below.

Age-Related Changes in Other Tests

There are certain other laboratory tests in which age-related changes occur. These cannot be included under the umbrella of "normal values," since their results are expressed in binary terms (i.e., positive or negative) rather than quantitative values. Among the most studied are the immunology/rheumatology tests—RF and ANA, both of which show an increased level of positivity in the elderly (Cavalieri et al., 1992; Wernick, 1989). This is probably related to the general overall increase of autoimmune activity in this age group (Makinodan, Kay, 1980). It does not appear to be a consequence of normal aging.

Urine culture is another test that shows an age-related phenomenon. A significant percentage of the elderly show asymptomatic bacteriuria (Mims, Norman, Yamamura, Yoshikawa, 1990; Sourander, 1966; Tronetti, Graceley & Boscia, 1990; Wolfson, Kolmanson, & Rubins, 1965). This finding is either transient or persistent and appears to be related to the general physical condition of the population studied, being more prevalent in institutionalized than noninstitutionalized groups (Mims et al., 1990; Tronetti et al., 1990). The exact explanation of this phenomenon is unclear.

A third test in this category is tuberculin reactivity. The elderly frequently show a loss of prior tuberculin sensitivity (Creditor, Smith, Gallai, Baumann, & Nelson, 1988; Grzybowski, 1965; Stead, 1983; Vorken, Grzybowski, & Allen, 1987). In addition, elderly individuals who are nonreactive to tuberculin are also frequently nonreactive to the commonly tested cutaneous recall antigens (*Candida albicans*, mumps, etc.) (Creditor et al., 1988; Vorken et al., 1987). This is not generally related to anergy, since those exposed to an infectious source or subjected to a booster test will frequently revert to positivity. This was illustrated by Creditor et al. (1988), who studied an elderly nursing home population after exposure to a case of active tuberculosis. Whether this represents general immune senescence is unclear.

EFFECT OF TECHNOLOGY ON LABORATORY INSTRUMENTATION AND METHODOLOGY

Recent decades have seen increasing automation in the clinical laboratory. Although various aspects of automation have in general had a positive effect on gerontological medical practice, this has not always been the case. Specific considerations are as follows.

Specimen Size

The newer instruments have tended to require less blood volume, minimizing blood loss through phlebotomy. Of the analyzers currently in use the largest and most automated hematology or chemistry analyzers can do a complete blood count or a multitest chemistry profile with as little as 0.5–1.0 ml of blood or serum. The smaller instruments may require specimens of 2–5 ml. However, the lower limit of phlebotomized hematology samples cannot be less than 2 ml of blood, since that amount is required in pediatric (small size) tubes for optimal anticoagulation. Although blood from a finger stick with volumes as low as 0.1–0.25 ml can be used in many modern hematology analyzers, factors such as safety and lack of adaptability to large numbers of patients preclude widespread hospital use of this technology. Therefore, further advances in reducing blood specimen size will have to await improvements in phlebotomy and specimen acquisition.

Loss of blood via phlebotomy is not a trivial consideration. A recent study by Joosten et al (Joosten, Hiele, Pelemans, & Haesen, 1992) showed that in an acute geriatric ward, patients were phlebotomized, on average, a little less than once per day. There was a weak but significant correlation between the amount of blood taken for phlebotomy and a decrease in hemoglobin levels between admission and discharge. In addition, 28% of the patients who were not anemic on admission became anemic. In most of these cases this was disease-related; however, three patients did have a mild unexplained anemia. Although the effect of phlebotomy per se may not be very clinically significant, it is still likely to have an additive adverse effect on disease-related anemia. In addition, the elderly are known to have a diminished hemopoetic response to stress and blood loss (Hirota, Okamura, & Kimura, 1988). This effect is compounded by illness.

Improved Accuracy of the Newer Analyzers and Methodologies

In recent decades there have been two technological factors contributing to improvements in analytical accuracy: (1) more sophisticated instrumentation in the performance of existing methodology and (2) the institution of newer, more refined techniques. The commonly used chemistry analyzers are an example of the first. The newer methodologies are exemplified by laser hematology analyzers and the use of polarization, chemoluminescence, and immunoassays in endocrinology, therapeutic drug monitoring, and toxicology.

Along with technology-associated improvements in testing accuracy, there have been improvements in timeliness. Each new succeeding generation of analyzers is as fast, if not faster, than its predecessors.

Expense

Although the cost of the newer more automated laboratory analyzers has increased appreciably, the actual expense of laboratory tests in terms of reagent costs has tended to either remain the same, increase, or decrease, depending on various factors. Technologies with increased reagent costs usually offer some special compensating feature. Examples include the analyzers which offer an extremely rapid turn-around time and emergency response capability; and immunoassay techniques that can detect extremely minute amounts of analyte. However, the basic issue is that even though the newer automated analyzers are usually more expensive than their predecessors, they make up for this in the long term by a savings on labor costs and frequently on reagent costs as well.

Another problem relating to instrumentation was the widespread use a few years ago of multichannel chemistry autoanalyzers that, with continuous flow technology, automatically furnished a battery of 18–20 tests on every specimen. This battery of tests was usually cheaper than a few tests ordered individually. As a holdover from this era, many clinicians were conditioned to reflexively order 6, 12, or 20 test profiles rather than discrete individual tests. The negative impact of this is that abnormal results on tests that are performed incidentally can leave the clinician in a quandary in regard to interpretation and follow-up. Many of these abnormal results might be expected to occur purely on the basis of statistical probability. Nevertheless, due to nonfamiliarity with analytical probabilities or age-related changes, perceived pressure from regulatory agencies, or threat of litigation, time and resources are often expended in the investigation of abnormalities of frequently marginal or no significance.

EFFECT OF LABORATORY TESTING AND TECHNOLOGY ON CLINICAL GERIATRIC DECISION MAKING

General Principles: Steps in Laboratory Testing

To assess the usefulness of specific laboratory tests in the geriatric population, it is first necessary to review the steps and strategies in clinical laboratory utilization. The three steps in laboratory usage are as follows: (1) test ordering; is the ordering of a specific laboratory test appropriate? (2) Test interpretation; what are the probabilities of any test result being significant, given the other clinical factors (history, physical exam, other tests) in any particular patient? (3) Follow-up; what should be done (if anything) in the way of follow-up of a particular test result? This includes diagnostic as well as possible therapeutic modalities.

Test Ordering

What are the prerequisites for efficient test ordering?

An awareness of the sensitivity and specificity of the test in question and thus its usefulness under the particular set of conditions. Sensitivity can be defined as the ability of a test to identify the greatest number of patients in the test population with disease, i.e., the positive group will be as large as possible and may include some false positives. There will therefore be as few false negatives as possible. Sensitivity can thus be calculated as the number of true positives divided by the total number of patients with disease (true positives plus false negatives) (Galen & Gambino, 1975; Rock, 1984; Wernick, 1989).

Specificity can be defined as the ability of a test (as much as possible) to identify only the patients in a tested population with disease (true positives); in other words to minimize the false positives. The negative group may therefore include some false negatives. This can thus be expressed as the number of true negatives divided by the total number of patients without disease (true negatives plus false positives). Since most tests show an area of overlap between patients with and without disease, the sensitivity and specificity of any test will not be represented by the same threshold.

Moreover, they will vary, depending on where the threshold (reference range) is drawn. If the sensitivity is maximized, the specificity is downgraded (more false positives), and vice versa.

An awareness of the clinical threshold of suspicion (pretest probability). This can be defined as the probability as to whether a given patient has the disease, and it is based upon such factors as history, physical findings, and prior testing. If the index of suspicion is already high and the test has a high specificity, a positive result will be confirmatory, a negative result clinically not very significant. With tests showing a high degree of sensitivity, a negative result will be much more clinically significant than a positive one.

The concept of clinical testing thresholds can be further refined (as proposed by Pauker and Kassirer [1980]) by recognizing two thresholds for each situation: a "testing threshold," which is a cutoff point below which the probability of disease is so remote that the test in question is not worth performing, and a "test treatment threshold," a cutoff point above which the probability of disease is so likely that it is not worth the expense and effort to perform the test (i.e., treatment can be initiated without the need for further testing). It is in the zone between the two thresholds that the test can give useful clinical information. In this model (Pauker & Kassirer, 1980) the zone between the two thresholds can be expanded if the test is low-risk or expense and reduced if the test in question contains a higher risk or expense.

In laboratory medicine, however, most tests are relatively inexpensive and involve only venipuncture, and are thus low-risk. Because of this, physicians, when in doubt, tend to order laboratory tests rather than hold back. This trend is also reinforced by defensive medicine/risk management pressures in today's climate of frequent malpractice litigation, pressures that tend to promote overutilization of laboratory resources. Also, the specificity and sensitivity of a given test must be separately considered when tests are ordered, since they tend to alter the thresholds asymmetrically (i.e., the test treatment threshold can be expanded upward if the test is highly sensitive, since a negative result will be highly significant, and the testing threshold can be expanded downward for a highly specific test, since a positive result in this case would be highly significant).

An awareness of the pretest prognosis (or life expectancy). This is based upon the patient's age and modified by prior indications of disease (Pauker & Kassirer, 1987). It would obviously not be advisable to initiate a workup to diagnose a disease that, if treated, would only minimally prolong life expectancy and/or subject the patient to stressful therapeutic modalities with considerable morbidity that the patient would poorly tolerate.

Test Interpretation

The interpretation of any test must be tempered by an awareness of the variables that can affect the result, as well as other factors.

The variables affecting test results. These consist of intraindividual, interindividual, and analytic variation (Galen & Gambino, 1975; Rock, 1984). Can test results be explained by these types of variations, rather than signifying disease? Different tests have different characteristic patterns of variation; in addition, factors such as age, sex, and test methodology are also important. In general, biologic variation is greater than analytic variation, and interindividual variation is greater than intraindividual variation. Intraindividual variation, or "biochemical individuality," is important to monitor because a drift from a previously recorded range of values can signify early disease, even though the test result in question is still within the accepted reference range (Rock, 1984).

Predictive value. In addition to sensitivity and specificity, each test result has a built-in predictive value that can be defined as the ability of a result to predict the true clinical state. This is expressed as true positives divided by all positives (true and false positives) × 100 for a positive test, and true negatives divided by all negatives × 100 for a negative test.

Degree of deviation from the threshold or reference range. Tests minimally beyond the cutoff or reference range should not be considered as clinically significant as those more clearly out of range (Wernick, 1989). On the other hand, deviations from a patient's previous norms can be clinically significant, even within the reference range (see above).

Followup

Posttest probability. The test result should enable the clinician to estimate the posttest probability (likelihood) of disease (Wernick, 1989), which can be expressed as true positives divided by all positives, as well as the change in probability (if any) due to the test result.

Decision tree/sensitivity analysis. These techniques are helpful in planning further diagnostic or therapeutic options (Pauker & Kassirer, 1980). As above, limitations of the geriatric patient due to decreased life expectancy and tolerability of stressful procedures should be considered.

Previous results. In any follow-up situation it is always important to plot a patient's course by comparing the current with any previous test values.

Purposes and Usefulness of Laboratory Testing

Although many of the factors associated with geriatric and general medical practice are similar, there are two that are unique to geriatrics. The geriatric patient has an underlying reduced prognosis in many, if not most situations, due to his/her shorter expected life span. Second, the geriatric patient, in many cases, has a reduced capacity to tolerate vigorous, stressful, or invasive diagnostic and therapeutic modalities due to his/her frequently impaired physical condition. Even elderly patients in excellent physical condition frequently respond poorly to such stresses as major surgery.

Laboratory tests are used for three general purposes: diagnosis of disease in symptomatic individuals, follow-up testing in patients with established disease to monitor the clinical course and prognosis of the individual patient, and screening of asymptomatic individuals to discover diseases at an early stage.

Diagnosis and Prognosis in Symptomatic Patients

In regard to diagnosis in symptomatic patients, since laboratory tests are for the most part low-risk/noninvasive, the geriatrician can be and should be just as aggressive as the general internist in using the laboratory for this purpose. In the case of the healthy elderly, the situation more closely resembles adult general medicine, since these patients have a longer life expectancy, many illnesses are life-threatening, therapeutic benefits are usually immediate, and patients are frequently fit enough to tolerate aggressive stressful therapeutic modalities. In the frail elderly, even in the case of incurable disease or disease in which definitive therapy cannot be tolerated, conservative or palliative therapy can make the patient more comfortable, improve the quality of life, and therefore make the diagnostic effort worthwhile.

Follow-up Testing in Patients with Established Disease

Follow-up testing is usually useful in the geriatric setting to keep the patient and/or family appraised of the patient's condition and to adjust conservative therapy when needed.

Screening

Screening asymptomatic geriatric patients is the most controversial and questionable of the uses of laboratory testing because life expectancy may be too short to derive considerable benefit from therapy, or patients are frequently not fit enough to tolerate stressful therapy. Even in the case of screening tests in the healthy elderly, the patients may not live long enough to benefit from early detection of diseases that may not become clinically manifest or life-threatening for several years. This topic is further discussed in the section on screening.

Several considerations for testing in the geriatric setting include the following. Factors favoring test usage are (1) severity of disease, (2) treatability of disease in relation to prolongation and quality of life, and (3) specificity of the test. Factors adverse to test usage include (1) frailty of the individual patient and (2) expense of the test. A pretest probability of disease at a level where the test is apt to be informative (Pauker & Kassirer, 1987) is also important.

USEFULNESS OF SPECIFIC LABORATORY TESTS

A summary of the usage of laboratory tests in geriatric medicine is given in Table 2.2 (Duthie & Abbasi, 1991; Kalchthaler & Rigor, 1980; Ochs, 1991; Rock, 1985; Wernick, 1989). It lists diseases important in geriatric medicine, tests used in diagnosis and follow-up, and their specificity.

From this table the following points should be cited. For the diagnosis of sepsis, a differential count is recommended, since some patients will not have leukocytosis, and the diagnosis must be supported by an elevated neutrophil and/or neutrophil band count (percent or absolute). Electrolytes are useful to exclude dehydration, which can also give a febrile response; however, dehydration can also be assessed by physical exam. For diabetes mellitus, a fasting blood sugar is usually adequate, although a 2-hour postprandial glucose may occasionally be necessary. Glycosolated hemoglobin levels are useful in monitoring long-term diabetic control. In thyroid function testing TSH value has the greatest sensitivity but is less specific for overt disease. T3, T4, and antibody (thyroglobulin or microsomal) levels are more significant, since they are apt to flag or confirm cases of overt disease. Arterial blood gases are of minor confirmatory importance in chronic obstructive pulmonary

TABLE 2.2   Usefulness of laboratory tests for diagnosis and follow up in the elderly

Disease	Test(s)	Test Specificity	Test Usage Dx/FU	Comment
Sepsis	WBC, Diff	+ + +	Dx	
	Electrolytes	+	Dx	Used to rule out dehydration
Diabetes Mel.	Fasting Bl. Glu.	+ + +	Dx/FU	
	Glyco. Hbg.	+ +	FU	
Thyroid Dis.	T_3, T_4	+ + +	Dx/FU	
	TSH	+ +	Dx/FU	Most sensitive, less useful
Chr. Obs. Pum. Dis.	Art. Bl. Gas	+	Dx/FU	Non lab tests more helpful
Osteo/Paget's	Ca, P	+	Dx/FU	Non lab tests more helpful
Liber Dis.	Enzymes/Alk. Phos.	+ +	Dx/FU	
Malignancy	Fecal Oc. Bl./	+	Dx	Controversial
	Pr. Sp. Ag.	+	Dx	in frail elderly
Rheumatology	ESR/RF	+	Dx/FU	
	ANA	(+ +)	Dx	SLE uncommon in aged
Nutritional Dis.	T Prot/Alb/Prealb	+ +	Dx/FU	
Cardiovascular Disease (risk)	Cholesterol/ lipids	+ +	Dx/FU	Controversial; little use in frail elderly
Myo. Infarct	CPK + LDH Iso	+ + +	Dx	
Neuro Dis.	Thy FT/Syph Ser/B_{12}	+	Dx	Neurological dis is occasionally only indication of B_{12} def.
Renal Dis.	BUN/Cr/Urinalysis	+ + +	Dx/FU	
Coagulation	PT/PTT	+ + +	Dx/FU	FU in anticoag therapy
Hemo (Anemia)	Hbg/Hct	+ + +	Dx/FU	
	B_{12}/Folate/ Retic/Fe studies	+ +	Dx/FU	Secondary tests after Hbg/Hct
Hemo (platelets)	Platelets	+ + +	Dx/FU	FU for chemotherapy
Tuberculosis	Tuberculin	+ + +	Dx/FU	
Fluid imbalance	Electrolytes	+ + +		

Dx/FU - Diagnosis/ Follow up

disease. Calcium and phosphorus levels play a minor role in the diagnosis and management of bone disease. Fecal occult blood and prostate-specific antigen are of little use in the workup of symptomatic patients; more will be said about them as screening tests. The rheumatology tests are nonspecific, since false positives are not infrequent in the nondiseased elderly (Wernick, 1989) (besides, disseminated lupus erythematosus is uncommon in the elderly). In assessing nutritional status, prealbumin is frequently more useful than total protein or albumin, since it reflects recent responses to therapy (Bernstein, Lenkhardt-Fairfield, Pleban & Rudolph, 1989; Winkler, Gerrior, Ponp, & Albina, 1989).

The use of tests for cholesterol in the elderly is controversial. There is some indication that it may be worthwhile monitoring and attempting to reduce cholesterol levels, at least in the healthy elderly (Kaiser & Morley, 1990). In the frail elderly, cholesterol and lipid levels are of little value. Laboratory testing has shown only a minor role in the workup of dementia; however, in the elderly, dementia may occasionally be the only manifestation of vitamin B^{12} deficiency. In assessing renal function, creatinine is usually more sensitive than BUN. In assessing anemia, it is important to differentiate iron deficiency anemia from the anemia of chronic disease. The former is usually due to underlying sources of occult bleeding and is frequently treatable (Katchthaler et al., 1980). Hemolytic and macrocytic anemias are infrequent in the elderly. Platelets are useful mainly for monitoring chemotherapy. The tuberculin test (PPD) is important in chronic care institutions to monitor conversions after unknowing exposure to an active case.

SCREENING TESTS

A screening test can be defined as a test performed in an asymptomatic individual to detect the unsuspected presence of disease. The strategy is to detect an incipient condition that can be treated at an early stage, before overt damage can be inflicted. Although screening is most often thought of as periodic (frequently yearly) testing in a healthy, disease-free population, it may also be confined to a single episode of testing. If it occurs in a population being admitted to a hospital or chronic care facility, it is more properly referred to as admission or preadmission screening. If the population is being evaluated in an ambulatory care setting for an unrelated symptomatology, the testing is referred to as "case finding." Since there are relatively few elderly with no diseases, most screening in the elderly really falls into this category. Since the elderly are prone to harbor appreciable asymptomatic as well as overt disease, screening should be more productive in this group than in young healthy adults.

In order for screening for a particular disease to be successful, a number of conditions must be fulfilled:

1. The condition in question must be relatively common and effective therapy readily available.

2. The test employed must be inexpensive and contain minimal risk. It must be as sensitive as possible without picking up an excessive number of false positives. This presents an inherent problem, in that current reference ranges are based on the fact that 95% of normals will fall within two standard deviations (2 SD). Conversely, 5% of normals will be outside the + 2 SD range, thus implying that if a large battery of tests is performed on normal healthy subjects, a significant number of false positives will occur (Ochs, 1991). When one also considers the fact that certain tests tend to be elevated or show a higher percentage of positivity in the healthy elderly, the problem of false positives is further compounded.

3. The strategy must be capable of either prolonging life or at least improving the quality of life at some time in the future. Therefore, the longer the life expectancy, the more effective screening should be. There is one qualifier, however. The disease in question should be prevalent at the age of the individuals screened (i.e., it would be useless to screen a 20–year-old population for colonic cancer).

Some other points about screening are pertinent. Screening must be defined in terms of the frequency of testing and the population tested. In a relatively healthy population, screening done on a one-time basis (or the first time) is apt to be more effective than subsequent testing, especially if tests are done very frequently. Screening will also be more effective if tailored to selected populations, such as blood glucose in the obese, thyroid function in elderly females (see below), or patients unable to provide an adequate history or voice complaints, such as patients with dementia.

The efficiency of screening in elderly individuals is also inversely related to the quality of health care monitoring they receive between screening episodes and the mental acuity and articulateness of the population. These factors are apt to make it more likely that intercurrent disease will be detected before the next round of screening.

Although the use of some screening tests has been widely ac-

TABLE 2.3 Usefulness of laboratory tests as screening tests in the elderly

Diease	Test(s)	Sensitivity	Usefulness	Comments
Diabetes Mel.	Fasting Bl. Glu.	+ +	+ + +	Sensitivity decreased with age
Diabetes Mel.	Glucose Tol. Test	+ + +	+ +	Too cumbersome for mass testing
Diabetes Mel.	Urinalysis	+	+	
Thyroid Dis.	TSH	+ + +	+ +	Most sensitive, however many questionable cases detected
Thyroid Dis.	T_3, T_4	+ +	+ + +	Confirmatory
Anemia	Hbg/Hct	+ + +	+ + +	
Fluid imbalance	Electrolytes	+ + +	+ +	
Renal Failure	BUN, Creatinine	+ +	+ + +	
Cardiovascular Risk	Cholesterol/ lipids	+ +	(+ +)	Controversial; not useful in frail elderly
Malignancy (colon)	Fecal occult blood	+ +	+ +	Not as useful in frail elderly; use with other modalities
Malignancy (prostate)	Prostate Sp. Ag.	+ +	+ +	Use with other modalities
Urinary tract Disease dis./Diabetes M	Urinalysis	+ +	+ +	Most useful in asymptomatic bacteriuria
Nutritional status	Total Protein Albumin	+ +	+	
Rheumatology	RF/ANA/ESR	+ +	+	False positives a problem
Liver disease	Enzymes, Bili., Alk. Phos	+ +	+	
Tuberculosis	Tuberculin	+ +	+ +	
Vitamin deficiency	Folate/B_{12}	+ + +	+	

cepted, others are more controversial. The frequency of screening of those tests acknowledged to be useful is still somewhat unsettled. It is not surprising, therefore, that there have been numerous publications on this subject (Cebal & Beck, 1987; Domoto, Ben, Wei, Pars & Komoroff, 1985; Joseph & Lytes, 1992; Kalchthaler et al., 1980; Levinstein, Ouslander, Rubinstein, & Forsythe, 1987; Wolf-Klein, Holt, Silverstone, Foley, & Spatz, 1985). A summary of apparent consensus is presented in Table 2.3.

In screening for diabetes mellitus, the fasting blood glucose is cheaper and quicker to perform, but its sensitivity decreases with age. The glucose tolerance test is suitable essentially as a confirmatory test, because it is more cumbersome to perform and less adaptable to large groups. Its usefulness for screening is improved when selected populations (i.e. the obese or those with a family history) are tested. In regard to thyroid function screening, TSH is the most sensitive test; however, it picks up a number of spurious or borderline cases, most of which do not progress to overt disease. A number of heterologous acute diseases also affect thyroid function, and this must be considered, especially when institutionalized patients are being tested. Thyroid function screening is, therefore, most effective in an elderly institutionalized female population, especially those with chronic nonspecific symptomatology (Helfand & Crapo, 1990; Joseph & Lytes, 1992; Levinstein et al., 1987). Anemia appears to be another condition amenable to screening. Most studies have shown a significant number of newly detected abnormal hemoglobin/hematocrit levels in the screened institutionalized elderly (Domoto et al., 1985; Joseph & Lytes, 1992; Levinstein et al., 1987; kalchthaler et al., 1980; Wolf-Klein et al., 1985). As in the area of diagnostic testing, many, if not most, cases of anemia detected by screening turn out to be iron deficiency anemia related to some source of occult bleeding. Many of these cases are treatable, as opposed to the anemia of chronic disease, the other major cause of anemia in the elderly. Electrolytes appear to be useful in detecting diverse causes of fluid imbalance, such as dehydration; overdiuresis, including hypokalemia secondary to diuretic use; and the inappropriate ADH syndrome (Levinstein et al., 1987). Most screening studies recommend the use of BUN/creatinine ratio to monitor renal function (Domoto et al., 1985; Levinstein et al., 1987; Wolf-Klein et al., 1985).

Screening for cholesterol in the healthy elderly yields a large percentage of abnormally high results (Fritzsche et al., 1990; Lowik et al., 1992). However, the beneficial effect of dietary alterations and therapy in this group is controversial (Kaiser & Morley, 1990). If it turns out to be beneficial, HDL may be more important than total cholesterol (Romm, Green, Reagan, & Rackley, 1991). In any event, cholesterol screening in the frail elderly may have a reverse rationale; that is, a lower cholesterol in this group may indicate a poorer prognosis excluding atherosclerotic cardiovascular disease (Fagard, et al., 1991; Noel et al., 1991).

Screening for malignancy includes two important laboratory tests: fecal occult blood (FOB) for colon cancer and prostate-specific antigen (PSA) for prostatic cancer. Although these tests have very limited specificity and sensitivity, they are still useful because they can pick up some lesions; they are easy to perform on a large-scale screening mode and are relatively inexpensive. Many publications abound.

FOB has become one of the pivotal tests in colonic cancer detection in spite of its poor sensitivity and specificity (Ahlquist et al., 1993; Alcorn, 1992; Allison, Feldman, & Tekawa, 1990; Mandel et al., 1989; Morris, Stellato, Guy, Gordon, & Berger, 1991). The reason is that it and the digital rectal exam complement each other, and as noted above they are the only tests that are relatively noninvasive, inexpensive, and suitable to large-scale screening. The digital rectal exam is useful only for the detection of low rectal lesions. FOB detects polyps as well as overt carcinomas, although the sensitivity for polyps is even lower than that for carcinomas. However in the elderly it is not as important to detect small polyps, since their evolution to carcinoma is likely to be longer then the remaining life span of the population tested. The specificity and thus the usefulness of the test appears to be further diminished in the frail and "elderly elderly," who are also known to have an increase in nonspecific occult bleeding (Klos, Drinka, & Goodwin, 1991).

The sensitivity and specificity of PSA is also poor. However, the alternative screening method, digital rectal exam, is more efficient for prostatic than for colon cancer. Therefore, most authors agree that PSA by itself has limited value as a screening tool, although it is useful when combined with digital examination and ultrasound, since it complements the results of these tests (Catalona et al., 1991; Cooner et al., 1990; Mettlin, Lee, Drago, Murphy et al., 1991; Oesterling, 1991). In the frail elderly, screening for colorectal and prostatic cancers is controversial. These patients, in most cases, probably could not tolerate definitive surgery if lesions were detected, and small or low-grade prostatic lesions, even if untreated, would not be the ultimate cause of death. However, palliative therapy could be initiated; prostatic lesions, if detected, could still be treated with castration or hormonal therapy, and a diverting colostomy could be performed before a colonic lesion caused obstruction.

In regard to other tests, urinalysis has been useful in some series, especially in the detection of asymptomatic bacteriuria (Ochs, 1991). However, the benefits of treating asymptomatic bacteriuria in the frail elderly are questionable. Nutritional status is best screened by mechanisms other than laboratory testing, although total protein and albumin may have a confirmatory role. The use of rheumatology tests for screening purposes is limited by the variable sensitivity and low specificity of these tests in the elderly; however, in certain situations, such as a very high ESR, they are almost certainly significant and should prompt a thorough investigation for malignancy and inflammatory disorders (Wernick, 1989). Some geriatric screening studies have recorded elevated liver enzymes, including alkaline phosphatase (Kampmann et al., 1975; Morgan, 1983; Tietz et al., 1984). However, most of these results appear to have had no direct clinical significance or ultimate benefit to the patient. It is, however, important to screen the institutionalized population for tuberculin sensitivity to monitor possible spread of infection if an active case should be detected, although, as noted above, the elderly tend to lose their sensitivity over time (Creditor et al., 1988; Grzybowski, 1965). Tests not listed in Table 2.3 have not so far been cited to show any beneficial clinical effect when used for screening in the elderly.

In summary, the consensus is to either discourage routine screening in the elderly altogether or recommend that it be limited to a small number of tests, such as FOB, CBC, glucose, electrolytes, BUN/creatinine, and perhaps urinalysis, thyroid function tests, and tuberculin sensitivity, the latter in the frail institutionalized elderly only. Also, measuring cholesterol levels in the healthy elderly may be useful. In general, the majority of screening tests are less useful in the frail institutionalized elderly, with the exception of tuberculin sensitivity (see above).

In most studies there was a very small percentage of clinical benefit in detecting unexpected abnormal results, even in cases of treatable disease. Furthermore, in some series, many of the newly detected abnormal results were not followed up by the patients' primary care physicians. In spite of the uncertainty about the usefulness for screening of some of these tests, the value of other tests for screening in the elderly is now widely accepted.

A POLL OF LABORATORY USAGE HABITS IN A GROUP OF PRACTICING GERIATRICIANS

In order to assess laboratory utilization in actual geriatric practice, a panel of 14 practicing internist/geriatricians were polled on the usefulness of diagnostic/follow-up tests in the frail elderly and screening tests in the healthy and frail elderly. The panel consisted of a mixture of junior and senior practitioners, some in private

TABLE 2.4   Usefulness of laboratory testing in defined geriatric clinical situations. A survey of 14 practicing academic and community geriatricians. percent of practitioners finding test useful.

Test	Active (Healthy) Population Screening	Frail (Nursing Home) Population	
		Screening	Diagnostic/Follow Up
CBC	86	100	100
Diff	50	64	100
Retic	7	14	71
Platelets	50	57	100
ESR	21	29	92
PT/PTT	14	43	92
Electrolytes	64	92	100
Ca/P	57	79	92
BUN/Cr	79	86	92
Uric Acid	29	36	92
Mg	14	64	71
Amylase	7	7	71
Fasting Glucose	86	86	92
Glu. Tol. Test	7	7	36
Gly. Hbg.	7	21	64
Cholesterol/lipids	57	29	71
LFT/Enzymes	29	57	92
Thy. Funct. Test	50	64	92
Folate/B_{12}	43	64	92
Protein/Alb	36	71	86
Prost. Sp. Ag	79	57	71
RF/ANA	7	7	64
Syph. Ser.	29	29	64
PPD	36	92	79
Urine Cult.	0	14	92
C. Diff Titer	7	14	79
Urinalysis	86	92	92
Fecal Occ. Blood	100	100	92
Iron Studies	0	7	86

practice, others mainly hospital-based. Findings are listed in Table 2.4.

In comparing Table 2.4 with the preceding sections on test usefulness and screening, a number of points become apparent.

The geriatricians felt that the vast majority of tests were justified for diagnostic/follow-up purposes, even in the frail elderly. This is concordant with views, expressed earlier in this chapter, that even in the frail elderly an aggressive diagnostic workup is justified in order to institute appropriate conservative therapy.

For most of the tests listed in Table 2.4, a higher proportion of

geriatricians felt that screening in the frail elderly was more useful than screening in the healthy elderly. This is contrary to views
generally expressed in the literature and in the preceding section
of this chapter and requires some comment. One possible explanation is that since the frail elderly are frequently poor historians (institutionalized patients often suffer from organic brain disease),
geriatricians feel that they cannot rely on them for accurate histories (sometimes no history at all), and therefore they tend to rely
more on laboratory screening tests to signal the appearance of new
pathology. The tendency to utilize screening more in the frail elderly was not universal, since this trend was reversed in PSA and
cholesterol testing. Also it was the general unequivocal consensus
that screening for cholesterol in the frail elderly is worthless.

The use of tests not generally accepted as screening tests were
endorsed for screening by only a low percentage of the geriatricians
(Table 2.4). Exceptions to this were liver function tests, folate/B^{12},
Ca/P, protein/albumin, and magnesium in the frail population,
where the majority of geriatricians endorsed screening in spite of
widely published views. In the case of folate/B^{12}, there may be a
persistent perception that it is necessary to test for these vitamin
deficiencies even though they appear to be relatively uncommon.
In the case of protein/albumin, the rationale is perhaps a need to
document objectively changes that are usually apparent on clinical
observation. In general, however, these cases perhaps illustrate the
point made previously that the availability of low-risk ubiquitous
laboratory testing encourages laboratory usage.

CONCLUSIONS

Modern laboratory technology has had both positive and negative
impacts on geriatric medicine, mostly the former. These include the
development of newer tests, greater accuracy, and smaller sample
size. On the negative side, the multitest panels occasionally produce unsolicited abnormal results, most of which are clinically insignificant. Nevertheless, these tests must be repeated and other
confirmatory tests frequently ordered before the abnormal result
can be safely disregarded.

In the elderly, some test values remain stabilized within established normal ranges, while others show age-related drift, sometimes within established reference ranges, sometimes going beyond
them. Most of the drift appears to be disease-related, although

some tests may show the effects of the normal aging process and others a combination of the two. However, the emphasis on this distinction is probably unwarranted, and the effects of normal aging and disease are most likely shades of a continuous spectrum. Moreover, some test results will be out of range due to intraindividual or analytical variation or due to the transitory effects of medication or intercurrent disease. These will most likely revert to normal upon retesting. All in all, the variations cited above do not justify creation of separate reference ranges for the elderly.

In regard to test usage, most diagnostic and follow-up tests appear appropriate, even in the frail elderly, since the risk of phlebotomy is minimal and accurate diagnosis and follow-up permits the institution of conservative therapy, which can make patients more comfortable and in many cases probably even prolong life. Finally, the use of laboratory testing for screening purposes is firmly established in geriatric practice. The number of tests useful for screening, however, is limited, and some tests appropriate in the healthy elderly may be inappropriate in the frail, chronically ill group. With other tests, the reverse apparently is true. A poll of geriatricians on the usefulness of specific laboratory testing shows general agreement with guidelines derived from published screening studies.

References

Ahlquist, D. A., Wieand, H. S., Mobrtel, C. G., McGill, D. B., Yoprinnzi, C. L., O'Connell, M. J., Maclliard, J. A., Gerstner, J. B., Pandya, K., & Effefson, R. D. Accuracy of fecal occult blood screening for colorectal neoplasia: A prospective study using hemocult and hemoquant tests. *JAMA, 269*; 10: 1262–1267. 1993.

Alcorn J. M. Colorectal cancer prevention: A primary care approach. *Geriatrics, 47*; 2: 24–30. 1992.

Allison, J. E., Feldman R., & Tekawa, I. S. Hemoccult screening in detecting colorectal neoplasm: Sensitivity, specificity and predictive value: Long term follow up in a large group practice setting. *Ann Intern Med, 112*; 5: 328–333. 1990.

Bernstein L. H., Lenkhardt-Fairfield C. J., Pleban W., & Rudolph R.: Usefulness of data on albumin and prealbumin concentrations in determining effectiveness of nutritional support. Clin Chem 35; 2: 271–274. 1989.

Blunt, B. A., Barrett-Connor, E., & Wingard, D. L. Evaluation of fasting plasma glucose as screening test for NIDDM in older adults. Rancho Bernardo Study. *Diabetes Care, 14*; 11: 989–993. 1991.

Broughton, D. L., & Taylor, R. Review: Deterioration of glucose tolerance with age: The role of insulin resistance. *Age & Aging, 20*; 3: 221–225. 1991.

Busby, M. J., Bellantoni, M. F., Tobin, J. O., Muller, D. C., Kafonek, S. D., Blackman, M. R., & Andres, R. Glucose tolerance in women: The effects of age, body composition, and sex hormones. *J Am Geriatr Soc, 40*; 5: 497–502. 1992.

Campion, E. W., de Labry, L. O., & Glynn, R. J. The effect of age on serum albumin in healthy males: Report from the normative aging study. *J Gerontol 43*; 1: M18–20. 1988.

Cape, R. D. T., & Shinton, N. K. Serum vitamin B_{12} concentration in the elderly. *Gerontol Clin, 3*; 163–172. 1961.

Caird F. I.: Problems of interpretations of laboratory findings in the old. Br Med J. *4*: 348. 1973.

Castro, O. L., Haddy, T. B., & Rana, S. R. Age and sex related blood cell values in healthy black Americans. *Public Health Reports, 102*; 2: 232–237. 1987.

Catalona, W. S., Smith, O. S., Ratliff T. L., Dodds, K. M., Caplen, D. E., Yuan, J. J. J., Petros, J. A., & Andriole, G. L. Measurement of prostate specific antigen in serum as a screening test for prostate cancer. *N Engl J Med, 324*; 17: 1156–1161. 1991.

Cavalieri, T. A., Chopra, A., & Bryman, R. N. When outside the norm is normal: Interpreting lab data in the aged. *Geriatrics 47*; 5: 66–70. 1992.

Cebal, R. D., & Beck, J. R. Biochemical profiles: Applications in ambulatory screening and preadmission testing of adults. *Ann Intern Med, 106*; 3: 403–413. 1987.

Coodley, E. L. Laboratory tests in the elderly. *Postgrad Med 85*; 1: 333–338. 1989.

Cooner, W. H., Mosley, B. R., Rutherford, C. L., Beard, J. H., Pond, H. S., Terry, W. J., Igel, T. C., & Kidd, D. D. Prostate cancer detection in a clinical urological practice by ultrasonography, digital rectal examination and prostate specific antigen. *J Urol, 143*; 1146–1154. 1990.

Cooper, J. K., & Gardner, C. Effect of aging on serum albumin. *J Am Geriatr Soc 37*; 11: 039–1042. 1989.

Crawford, J., Eye-Boland, M. K., Harvey, B. S., & Cohen, J. Clinical utility of erythrocyte sedimentation rate and plasma protein analysis in the elderly. *Am J Med 82*; 2: 239–246. 1987.

Creditor, M. C., Smith, E. C., Gallai, J. B., Baumann, M., & Nelson, K. E. Tuberculosis, tuberculin reactivity and delayed cutaneous hypersensitivity in nursing home residents. *J Gerontology Medical Sci, 43*; 4: M97–100. 1988.

Domoto, K., Ben, R., Wei, J. Y., Pass, T. M., & Komoroff, A. L. Yield of routine annual laboratory screening in the institutionalized elderly. *Am J Public Health, 75*; 3: 243–245. 1985.

Drinka, P. J., Nolten, W. E., Vocks, S. K., & Langer, E. H. Follow-up of mild hypothyroidism in a nursing home. *J Am Geriatr Soc 39*; 3: 264–266. 1991.

Drinka, P. J., & Goodwin, J. S. Prevalence and consequences of vitamin deficiency in the nursing home: A critical review. *J Am Geriatr Soc, 39*; 10: 1008–1017. 1991.

Duthie, E. H., & Abbasi, A. A. Laboratory testing: Current recommendations for older adults. *Geriatrics, 46*; 10: 41–50. 1991.

Dybkaer, R., Lauritzen, M., & Krakauer, R. Relative reference values for clinical, chemical and haematological quantities in "healthy" elderly people. *Acta Med Scand, 209*; 1-2: 1-9. 1981.

Fagard, R. et al. Serum cholesterol levels and survival in elderly hypertensive patients: Analysis of data from the European Working Party on high blood pressure in the elderly. *Am J Med, 90*; 3A: 62S-63S. 1991.

Fritzsche, V., Tracy, T., Speirs J., & Glueck, C. J. Cholesterol screening in 5,719 self-referred elderly subjects. *J Gerontol, 45*; 6: M198-202. 1990.

Galen, R. S., & Gambino, S. R. *Beyond normality: The predictive value and efficiency of medical diagnosis.* New York: Wiley. 1975.

Gambert, S. R., Csuka, M. E., Duthie, E. H., & Tiegs, R. Interpretation of laboratory results in the elderly. *Postgrad Med 72*; 3: 147-152. 1982.

Gersovitz, M., Munroe, H. N., Udall, J., & Young, V. R. Albumin synthesis in young and elderly subjects using a new stable isotope methodology response to level of protein intake. *Metabolism—, 29*; 11: 1075-1086. 1980.

Greenblatt, O. J. Reduced serum albumin concentration in the elderly: A report from the Boston Collaborative Drug Surveillance Program. *J Am Geriatr Soc, 27*; 1: 20-22. 1979.

Griffiths, R. A., Good, W. R., Watson, N. P., O'Donnell, H. F., Fell, P. J., & Shakespeare, J. M. Normal erythrocyte sedimentation rate in the elderly. *B Med J, 289*; 6447: 724-725. 1984.

Grzybowski, S. Ontario studies on tuberculin sensitivity. *Can J. Public Health, 56*; 5: 181-192. 1965.

Hale, W. E., Stewart, R. B., & Marks, R. G. Hematology and biochemistry values in an ambulatory elderly population: An analysis of the effects of age, sex and drugs. *Age & Aging, 12*; 4: 275-284. 1983.

Hamilton, P. J., Dawson, A. A., Ogston, D. D., & Douglas, A. S. The effect of age on the fibrinolytic enzyme system. *J Clin Pathol, 27*; 4: 326-329. 1974.

Hanger, H. C., Sainsbury, M. B., Gilchrist, N. L., Beard, M. E. J., & Duncan, J. M.: A community study of vitamin B[12] and folate levels in the elderly. *J Am Geriatr Soc, 39*; 12: 1155-1159. 1991.

Helfand, M., & Crapo, L. M. Screening for thyroid disease. *Ann Intern Med 112*; 11: 840-849. 1990.

Herrmann, J., Heinen, E., Kroll, H. J., Rudorff, K. H., & Kruskemper, H. L. Thyroid function and thyroid hormone metabolism in elderly people: Low T[3] syndrome in old age? *Klin Wochenschr, 59*; 315-323. 1981.

Hirota, Y., Okamura, S., & Kimura, N. Hematopoesis in the aged as studied by in vitro colony assay. *Eur J Hematol, 40*; 1: 83-90. 1988.

Htoo, M. S. H., Kofkoff, R. L., & Freedman, M. L.: Erythrocyte parameters in the elderly: An argument against new geriatric normal values. *J Am Geriatr Soc, 27*; 27: 547-551. 1979.

Jernigan, J. A., Gudat J. C., Blake J. L., Bowen L. and Lezotte D.C.: Reference values for blood findings in relatively fit elderly persons. *J Am Geriatr Soc 28*; 7: 308-314. 1980.

Joosten E., Hiele, M., Pelemans, W., & Haesen E. Blood loss from diagnostic laboratory tests in elderly patients. *J Am Geriatr Soc, 40*: 3: 298. 1992.

Joseph, C., & Lytes, Y. Routine laboratory assessment of nursing home patients. *J Am Geriatr Soc, 40*; 1: 98–100. 1992.

Kaiser, F. E., & Morley, J. E. Cholesterol can be lowered in older persons. Should we care? *J Am Geriatr Soc, 39*; 1: 84–85. 1990.

Kalchthaler, T., & Rigor Tan, M. E. Anemia in institutionalized elderly patients. *J Am Geriatr Soc, 28*; 3: 108–113. 1980.

Kampmann, J. P., Sinding, J., & Moller-Jergensen, I. Effect of age on liver function. *Geriatrics, 30*; 8: 91–95. 1975.

Kashyap, M. L. Hyperlipidemia: Current recommendations and methods for making an accurate diagnosis. *Mod Med, 55*; 2: 56–60. 1987.

Keating, F. R., Jones, J. D., Elveback, C. R., & Randall, R. V. The relation of age and sex to distribution of values in healthy adults of serum calcium, inorganic phosphorus, magnesium, alkaline phosphatase, total protein, albumin and blood urea. *J Lab & Clin Med, 73*; 5: 825–834. 1969.

Klos, S. E., Drinka, P., & Goodwin, J. S. The utilization of fecal occult blood testing in the institutionalized elderly. *J Am Geriatr Soc, 39*; 12: 1169–1173. 1991.

Lehtonen, L., Eskola, J., Vainio, O., & Lehtonen, A. Changes in lymphocyte subsets and immune competence in very advanced age. *J Gerontol, 45*; 3: M108–112. 1990.

Leto, S., Kiergst, M. J., & Barrows, C. H. The effect of age and protein deprivation on the sulfhydryl content of serum albumin. *J Gerontol, 25*; 1: 4–8. 1970.

Levinstein, M. R., Ouslander, J. G., Rubinstein, L. Z., & Forsythe, S. B. Yield of routine annual laboratory tests in a skilled nursing home population. *JAMA, 258*; 14: 1909–1915. 1987.

Lowik, M. R. H., Wedel, M., Kok, F. J., Odink, J., Westenbrink, S., & Meulmeester, J. F. Nutrition and serum cholesterol levels among elderly men and women (Dutch nutrition surveillance system). *J Gerontol, 46*; 1: M23–28. 1991.

Makinodan, T., & Kay, M. B. Age influence on the immune system. *Adv Immunol, 29*; 2: 287–327. 1980.

Mandel, J. S., Bond, J. H., Bradley, M., Snover, D. C., Church, T. R., Williams, S., Watt, G., Schuman, L. M., Ederer, F., & Gilbertsen, V. Sensitivity, specificity and positive predictivity of the Hemoccult test in screening for colorectal cancers. *Gastroenterology, 97*; 3: 597–600. 1989.

Mattila, K. S., Knusela, V., & Palliniemi, T. T. Haematological laboratory findings in the elderly: Influence of age and sex. *Scand J Clin Lab Invest, 46*; 5: 411–415. 1986.

Mayer, J., & Necheler, H. Studies in old age. IV The clinical significance of salivary, gastric and pancreatic secretion in the aged. *JAMA, 115*; 24: 2050–2053. 1940.

Meade, T. W., Chahrabarti, R., Haines, A. P., North, W. R. S. & Sterling, Y. Characteristics affecting fibrinolytic activity and plasma fibrinogen concentrations. *Brit Med J 1*; 6157: 153–156. 1979.

Mettlin, C., Lee, F., Drago, J., & Murphy, G. P., et al. The American Cancer Society National Prostate Cancer Detection Project. Findings on the detection of early prostate cancer in 2,425 men. *Cancer, 67*; 12: 2949–2958. 1991.

Mims, A. D., Norman, D. C., Yamamura, R. H., & Yoshikawa, T. T. Clinically inapparent (asymptomatic) bacteriuria in ambulatory elderly men: Epidemiological, clinical and microbiological findings. *J Am Geriatr Soc, 39*; 11: 1209–1214. 1990.

Morgan, D. B. The impact of aging—present and future. *Ann Clin Biochem, 20*; 257–261. 1983.

Morris, J. B., Stellato, T. A., Guy, B. B., Gordon, N. H., & Berger, N. A. A critical analysis of the largest reported mass fecal occult blood screening program in the United States. *Am J Surg, 161*; 1: 101–106. 1991.

Munro, H. N., McGandy, R. B., Harty, S. C., Russell, R. M., Jacob, R. A., & Otradovec, M. A. Protein nutriture of a group of free-living elderly. *Am J Clin Nutr, 46*; 4: 586–592. 1987.

Myers, A. M., Saunders, C. R. G., & Chalmers, D. G.: The haemoglobin level of fit elderly people. *Lancet 2*; 7: 261–263. 1968.

Nilsson-Ehle, H., Jagenburg, R., Landahl, S., Svanborg, A., & Westin, J. Hematological abnormalities and reference intervals in the elderly. *Acta Med Scand, 224*; 6: 595–604. 1988.

Noel, M., Smith, T. K., & Ettinger, W. H . Characteristics and outcomes of hospitalized older patients who develop hypocholesterolemia. *J Am Geriatr Soc, 39*; 5: 455–461. 1991.

Ochs, M. Selecting routine outpatient tests for older adults. *Geriatrics, 46*; 11: 39–50. 1991.

Oesterling, J. E. Prostate specific antigen: A critical assessment of the most useful tumor marker for adenocarcinoma of the prostate. *J Urol, 145*; 5: 907–923. 1991.

Orwoll, E. S., Weigel, R. M., Oviatt, S. K., Meier, D. E., & McClung, M. R. Serum protein concentrations and bone mineral content in aging normal men. *Am J Clin Nutr, 46*; 4: 614–621. 1987.

Pauker, S. G., & Kassirer, M. D. Medical progress: Decision analysis. *N Engl J Med, 316*; 5: 250–258. 1987.

Pauker, S. G., & Kassirer, J. P. Special article: The threshold to clinical decision making. *N Engl J Med, 302*; 20: 1109–1117. 1980.

Rock, R. C.: Effects of age on common laboratory tests. *Geriatrics, 39*; 6: 57–60. 1984.

Rock, R. C. Interpreting laboratory tests: A basic approach. *Geriatrics, 39*; 1: 48–54. 1984b.

Rock, R. C. Interpreting thyroid tests in the elderly: Updated guidelines. *Geriatrics, 40*; 12: 61–68. 1985.

Romm, P. A., Green, C. E., Reagan K., & Rackley, C. E.: Relation of serum lipoprotein cholesterol levels to presence and severity of angiographic coronary artery disease. *Am J Cardiol, 67*; 3: 479–483. 1991.

Runnels, B. L., Garry, P. J., Hunt, W. C., & Standefer, J. C. Thyroid function in a healthy elderly population: Implications for clinical evaluation. *J Gerontol, 46*; 1: B39–44. 1991.

Salive, M. E., Cornini-Hantley, J., Guralnik, J. M., Phillips, C. L., Wallace, R. B., Ostfeld, A. M., & Cohen, H. J. Anemia and hemoglobin levels in older persons: Relationships with age, gender and health status. *J Am Geriatr Soc, 40*; 5: 489–496. 1992.

Shearn, M. A., & Kang, J. V. Effect of age and sex on the erythrocyte sedimentation rate. *J Rheumatol, 13*; 2: 297–298. 1986.

Shibata, H., Haga, H., Eleno, M., Nagai, H., Yasumura, S., & Koyano, W. Longitudinal changes of serum albumin in elderly people living in the community. *Age Aging, 20*; 6: 417–420. 1991.

Shimokata, H., Muller, D. C., Fleg, J. L., Sorkin, J., Ziemba, A. W., & Andres, R. Age as independent determinant of glucose tolerance. *Diabetes, 40*; 1: 44–51. 1991.

Sorva, A., Valvanne, J., & Tilvis, R. S. Serum ionized calcium and the presence of primary hyperthyroidism in age cohorts of 75, 80 and 85 years. *J Intern Med, 231*; 3: 309–312. 1992.

Sourander, L. B. Urinary tract infection in the aged. *Ann Med Intern Fenn, 55* (Suppl 45): 7. 1966.

Sparrow, D., Row, J. W., & Silbert, J. E. Cross-sectional and longitudinal changes in the erythrocyte sedimentation rate in men. *J Gerontol, 36*; 2: 180–184. 1981.

Stead, W. W. Medical perspective—does the risk of tuberculosis increase in old age? *J Infect Dis, 147*; 5: 951–955. 1983.

Sundbeck, G., Lundberg, P. A., Lindstedt, G., Jagenburg, R., & Eden S. Incidence and prevalence of thyroid disease in elderly women: Results from the longitudinal population study of elderly people in Gothenburg, Sweden. *Age Aging, 20*; 4: 291–298. 1991.

Tietz, N. W., Wekstein, D. R., Shuey, D. F., & Brauer, G. A. A two-year longitudinal reference range study for selected serum enzymes in a population more than 60 years of age. *J Am Geriatr Soc, 32*; 8: 563–570. 1984.

Timiras, M. L., & Brownstein H. Prevalence of anemia and correlation of hemoglobin with age in a geriatric screening clinic population. *J Am Geriatr Soc, 35*; 7: 639–643. 1987.

Tronetti, P. S., Graceley, E. J., & Boscia, J. A. Lack of association between medication use and the presence or absence of bacteriuria in elderly women. *J Am Geriatr Soc, 38*; 11: 1199–1202. 1990.

Vorken, E., Grzybowski, S., & Allen, E. A. Significance of the tuberculin test in the elderly. *Chest, 92*; 2: 237–240. 1987.

Wernick, R. Avoiding laboratory test misinterpretation in geriatric rheumatology. *Geriatrics, 44*; 2: 61–80. 1989.

Winkler, M. F., Gerrior, S. A., Ponp, A., & Albina, J. E. Use of retinal binding protein and prealbumin as indicators of the response to nutrition therapy. *Perspectives in Practice, 89*; 5:684–687. 1989.

Wiske, P. S., Epstein, S., Bell, N. H., Queener, S. F., Edmondson, I. E., & Johnstone, C. C. Increases in immunoreactive parathyroid hormone with age. *N Engl J Med, 300*; 25: 1419–1421. 1979.

Wolf-Klein, G. P., Holt, T., Silverstone, F. A., Foley, C. J., & Spatz, M. Efficiency of routine annual studies in the care of elderly patients. *J Am Geriatr Soc, 33*; 5: 325–329. 1985.

Wolfson, S. A., Kolmanson, G. M., & Rubins, M. E. Epidemiology of bacteriuria in a predominantly geriatric male population. *Am J Med Sci,* *250*;168;38; 86 1965.

Zauber, N. P., & Zauber, A. G. Hematologic data of healthy very old people. *JAMA, 257*; 16: 2181–2184. 1987.

Chapter Three

Prophylactic (Preventive) Therapies in Old Age

Lawrence J. Kerzner and Spencer Van B. Wilking

Life table graphs depicting survivors in populations of developing countries plotted against age have shifted to the right during this past century without a concomitant prolongation of life span (Hayflick, 1976; Schneider, 1985). This has resulted in a steepened slope of descent in old age and has suggested that diminishing the impact of debilities associated with chronic illnesses, or delaying their onset, could theoretically result in an ultimate rectangular curve. Functional limitations would be compressed into fewer years, and death in the population would uniformly occur at a given age (Fries, 1980). Based on this observation, a measurement of "active life expectancy" has been proposed to illustrate the expected duration of functional well-being, the end-point of which is defined by onset of dependency in activities of daily living (Katz et al., 1983). The term "successful aging" considers the biological effects of age separate and distinct from the impact of intercurrent disease and environmental stress, as occurs in "usual" aging (Rowe & Kahn, 1987). Diminished death rates at younger ages have resulted in an overall older but more functionally impaired population, focusing attention on the need to develop more effective techniques that are targeted at preventing and delaying the onset of chronic debilities (Stout & Crawford, 1988; Williams & Hadler, 1983).

Prophylactic interventions have as their primary purpose preventive rather than remedial outcomes. In contrast to interventions directed at improving symptomatic debility as a consequence of acute or chronic illness, or other functional limitations, prophylactic measures are designed to effect some future benefit. Table 3.1 identifies a nosology of morbid events responsible for significant debility in the elderly, organized by underlying pathophysiologic processes that might be amenable to prophylactic intervention, location of health care provision where clinical decisions need to be made regarding such interventions, and the type of interventions that have been proposed as being effective. "Primary prevention" (1°) includes those interventions designed to prevent or lessen the likelihood of a disease developing. "Secondary prevention" (2°) encompasses interventions targeted at preventing the symptomatic manifestation of disease once the underlying pathophysiologic process is established. Tertiary prevention (3°) implies prevention of subsequent debility after a disease process has become symptomatic. Immunization against certain infectious diseases (influenza, pneumococcal pneumonia, tetanus) are good illustrations of primary preventive therapy. In practical terms, however, most interventions are not usually fully characterized by any single level of prevention; they may exhibit features characteristic of all three at the same time. This chapter will focus attention on preventing morbidity as a consequence of preexisting illness.

Specific loci of health care delivery may bear particular relevance for preventive efforts, depending on the type of problem considered as potentially preventable and the location where patients exhibit a high prevalence of predisposing factors. Increasingly complex medical care decisions are being made in home care and long-term care institutional settings, bringing them clearly into the arena of medical technology evaluation.

Since future circumstances are affected by numerous, frequently unpredictable variables, the wisdom of initiating prophylactic interventions must be subject to analysis that carefully weighs their potential for current and future liabilities. Cape's (1978) conceptualization of clinical problems in geriatric care as the intersection of five commonly occurring problematic areas—falls, incontinence, confusion, homeostatic dysregulation and iatrogenesis—highlights the observation that adverse effects of medical interventions are part of the frequent syndromic presentation of clinical problems in the elderly and underscores the frequency with which well-intentioned interventions may be responsible for adverse clinical effects. Since Steel (Steel, Gertman, Crescenzi, & Anderson, 1981) reported

TABLE 3.1 Nosology of Morbid Events Responsible for Significant Debility

Prophylaxis for or Prevention of Morbid Event of Special Relevance to the Elderly	Target	Locus of Clinical Decision	Type of Prevention	Potential Interventions
1. Bone fracture	Osteoporosis	O,L	1°	Diet (calcium intake), weightbearing exercise, smoking cessation.
		O,L	2°	Estrogen replacement, calcium, calcitriol weightbearing exercise.
		O,L	3°	Estrogen replacement, biphosphonates, calcitriol, calcium, calcitonin, fluoride.
2. Lower extremity deep venous thrombophlebitis, pulmonary embolus	Lower extremity deep venous thrombophlebitis	H,L	1°	Subcutaneous low dose (low molecular weight) heparin, low dose warfarin, mechanical venous compression.
		H	2°	Therapeutic anticoagulation, inferior vena cava interruption.
		H	3°	Therapeutic anticoagulation, inferior vena cava interruption.
3. Cardiovascular events	Isolated Systolic Hypertension	O	2°	Antihypertensive medications
4. Stroke	Carotid artery atherothrombosis	O,L,H	2°	Aspirin, ticlopidine, warfarin, Carotid endarterectomy, antihypertensive medication
		O,L,H	3°	
5. Symptomatic urinary tract infection	Asymptomatic bacteriuria	L,O	2°	Antibiotics
6. Falls and associated injuries	Gait abnormality - cognitive deficits	L	2°	Protective device (restraints), sedating medicines
			3°	
7. Active tuberculosis	Latent tuberculosis	L,O	2°	Antitubercular antibiotics, TB skin test screening
8. Pneumococcal pneumonia, tetanus, influenza	Bacterial infection or intoxication, viral infection	O,L,H	1°	Immunization
9. Recurrent aspiration pneumonia	Oral-tracheal aspiration	L,H	3°	Improved feeding techniques, preventing constipation related ileus.

L = Long Term Care   O = Outpatient Office   H = Hospital

that 36% of 815 consecutive patients admitted to a general medical service over a 5-month period experienced an iatrogenic illness, 9% of which were considered life-threatening or produced considerable debility, additional reports have confirmed at least a 25%–50% iatrogenic illness rate during acute hospitalization (Davis, Shapiro, & Kane, 1984; Jahnigen, Hannon, Laxson, & La Force, 1982; Lefevre et al., 1992; Steel et al., 1981). Adverse drug reactions in the elderly underlie approximately 5%–10% of admissions to acute hospitals (Colt & Shapiro, 1989; Lakshmanan, Hershey, & Breslan, 1986). These observations point out that any intervention should be carefully considered with respect to potential adverse effect.

INFORMED CONSENT

Concepts of informed consent lie at the heart of the doctor-patient relationship. These have been articulated to include ensuring patient understanding of the proposed treatment, risks and benefits of what is proposed, description of the alternatives, possible outcomes of no treatment, probability of success (and what that means), details of recuperation, and any other information the patient may determine to be important (Annas, 1989). The patient must have the capacity to decide the issue, meaning that the patient must be able to understand the nature of the information needed to give consent. It becomes clear that interventions undertaken as preventive in nature bear particular relevance to the "benefits" and "likely result if no treatment" aspects. A careful understanding of the natural history of the underlying pathophysiologic processes one is attempting to influence, as well as the existence of or potential for intercurrent illness and debility, help patients respond to the "possible outcome of no treatment" section. Detailed understanding of potential benefits originates in interventional or other forms of observational research (as does risk). However, our desire to embrace prophylactic (temporal reorganizational) strategies is frequently tempered by the recognition, especially in the setting of already existing debilities or chronic diseases, that the limitations, potential risks, and added requirements imposed by such proposals may weigh very heavily in our patients' perceptions against overall benefit. Considering that those over 65 constitute 12.5% of the U.S. population yet receive 25% of all prescription drugs, that home-dwelling elderly take an average of 4.5 prescribed medicines per year, and that both physicians and patients are increasingly aware of the potential problems associated with polypharmacy, it is not surprising that adding only one more medicine or additional need for medical care intervention may be viewed by the elderly person as untenable.

Normal psychological development in old age includes the concepts of self-acceptance and ego integrity. Enhanced attention to review of life events fostering psychological consolidation of who the person "is" and a greater acceptance of functional debility allows for a relative diminution of energy directed toward planning for future events. While the medical care provider may view with frustration the forgoing of treatment designed to prevent a "bad" outcome, respect for each persons individual assessment of his or her own desires is paramount and may provide insight into other potential avenues for therapeutic direction.

We should note, however, that well-validated measurements of patients' functional state, well-being, and health perception are increasingly being applied to populations receiving various treatment modalities, providing objective insight into what was previously understood as an entirely subjective and anecdotally characterized area: self-described quality of life determinations. For example, in one report the requirements for taking medicine and enhanced monitoring of warfarin therapy used as a prophylaxis for arterial emboli in patients with atrial fibrillation did not adversely affect these quality of life measures (Lancaster et al., 1991; Hirsch, 1991b). Since we now have the tools to quantify how populations of patients perceive particular interventions with respect to impact on quality of life, we will increasingly be better able to understand and communicate this aspect of benefits and burdens of prophylactic therapy (Kutner, Nixon, & Silverstone, 1991).

PREVENTION OF OSTEOPOROSIS IN OLD AGE

Bone fractures in the elderly contribute very substantially to functional dependence, debility, health care costs, and death. Osteoporosis is the most significant underlying risk factor for bone fracture to occur with any given degree of mechanical stress. While improving gait abnormalities and preventing falls are likely to decrease fractures, causing a decrease in the progression of bone loss that occurs as a concomitant of aging may also diminish the prevalence of bone fractures in any specific age group. Analysis of risk factors may help determine which persons are at greatest risk of bone thinning in perimenopausal years and in advanced old age, as well as identify those in whom osteoporosis is likely to have already significantly progressed. Predisposing factors include family history of osteoporosis and fractures, diet, smoking, body frame and size, medicines, underlying diseases associated with osteoporosis, degree of physical activity, and age at menopause (natural or surgical).

The cellular pathophysiology of perimenopausal bone loss is a consequence of estrogen withdrawal and relates to enhanced osteoclastic bone resorption (Riggs & Melton, 1992). Osteoblastic bone deposition is increased as well but to a lesser degree than resorption. The net overall effect is a loss of bone. This rapid phase of bone loss (Type I) persists for 5 years after normal or surgically induced menopause and is responsible for up to 3% of bone loss per year. A consequence of rapid perimenopausal bone loss is an earlier onset of symptomatic osteoporosis in women compared to men. Bone loss that develops with advanced age (Type II) is related to osteoclastic bone resorption, proceeding at the rate associated with normal bone remodeling but with marked diminished osteoblastic bone accretion. The progression of Type II bone loss in men is such that by the ninth decade of life osteoporosis is equally severe in both sexes.

Measurements of bone density via single photon absorption densitometry, dual energy photon absorption densitometry, dual energy x-ray absorption densitometry, and quantitative computer tomography have been proposed for osteoporosis screening, as well as for providing serial measurements of those who have been identified as being at high risk (Sartoris, & Resnick, 1990). Difficulties in distinguishing between cortical and trabecular bone density, limitations of analysis of bone density to peripheral sites using single photon methods, radiation associated with computer tomography, and cost are technical limitations in this technology's current broad applicability. While there may be a relationship between appendicular skeletal density and hip fractures, there is a great overlap between those with and without fracture (Cummings et al., 1990; Johnston, Slemenda, & Melton, 1991). Dual photon, dual energy x-ray absorbed densitometry and quantitative computer tomographic techniques can measure bone density at the hip, but these areas have been available for too short a time to develop an intimate understanding of their long-term accuracy in predicting hip fracture.

Partly as a consequence of the limitation of bone density measuring techniques, as well as limitations in our understanding of the full range of effects of proposed therapeutic options, bone density measurements used as screening tools for osteoporosis have not been recommended as a public health initiative (Melton, Eddy, & Johnston, 1990). However, if treatment with estrogen is being considered for a specific patient for primary prevention of osteoporosis (by delaying its onset) or for secondary or tertiary prevention of symptomatic debility (fracture) as a consequence of osteoporosis, bone density determined to be in the lower one-third of age-matched populations may be helpful information.

Potential prophylactic interventions include the following.

Estrogen

Estrogen's effect on the skeleton is as an antiresorptive agent. Treatment with estrogen in perimenopausal years inhibits osteoclastic stimulation that occurs as a consequence of estrogen withdrawal, thereby preventing the immediate rapid phase of bone loss. It has been pointed out that perimenopausal use of estrogen to effect primary prophylaxis of osteoporosis should be continued for at least 5–10 years so as to sufficiently delay the onset of rapid bone loss and subsequent reduction of bone mass beyond the fracture threshold to an age at which other causes of morbidity and mortality play a more significant role. Data from the Framingham Osteoporosis Study identified a waning beneficial effect on primary prophylaxis of osteoporosis conferred by at least seven years of prior estrogen therapy in women over 75 years old and suggests consideration of lifelong prophylactic treatment (Felson et al., 1993).

The beneficial effect of estrogen on bone is accompanied by a myriad of other hormonal and tissue effects. Estrogen alone decreases the risk for coronary artery disease, may slightly increase the risk of breast cancer, and clearly increases the risk of uterine cancer (Henrich, 1992). An analysis that translated relative risks to absolute risks by considering actual prevalence of morbid events indicated that by using estrogen between ages 65 and 74 years there would be a 0.36% absolute reduction in death from hip fracture, a 0.30% absolute increase in the risk of death from breast cancer, a 2.4% absolute reduction in the risk of death from ischemic heart disease, and a 2.4% increase in the absolute risk of death from endometrial carcinoma (Goldman & Tosteson, 1991). However, since it has been suggested that uterine cancer related to estrogen use is more rapidly identified and cured via surgery than naturally occurring disease, because of enhanced screening and an increased awareness of the potential problem, the actual increase in absolute risk of death from endometrial carcinoma may indeed be much less. Adding medroxyprogesterone, 5 mg daily, has the effect of causing endometrial involution which is thought to negate entirely the enhanced risk of endometrial carcinoma brought about by unopposed estrogen. While the marked reduction in death from cardiovascular causes overshadows all other enhanced risks, the reversal by progesterone of the beneficial HDL/LDL ratio (Walsh et al., 1991) induced by estrogen is likely to bring about some reduction in cardiovascular benefit during combined therapy. Guidelines for counseling postmenopausal women regarding preventive hormonal therapy have been promulgated (American College of Physicians, 1992; Grady, Ruben, & Petitti, 1992). Clinicians should consider that while the increase in risk of death as a consequence of breast cancer is equaled by the reduction in risk of death from hip fracture, the patient's subjective interpretation of that risk–benefit ratio is likely to weigh against estrogen therapy. A randomized controlled trial of estrogen replacement therapy will be critical in helping to define more clearly the specific benefits and potential liabilities of postmenopausal estrogen use.

Estrogen administered orally or transdermally also may be helpful in tertiary prophylaxis of bone fractures in the elderly via a beneficial effect on established osteoporosis of old age (Ott, 1992). Estrogen-induced blockade of bone resorption results in an overshoot of bone formation as a consequence of continued osteoblastic bone accretion and may result in a 5%–10% increase in bone density when measured over 1 year and a lower rate of new vertebral fractures (Lufken, Wahner, & O'Fallon, 1991).

Biphosphonates

Biphosphonates impair bone resorption by adhering to bone crystals and inhibiting osteoclastic activity. Cyclic administration of etidronate and calcium have been used as tertiary prophylaxis for fractures by stabilizing bone loss and causing small increases in spinal mass (Storm, 1990; Watts et al., 1990). Decreased numbers of vertebral compression fractures have resulted when cyclic etidronate and calcium were given for a 2 year period in patients with postmenopausal osteoporosis and preexisting spinal compression fractures.

Calcium

Obligate calcium losses in urine and stool result in a net calcium loss from bone if sufficient dietary intake and absorption is not maintained. Evidence supporting enhancement of bone mass in premenopausal women given 1500 mg calcium supplement daily suggest a primary prophylactic effect. Dietary calcium supplementation in postmenopausal women has secondary and tertiary preventive value as well. When controlled for the rapid bone loss consequent to physiologic peri-menopausal estrogen withdrawal, 1000 mg per day calcium supplement significantly reduced bone loss determined via dual energy x-ray absorptiometry at axial and appendicular sites over 2 years (Reid, Ames, Evans, Gamble, & Sharpe, 1993). Dosages of 800 IU vitamin D_3 and 1200 mg per day elemental calcium supplementation compared to placebo resulted in a similarly measured increase in proximal femur bone density and a significant decrease in the subsequent hip and non-vertebral fracture rate over an 18-month period (Chapuy et al., 1992).

Distinguishing a secondary from a tertiary preventive effect is not possible from this study because women who previously sustained fractures were included. While vitamin D effects on bone mineralization independent of an effect on promotion of calcium absorption probably played a role, it has been pointed out that at least some of its effect was via calcium, which argues strongly for calcium supplementation (Heaney, 1993). Elemental calcium supplementation, 1500 mg per day, for postmenopausal women has been suggested (Office of Medical Applications, 1984). Exercise regimens plus calcium have demonstrated a slower rate of bone loss in secondary preventive studies (Prince et al., 1991).

Calcitriol (1–25 dihydroxy vitamin D_3)

Calcitriol (1–25 dihydroxy vitamin D_3) has also been demonstrated as having tertiary prophylactic value in experimental protocols (Gallagher & Goldgard, 1990; Tilyard, Spears, & Thompson, 1992). The need for careful metabolic follow-up during treatment with calcitriol limits its general applicability and is currently regarded as experimental (Chestnut, 1992).

Fluoride and Parathyroid Hormone

Sodium fluoride and parathyroid hormone have been used in experimental models to attempt osteoblastic bone stimulation. Sodium fluoride has been associated with decreased quality of bone and an unacceptable rate of gastrointestinal side effects.

Calcitonin

Parenteral calcitonin has antiresorptive properties that can transiently increase vertebral bone mass in women with postmenopausal osteoporosis. Its expense and need for administration via parenteral injection have precluded extensive clinical and field evaluation.

PROPHYLAXIS AGAINST LOWER-EXTREMITY DEEP VENOUS THROMBOPHLEBITIS AND PULMONARY EMBOLUS

The importance of identifying an optimal prophylactic approach against lower-extremity deep venous thrombophlebitis and pulmonary embolus is underscored by the observation that 300,000–600,000 hospitalizations in the United States per year are associated with these problems and that 50,000 deaths per year are due to pulmonary embolus. Even more people experience some degree of debility as a consequence of chronic venous insufficiency. Rational clinical approaches to these problems have been articulated by the World Health Organization, the NIH Office of Medical Applications of Research, and others (Goldhaber & Morpurgo, 1992; Hyers, Hull, & Weg, 1992; Office of Medical Applications, 1986). Since advanced age is a major risk factor predisposing to venous thrombosis and thromboembolism, understanding the extent to which prophylactic interventions are under- or overutilized in the elderly is relevant. It has been suggested that virtually all hospitalized adult patients, particular after major surgery should receive prophylactic measures directed against venous thromboembolism. This would include pharmacologic, nonpharmacologic, and combined interventions. Graded compression stockings extending to midthigh have been considered a basic primary prophylaxis among low-risk patients and should be used, except for those who have compromised peripheral arterial circulation. Intermittent pneumatic compression also provides primary prophylaxis. Inferior vena cava interruption has been used as primary prophylaxis against pulmonary emboli in patients at extreme high risk and as secondary and tertiary prophylaxis in those in whom anticoagulation has failed or is contraindicated. Pharmacologic interventions have focused on low dose heparin, low-molecular-weight fractionated heparin, dose-adjusted warfarin, minidose warfarin, and aspirin.

Despite a volume of medical literature detailing consensus regarding potential risks, clinical use of potentially effective prophylactic measures in high-risk situations may be less than optimal. In 2,017 high-risk patients identified in 16 short-stay hospitals, prophylaxis was given in 32% with large interhospital degree of variability (Anderson et al., 1991). The five leading high-risk situations in this group were considered to be advanced age, surgery, obesity, cancer, and congestive heart failure. This study excluded graded elastic compression as acceptable prophylaxis because the patients were considered high risk.

Observations of underprescription of prophylaxis contrasts with concerns regarding overuse, especially with respect to optimal duration of subcutaneous heparin. Based on a 13% prevalence of lower-extremity venous thrombosis identified via fibrinogen scanning in hospitalized, non-acutely ill patients, recommendations have been made for continuous prophylaxis (Kierkegaard et al., 1987). It must be recognized, however, that study populations were invariably hospitalized patients. Since hospital care is likely to serve as a marker for recent acute illness and a consequent inflammatory response–related activation of coagulation factors, extrapolation of the prevalence of phlebitis determined in this population may not be referable to a nonhospitalized group. Doing so may result in an overestimate of phlebitis risk and be a stimulus for overprescription of pharmacological prophylaxis. A bed-bound or bed-to-chair level of activity, without other phlebitis risk factors, may not carry a high positive predictive value in identifying those at high risk. Understanding the locus of care as a marker for other potential risk factors is further blurred because, increasingly, patients with acute illness are cared for in long-term care and home care settings. The question of how long to continue subcutaneous heparin prophylaxis initiated during acute illness that has since resolved, with the person remaining relatively immobile and now cared for in a nonhospital setting, is raised. Continuous prophylaxis has been suggested for high-risk patients during the first month after hospital discharge (Goldhaber & Morpurgo, 1992).

Potential liabilities of heparin prophylaxis in nonsurgical patients include the need for twice-daily subcutaneous injection, resulting in progressive patient discomfort and injection site hematomas. Patients who are able to vocalize concern are very rarely able to tolerate 1 month of therapy. The twice-daily injection also identifies a requirement for skilled nursing care, which has great implications for the locus of the care to provide proper professional staff personnel and training at enhanced cost. Indeed the NIH consensus conference concluded with a call for randomized clinical trials focusing on determining which patients truly need prophylactic therapy and avoiding special high-risk circumstances (Office of Medical Applications, 1986).

Standard pharmacologic prophylactic intervention in nonsurgical patients consists of administering unfractionated heparin subcutaneously in low doses, 5,000 units every 8–12 hours. Commercial heparin is a heterogeneous (molecular weight 3,000–30,0000, mean 15,000) mixture of molecules prepared from porcine intestinal mucosa or bovine lung tissue (Hirsh, 1991a). Only one-third of the heparin mixture is active as an anticoagulant. Low-molecular-weight heparin fractionations (molecular weight 4,000–6,500) have greater half-life and biological availability than does standard heparin. Once-daily subcutaneous administration of low-molecular-weight heparin was at least as effective as continuous intravenous infusion of unfractionated heparin in the treatment of proximal deep vein thrombosis and appeared to be associated with a decrease in early hemorrhagic complications (Hull et al., 1992). Extrapolation of this information may help design effective once daily subcutaneous therapeutic and prophylactic regimens that might be more amenable to long-term care and home care settings (Salzman, 1992). While very low dose warfarin regimens (INR 1.5) have been suggested, the need for prothrombin time monitoring complicates this regimen and discourages its widespread applicability, especially in long-term care settings. Self-monitoring of prothrombin times via whole-blood finger stick determination may allow for enhanced acceptability of these regimens (Hyers et al., 1992).

ISOLATED SYSTOLIC HYPERTENSION

Blood pressure values reflect the characteristics of a continuous variable such that the relative risk of morbidity or mortality from atherothrombotic disease, whether cardiovascular or cerebrovascular, increases with elevations of either the systolic component, the diastolic component, or both. The prevalence of hypertension is high in an ever expanding elderly population. For instance, the National Health And Nutrition Examination Survey found that 63% of individuals aged 65–74 years have blood pressure with either systolic or diastolic pressures in excess of 140/90 mmHg (Working Group, 1986).

While the ramifications of diastolic blood pressure elevation have long been evident to the medical community in terms of increased relative risks for stroke, coronary artery, and peripheral vascular disease (Veterans Administration, 1970), the recognition that isolated systolic hypertension (ISH) is a highly prevalent and morbid condition amenable to treatment has been poorly recognized until recently. Elevations of systolic blood pressure greater than 160 mmHg with a diastolic pressure less than 90 mmHg is the most common form of hypertension in the elderly, affecting 57% of elderly men and 65% of elderly women (Wilking et al., 1988). Furthermore, ISH has an appreciable morbidity and mortality associated with it. Data from the Framingham Heart Study show that ISH contributes a twofold increase in all causes of cardiovascular disease mortality among elderly men and threefold increase in cardiovascular disease rates among elderly women. In addition, the incidence rates for coronary heart disease and stroke are increased 2.5 times in both men and women with ISH when compared with a normotensive cohort. Despite these ominous results, however, prophylactic treatment of ISH was not attempted because questions about efficacy of pharmacological intervention added to concerns that drug side effects would be too extensive to justify their use in an elderly population.

Fortunately, the Systolic Hypertension in Elderly Program, a multicenter, prospective, placebo-controlled study, conducted over a 5-year period helped to answer the question of whether treatment of ISH was safe, effective, and feasible in functionally unimpaired patients. The results revealed that a treatment regimen of either low-dose chlorthalidone alone or combined with atenolol up to 50 mg reduced incidence of nonfatal and fatal stroke by 36% over the 5-year study period (SHEP, 1991). This regimen also reduced the rate of nonfatal myocardial infarction and all cause coronary deaths by 25% in the same 5-year period. A high proportion of the study population achieved appropriate reductions in systolic blood pressure over the course of the study, and evaluation of side effects revealed no significant difference between the placebo and treatment groups in terms of significant complications from treatment.

The SHEP study therefore demonstrated that not only was ISH a prevalent and morbid condition but that for many elderly people appropriate blood pressure reduction is feasible and that this reduction confers a significant benefit in terms of protection from stroke and coronary disease.

Thus, hypertension in general and ISH in particular are common disorders amenable to prevention at the secondary level because once established as disease entities their cerebrovascular and cardiovascular sequelae can be palliated or removed. Clearly, antihypertensive interventions in the form of nonpharmacologic or pharmacologic modalities are absolutely necessary to combat all forms of elevated blood pressure in an increasing elderly population that can ill afford the devastating consequences of a stroke or coronary event. Perhaps in no other area of medicine could the adage of an ounce of prevention being worth a pound of cure be more pertinent and profound than in regard to the vigorous identification and treatment of abnormal blood pressure elevations in the elderly.

PREVENTION OF STROKE

The progressive decreased incidence of stroke to 6% per year during the past two decades is testimony to the beneficial primary preventive effects of enhanced population-wide control of hypertension and its contribution to atherosclerotic craniovascular disease. Once carotid artery atherscleorosis is established, progression of the disease results in ulcerative plaque formation, micro- and macroarterial emboli, progressive arterial occlusion, and subsequent ipsilateral brain infarction. With respect to pharmacological prevention of stroke or myocardial infarction, medical literature invariably confuses the terms *secondary prevention* with *primary* and *tertiary prevention* with *secondary* (Rothrock & Hart, 1991). By way of example, prevention of myocardial infarction by aspirin, in the "Physician's Study," has been considered a primary preventive effect (Steering Committee, 1989). However, when viewed from the perspective of underlying pathophysiology, aspirin's effect on diminishing the likelihood of coronary artery thrombosis as a consequence of coronary atherosclerosis is clearly understood as a form of secondary prevention. (Asymptomatic coronary artery disease is already present; symptomatic disease is prevented). Similarly, the diminished risk of stroke in patients with carotid artery–related transient ischemic attacks (TIAs) treated with aspirin, identified in the literature as secondary prevention, is clearly recognized as tertiary prevention since symptoms of the underlying disease are already present (Grotta, 1987; Lekstrom & Bell, 1991).

The role of carotid endarterectomy in preventing stroke, the subject of intense investigation, has recently been brought more clearly into focus (North American Symptomatic, Carotid Endarterectomy Trial Collaborators, 1991). This study was designed to evaluate the tertiary preventive effects of carotid endarterectomy on subsequent ipsilateral stroke in patients already experiencing carotid distribution TIAs or nondisabling stroke. Patients with these symptoms were randomly assigned to continued medical therapy or carotid artery surgery by surgeons and hospitals meeting strict performance standards. Whether randomized to medical or surgical treatment, almost all patients received an antithrombotic medicine. Patients were excluded if they had underlying an illness that was considered to reduce their 5-year chance of survival to less than 50% or had had a recent myocardial infarction, cognitive impairment, uncontrolled diabetes, severe hypertension, or other major organ dysfunction. Interim analysis of the data in December 1990 identified such beneficial effects for those with high-grade stenosis (70%–99% occlusion), in terms of subsequent stroke and death from any cause, that continued entry of this category of patient into the study was discontinued (U.S. Department of Health and Human Services, 1990). Outcome for patients with moderate (30%–69%) degrees of stenosis has not yet indicated a clear benefit (Barnett et al., 1992). With respect to carotid endarterectomy performed on asymptomatic patients with even severe carotid stenosis (secondary prevention), data are as yet insufficient to clearly demonstrate benefit (Barnett & Haines, 1993, Hobson et al., 1993).

SYMPTOMATIC URINARY TRACT INFECTION

Asymptomatic bacteriuria is identified with increased prevalence directly related to age and degree of functional impairment. Hypothesizing that antibiotic treatment would decrease the subsequent incidence of symptomatic urinary infection, renal impairment or hypertension would suggest that there exists a beneficial secondary preventive effect (asymptomatic disease is already present; symptoms would be prevented). The natural history of asymptomatic bacteriuria, however, runs counter to that argument.

In elderly men and women it is not associated with symptomatic infection or progressive renal impairment, though it may be a marker for advanced debility that is reflected in an increased non-urinary infection-related mortality (Dontas, Kasviki-Charvati, & Papanayiotou, 1981; Nicolle, Bjonson, Harding, & MacDonnell, 1987; Nicolle, Mayhew, & Bryan, 1983). The presence or absence of pyuria with bacteriuria does not alter these observations. Antibiotic treatment frequently results only in relapse of infection, signifying that whatever beneficial effects of antibiotic treatment exist, they are only transient.

This contrasts with the clinical course of asymptomatic bacteriuria in those with known obstructive uropathy, children, and pregnant women, in whom sequelae may be significant. Evaluation of urinary tract structure and function, as well as attempts at antibiotic eradication of bacteriuria, may be warranted in these instances. These observations point out that the management approach to asymptomatic bacteriuria in frail, elderly people should in general not include attempting secondary prevention of symptomatic infection via antibiotic therapy unless deficits in local (obstructive uropathy) or systemic host defenses are identified (Zhanel, Harding, & Guay, 1990).

TUBERCULOSIS

Tuberculin (PPD) skin testing is the major technique used to screen populations for active or latent tuberculosis infection and to identify those who may benefit from prophylactic therapy. The declining prevalence of PPD skin test reactivity with age, identified in cross-sectional population surveys, is counter to the observation that many elderly people lived during a time when exposure to TB was virtually ubiquitous; they would be expected to exhibit a high rate of reactivity. This has led to the question "Where did all the reactors go?" (Stead & Lofgren, 1983). It is clear that those who were exposed many years previously may have successfully contained the infection with subsequent waning of PPD reactivity. The "booster effect" is thought to be a measure of this diminishing degree of lymphocyte sensitization. It is identified when an initial PPD skin test results in less than 10 mm induration, and a second test performed a few weeks after the first results in a greater than 10 mm induration (positive test). This occurs in about 5%–10% of elderly people living in long-term care facilities (Price & Rutala,

1987). Its major significance lies in identifying with as great degree a sensitivity as possible those who have been previously exposed and in avoiding misinterpretation of subsequent positive skin tests as representing new conversions. Lessening the numbers of false-positive conversions will lead to a more accurate estimate of new infections and limit the number of people erroneously considered at high risk of developing active TB. Fewer will need to be treated with isoniazid (INH), and less drug toxicity will ensue. As a consequence, two-step TB skin testing is frequently recommended upon admission to long-term care facilities.

Public health guidelines for interpreting skin test reactivity with respect to need for prophylactic therapy is based on the presence or absence of host risk factors for developing active disease, whether the person belongs to a group identified as exhibiting a high incidence of disease, and age (Centers for Disease Control, 1990). Residents of long-term care facilities are considered within the high-incidence group because the rates of active TB rise exponentially with age and the close living quarters of long-term care environments facilitate spread. Medical risk factors include chest x-ray evidence of old TB, recent contact with tuberculosis, HIV infection, immunosuppressive medicines or diseases, chronic renal failure, diabetes mellitus, weight less than 10% of ideal, silicosis, gastrectomy, jejunolileal bypass, and other malignancies. For those with greater than 10 mm induration and no medical risk factors, age 35 has been traditionally considered the maximum for institution of INH prophylaxis. This historically derived cutoff represents prior experience with INH-related hepatitis and death from cirrhosis. Reevaluation of this problem has pointed out the benefits of preventing even small numbers of active cases, especially in long-term care settings. The risk of hepatitis and death from cirrhosis may have been significantly overestimated and can be mitigated by close follow-up (Comstock, 1986; Rose, Schecter, & Silver, 1986). Other authors have concluded that the risk of hepatitis to benefit in preventing active disease in this group may be marginal (Stead, To, Harrison, & Abraham, 1987).

FALLS AND ASSOCIATED INJURY

Cape's (1978) conceptualization of intersecting common geriatric syndromes bears special relevance to the problems of falls and associated injury. Physical and psychological morbidity as a consequence of a single or multiple falls is tremendous, as is cost and potential for death (Tinetti & Speechley, 1989). Attention focused on understanding multiple, frequently simultaneously occurring risk factors for falls has allowed development of a risk index that predicted rates of falling for people newly admitted to nursing homes (Tinetti, Williams, & Mayewski, 1986). That lessened risk of falling can be obtained by mitigating risk factors make good sense. Do mechanical restraints prevent falls, and do restraint-free long-term care environments provide less risk for fall-related injuries? A 1-year study of mechanical restraint use in 12 nursing facilities pointed out their lack of efficacy in preventing fall-related injury and suggested that there may actually have been an increase (Tinetti, Liu, & Ginter, 1992).

RECURRENT ASPIRATION PNEUMONIA

Physicians caring for debilitated patients in long-term care or hospital settings recognize that recurrent aspiration pneumonia is a frequently occurring syndrome that contributes significantly to morbidity and mortality. Cognitive and swallowing impairments, as well as difficulty in maintaining adequate bronchopulmonary toilet, are well-recognized predisposing conditions; patients who experience recurrent pneumonia should be evaluated for remedial factors. We have cared for patients who exhibit a syndrome of recurrent pneumonia that we believe is related to either clinically or subclinically recognized gastroesophageal-oral regurgitation as a result of constipation. Such patients have underlying dementing illnesses, multiple strokes, or movement disorders that result in significant immobility. They may be orally or enterally fed. Evaluation for fever, tachypnea, cough, or altered mental state identifies, in addition to pneumonia (usually in the right lower lobe), abdominal distension with or without tenderness, absence of peritoneal signs, and normal or high-pitch bowel sounds. Vomiting may or may not be recognized. Review of bowel movement history may or may not identify limited bowel movements prior to the event.

Antibiotic treatment as well as supplemental measures directed at the respiratory tract infection may allow improvement. Recurrence of pneumonia, prompting a search for remediable causes, calls enhanced attention to the distended abdomen and the potential role of faulty gastrointestinal motility. Plain film x-ray of the abdomen identifies copious stool with or without signs of ileus.

Treatment with enemas to effect large bowel cleanout and maintenance of stool passage and decreased abdominal distension has allowed a reduction in frequency or resolution of pneumonia recurrences entirely. We postulate that increased intraabdominal pressure as a consequence of constipation results in distension, mild ileus, and clinical or subclinical vomiting, with resulting aspiration pneumonia. Clear-cut limitation in stool passage may not be recognized since there may be fecal impaction and stool leakage around the impaction. On the basis of these observations we believe that maintenance of adequate stool flow is critical as a secondary or tertiary prophylaxis for this form of recurrent aspiration pneumonia.

SUMMARY

Understanding the targets of proposed "treatments" as amelioration of current symptoms (either by addressing underlying pathophysiologic processes or by directly impacting the symptom itself) or as prevention of some future debility can more clearly bring into focus the potential benefits and liabilities of what is proposed. While enhanced primary preventive efforts are desirable at all ages (Manson et al., 1992; U.S. Department of Health and Human Services, 1990), secondary and tertiary prevention bear special relevance in old age because of already established pathophysiologic processes and underscore the observation that optimal management of chronic illness is integral to medical care of elderly patients.

References

American College of Physicians. Guidelines for counselling postmenopausal women about preventive hormone therapy. *Ann Intern Med, 117*: 1038–1041. 1992.

Anderson, F., Wheeler, B., Goldberg, R., Hosmer, D., Forcier, A., & Patwardhan, N. Physician practices in the prevention of venous thromboembolism. *Ann Intern Med, 115*: 591–595. 1991.

Annas, G. J. *The rights of patients* (2nd ed.). 1989 Southern Illinois University Press, Carbondale and Edwardsville. 1989.

Barnett, H., & Haines, S. North American symptomatic carotid endarterectomy collaborators. Beneficial effect of carotid endarterectomy in symptomatic patients with high grade carotid stenosis. *N Engl J Med, 325*: 445–453. 1990.

Barnett, H. J. M., Barnes, R. W., Clagett, G.P., Ferguson, G.G., Robertson, J. T., Walker, P. M. Symptomatic carotid artery stenosis: A solvable problem:

North American symptomatic carotid endarterectomy trial. *Stroke, 23*: 1048–1053. 1992.

Barnett, H. J. M., & Haines, S. J. Carotid endarterectomy for asymptomatic carotid stenosis. *N Engl J Med, 328*: 276–278. 1993.

Becker, P., McVey, L., Saltz, C., Feussner, J., & Cohn, H. Hospital-acquired complications in a randomized controlled clinical trial of a geriatric consultation team. *JAMA, 257*: 2313–2317. 1987.

Cape, R. Aging, its complex management. Hagerstown, MD: Harper and Row. 1978.

Centers for Disease Control. Screening for tuberculosis and tuberculosis infection and the use of preventive therapy for tuberculosis infection in the United Sates. *MMWR, 39*: 1–12. 1990.

Chapuy, M., Arlot, M., Duboeuf, F., Brun, J., Crouzet, B., Arnand, S., Delmas, P., Meunier, P.: Vitamin D_3 and calcium to prevent hip fractures in elderly women. *N Engl J Med, 327*: 1637–1642. 1992.

Chestnut, C. H. Osteoporosis and its treatment. *N Engl J Med, 326*: 406–407. 1992.

Colt, H., & Shapiro, A. Drug-induced illness as a cause for admission to a community hospital. *J Amer Ger Soc, 37*: 323–326. 1989.

Comstock, G. Prevention of tuberculosis among tuberculin reactors: maximizing benefits, minimizing risks. *JAMA, 256*: 2729–2730. 1986.

Cummings, S. R., & Black, D. M., & Nevitt, M. C., et al. Appendicular bone density and age predict hip fracture in women. *JAMA, 263*: 665–668. 1990.

Davis, J., Shapiro, M., & Kane, R. Level of care and complications among geriatric patients discharged from the medical service of a teaching hospital. *J Amer Ger Soc, 32*: 427–430. 1984.

Dontas, A. S., Kasviki-Charvati, P., & Papanayiotou, P. Bacteriuria and survival in old age. *N Engl J Med, 304*: 939–943. 1981.

Felson, D. T., Zhang, Y., Hannan, M., Kiel, D. P., Wilson, P., & Anderson, J. (1993). The effect of postmenopausal estrogen therapy on bone density in elderly women. *New England Journal of Medicine, 329*, 1141–1146.

Fries, J. F. Aging, natural death and the compression of morbidity. *N Engl J Med, 303*: 130–135. 1980.

Gallagher, J. C., & Goldgard, D. Treatment of postmenopausal osteoporosis with high doses of synthetic calcitriol. *Ann Intern Med, 113*: 649–654. 1990.

Goldhaber, S., & Morpurgo, M. Diagnosis, treatment, and prevention of pulmonary embolism. *JAMA, 268*: 1727–1733. 1992.

Goldman, L., & Tosteson, A. N. Uncertainty about postmenopausal estrogen—time for action not debate. *N Engl J Med, 325*: 800–802. 1991.

Grady, D., Ruben, S. M., & Petitti, D. B. Hormone therapy to prevent disease and prolong life in postmenopausal women. *Ann Intern Med, 117*: 1016–1037. 1992.

Grotta, J. Current medical and surgical therapy for cerebrascular disease. *N Engl J Med, 317*: 1505–1516. 1987.

Hayflick, L. The cell biology of human aging. *N Engl J Med, 295*: 1302–1308. 1976.

Heaney, R. Thinking straight about calcium. *N Engl J Med, 328*: 503–505. 1993.

Henrich J. B.: The postmenopausal estrogen/breast cancer controversy. JAMA. 268: 1900–02. 1992.

Hirsh, J. Heparin. *N Engl J Med, 324*: 1565–1574. 1991.

Hirsh, J. Influence on low-intensity warfarin treatment on patients' perceptions of quality of life. *Arch Intern Med, 151*: 1921–1922. 1991.

Hobson, R. W., Weiss, D. G., Fields, W., Goldstone, J., Moore, W., Towne, J., Wright, C., & the Veterans Affairs Cooperative Study Group Efficacy of carotid endarterectomy for asymptomatic carotid stenosis. *N Engl J Med, 328*: 221–227. 1993.

Hull, R., Raskob, G., Pineo, G., & Green, D., et al. Sucutaneous low-molecular weight heparin compared with continuous intravenous heparin in the treatment of proximal vein thrombosis. *N Engl J Med, 326*: 975–982. 1992.

Hyers, T., Hull, R., & Weg, J. Anti-thrombotic therapy for venous thromboembolic disease. *Chest, 102*: 408S-421S. 1992.

Jahnigen, D., Hannon, C., Laxson, L., & La Force, F. Iatrogenic disease in hospitalized elderly veterans. *J Amer Ger Soc, 29*: 387–390. 1982.

Johnston, C. C., Slemenda, C. W., & Melton L. J. Clinical use of bone densitometry. *N Engl J Med, 324*: 1105–09. 1991.

Katz, S., Branch, L. G., Branson, M. H., Papsidero, J., Beck, J., & Greer, D. Active life expectancy. *N Engl J Med, 309*: 1218–1224. 1983.

Kierkegaard, A., Norgren, H., Olsson, C., Cestenfors, J., Persson, G., & Perrson, S. Incidence of deep vein thrombosis in bedridden non-surgical patients. *Acta Med Scand, 222*: 409–414. 1987.

Kutner, M., Nixon, G., & Silverstone, F. Physicians' attitudes towards oral anticoagulants and antiplatelet agents for stroke prevention in elderly patients with atrial fibrillation. *Arch Intern Med, 151*: 1950–1953. 1991.

Lakshmanan, M.C., Hershey, C. O., & Breslan, D. Hospital admissions caused by iatrogenic disease. *Arch Intern Med, 146*: 1931–1934. 1986.

Lancaster, T., Singer, D., Sheehan, M., Oertel, H., Maraventano, S., Hughes, R., & Kistler, P. Boston area anticoagulation trial for atrial fibrillation investigators: The impact of long-term warfarin therapy on quality of life. *Arch Intern Med, 151*: 1944–1949. 1991.

Lefevre, F., Feinglass, J., Potts, S., Soglin, L., Yarnold, P., Martin, G., & Webster J. Iatrogenic complications in high-risk, elderly patients. *Arch Intern Med, 152*: 2075–2080. 1992.

Lekstrom, J. A., & Bell, W. R. Aspirin in the prevention of thrombosis. *Medicine, 70*: 161–178. 1991.

Lufken, E. G., Wahner, H. W., & O'Fallon, W. M. Treatment of postmenopausal osteoporosis with transdermal estrogen. *Ann Intern Med, 117*: 1–9. 1991.

Manson, J., Tosteson, H., Ridker, P., Satterfield, S., Hebert, P., O'Connor, G., Buring, J., & Hennekens, C. The primary prevention of myocardial infarction. *N Engl J Med, 326*: 1406–1416. 1992.

Melton, L. J., Eddy, D. M., & Johnston, C. C. Screening for osteoporosis. *Ann Intern Med, 112*: 516–528. 1990.

Nicolle, L., Bjonson, J., Harding, G., & MacDonell, J. Bacteriuria in elderly institionalized men. *N Engl J Med, 309*: 1420–1425. 1983.

Nicolle, L., Mayhew, W., & Bryan, L. Prospective randomized comparison of therapy and no therapy for asymptomatic bacteriuria in institutionalized elderly women. *Am J Med, 83*: 27–33. 1987.

North American Symptomatic Carotid Endarterectomy Trial Collaborators. Beneficial effect of carotid endarterectomy in symptomatic patients with high grade carotid stenosis. *N Engl J Med, 325*: 445–453. 1991.

Office of Medical Applications of Research, National Institute of Health. Osteoporosis. *JAMA, 252*: 799–802. 1984.

Office of Medical Applications of Research, National Institute of Health. Prevention of venous thrombosis and pulmonary embolism. *JAMA, 256*: 744–749. 1986.

Ott, S. N. Estrogen therapy for osteoporosis—even in the elderly. *Ann Intern Med, 117*: 85–86. 1992.

Price, L., & Rutala, W. Tuberculosis screening in the long-term care setting. *Infec Control, 8*: 353–356. 1987.

Prince, R. L., Smith, M., Dick, I. M., Price, R., Webb, P., Henderson, N., & Harris, M. Prevention of postmenopausal osteoporosis. *N Engl J Med, 325*: 1191–1195. 1991.

Reid, I., Ames, R., Evans, M., Gamble, G., & Sharpe, S. Effect of calcium supplementation on bone loss in postmenopausal women. *N Engl J Med, 328*: 460–464. 1993.

Riggs, B. L., & Melton, L. J. The prevention and treatment of osteoporosis. *N Engl J Med, 327*: 620–627. 1992.

Rose, D., Schechter, C., & Silver, A. The age threshold for isoniazid chemoprophylaxis: A decision analysis for low-risk tuberculin reactors. *JAMA, 256*: 2709–2713. 1986.

Rothrock, J., & Hart, R. Antithrombotic therapy cerebrovascular disease. *Ann Intern Med, 115*: 885–895. 1991.

Rowe, J. W., & Kahn, R. L. Human aging: Usual and successful. *Science, 237*: 143–149. 1987.

Salzman, E. Low molecular weight heparin and other new antithrombotic drugs. *N Engl J Med, 326*: 1017–1019. 1992.

Sartoris, D., & Resnick, D. Current and innovative methods for noninvasive bone densitometry. *Radiology Clin of N.A., 28*: 257–278. 1990.

Schneider, E. L., & Reed, J. D. Life extension. *N. Engl J Med, 312*: 1159–1168. 1985.

SHEP Cooperative Research Group. Prevention of stroke by antihypertensive drug treatment in older persons with isolated systolic hypertension. *JAMA, 265*: 3255–3264. 1991.

Stead, W. W., & Lofgren, J. Does the risk of tuberculosis increase in old age? *J Inf Dis, 147*: 951–955. 1983.

Stead, W., To, T., Harrison, R., & Abraham, J. Benefit-risk considerations in preventive treatment for tuberculosis in elderly persons. *Ann Intern Med, 107*: 843–845. 1987.

Steel, K., Gertman, P. M., Crescenzi, C., & Anderson, J. Iatrogenic illness on a general medical service at a university hospital. *N Engl J Med, 304*: 638–642. 1981.

Steering Committee of the Physicians' Health Study Research Groups. Final report on the aspirin component of the ongoing physicians health study. *N Engl J Med, 321*: 124–135. 1989.

Storm, T., Thamsborg, G., & Steiniche, T., et al. The effect of intermittent cyclical etidronate therapy on bone mass and fracture rate in women with postmenopausal osteoporosis. *N Engl J Med, 322*: 1265–1271. 1990.

Stout, R. W., & Crawford V. Active-life expectancy and terminal dependency: Trends in long-term geriatric care over 33 years. *Lancet 1*, February 6, 281–283. 1988.

Tilyard, M. W., Spears, G. F., & Thomson, J. Treatment of postmenopausal osteoporosis with calcitriol or calcium. *N Engl J Med, 326*: 357–362. 1992.

Tinetti, M., Liu, W., & Ginter, S. Mechanical restraint use and fall-related injuries among residents of skilled nursing facilities. *Ann Intern Med, 116*: 369–374. 1992.

Tinetti, M. E., & Speechley, M. Prevention of falls among of the elderly. *N Eng J Med, 320*: 1055–1059. 1989.

Tinetti, M. E., Williams, T. F., & Mayewski, R. Fall risk index for elderly patients based on number of chronic debilities. *Am J Med, 80*: 429–434. 1986.

U.S. Dept of Health and Human Services, Office of Technology Assessment. *Carotid endarterectomy.* 1990.

U.S. Department of Health and Human Services. *Healthy People 2000.* U.S. Government Printing Office. 1990.

Veterans Administration Cooperative Study Group on Antihypertensive Agents: Effects of treatment on morbidity in hypertension, II: Results in patients with diastolic blood pressure averaging 90 through 114 mmHg. *JAMA, 213*: 1143–1152. 1970.

Walsh, B. W., Schiff, I., Rosner, B., Greenberg, L., Ravinkar, V., & Sacks, F. The effects of postmenopausal estrogen replacement on the concentrations and metabolism of plasma lipoproteins. *N Engl J Med, 325*: 1196–1204. 1991.

Watts, B. N., Harris, T. S., & Genant, H. K., et al. Intermittent cyclical etidronate treatment of postmenopausal osteoporosis. *N Engl J Med, 323*: 73–79. 1990.

Wilking, S.V.B., et al. Determinants of isolated systolic hypertension. *JAMA, 260*: 3451–3455. 1988.

Williams, M. E., & Hadler, N. M. The illness as the focus of geriatric medicine. *N Engl J Med, 308*: 1357–1360. 1983.

Working Group on Hypertension in the Elderly: Statement on hypertension in the elderly. *JAMA, 256*: 70–74. 1986.

Zhanel, G., Harding, G., Guay, D. Asymptomatic bacteriuria, which patients should be treated? *Arch Intern Med, 150*: 1389–1396. 1990.

Chapter Four

Defensive Medicine in Geriatric Practice

Marshall B. Kapp

Considerations of clinical efficacy, humane and compassionate care, and health care cost containment dictate that advanced diagnostic and therapeutic technologies be used rationally in treating older patients. Many physicians are under the impression, however, that legal requirements, as embodied in the threat of medical malpractice lawsuits, sometimes interfere with their freedom to take the most rational approaches to patient management (Institute of Medicine, 1990a). This chapter aims to disabuse the reader of the misperception that defensive medicine in the care of older patients must be a necessarily negative and counterproductive phenomenon.

ELEMENTS OF MEDICAL MALPRACTICE

A basic understanding of defensive medicine compels an initial familiarity with that which is purportedly being defended against, namely, the subject of medical liability and particularly the medical malpractice lawsuit (Fiscina, Doumil, & Sharpe, 1991). A relatively small number of lawsuits brought by or on behalf of patients are predicated on a theory of violation of contract, usually where a physician's promise of a particular result (e.g., "If you undergo this vasectomy, you will never impregnate anyone again") does not come true, perhaps despite the fact that the physician delivered excellent technical care. Most malpractice actions, though, are based on a theory of tort, which means a civil wrong caused by the violation of a duty stemming from something other than a contract; within the physician/patient relationship, a tort is committed by violation of the physician's fiduciary or trust obligation to always act in the patient's best interests.

A small percentage of the tort actions brought against physicians allege intentional wrongdoing, such as battery for physically invading the patient's bodily integrity by doing some procedure without appropriate permission. However, the lion's share of medical malpractice cases are founded on a theory of negligence, or unintentional deviation from accepted medical standards. Medical negligence may occur through failure properly to inform the patient, or the proxy decision maker for a mentally incompetent patient, of information necessary for a truly informed, voluntary consent to a medical intervention (Rozovsky, 1991). Negligence may take place also through poor-quality, professionally unacceptable rendition of patient care. Many plaintiffs' complaints in medical malpractice cases allege both lack of adequate informed consent *and* the substandard performance of patient care.

In any negligence action, including one arising from a medical scenario, the plaintiff who initiates the claim must prove the presence of four elements in order to succeed. The plaintiff's inability to meet the burden of proof—convincing the jury by a preponderance of the evidence—regarding any one of these elements warrants dismissal of the case.

First, the plaintiff must show that the physician owed the patient a duty of due care; this responsibility is established by virtue of the existence of a physician/patient diagnostic or therapeutic relationship. The duty or standard of care owed is that degree of knowledge and skill that would be possessed and practiced by competent, prudent professional peers under similar circumstances. Second, since the current American malpractice system is based on the concept of fault, the plaintiff must show that the physician violated or breached the acceptable standard of care.

The third thing that a successful malpractice plaintiff must establish is that physical and/or emotional damage or injury was suffered. Finally, proving the element of causation is essential. Specifically, the plaintiff must convince the jury that the injury incurred was directly or proximately brought about by the defendant's violation of duty, that is, that "but for" (*sine qua non*) the defendant's negligence the injury would not have happened and furthermore that there were no other intervening, superseding, unforeseeable factors that would explain the injury.

OLDER PATIENTS AS MALPRACTICE PLAINTIFFS

With these basic elements of a successful medical malpractice claim in mind, it is easier to appreciate why older persons and their representatives are quite underrepresented as plaintiffs in the contemporary American medical litigation scene. Studies have shown that older patients and those acting on their behalf initiate lawsuits against physicians and other health care providers much less frequently than would be expected statistically on the basis of the elderly percentage of the general population or the rates at which older persons utilize the health care delivery system (Kapp, 1989; Sager, Voeks, Drinka, Langer, & Grimstad, 1990). This relatively low rate of invoking the legal process is not attributable to better medical care for the elderly; in fact, this lesser utilization of legal remedies occurs despite credible evidence that older patients are at higher risk than those in other age groups for suffering negligently inflicted injuries while undergoing medical care (Brennan et al., 1991).

There are several potential explanations for these data. First, the nature of the American legal system works to keep down the number and size of tort claims brought by or on behalf of older persons involving allegations of personal injury generally and medical malpractice specifically (Kapp, 1991a). For one thing, recoverable monetary damages for older plaintiffs usually are small, since large amounts of future lost wages or additional out-of-pocket medical expenses tend not to be easily provable. Furthermore, frequently it is difficult to prove that the health care provider's negligence was the proximate cause of injury for a patient who was frail and debilitated even before the alleged wrongdoing took place. Moreover, an older plaintiff who is severely compromised physically and mentally may not make a persuasive or credible witness on his or her own behalf, and sufficient supporting evidence from other sources may be difficult to uncover and to present. Indeed, the lawsuit may outlive the plaintiff. Where the older person lacks the physical or mental wherewithal to initiate and prosecute a civil claim personally, there frequently is not available a willing, capable family member or friend to advocate on the injured party's behalf in gaining access to the legal system.

Even assuming the other hurdles could be overcome, many potential plaintiffs who have received large amounts of health care funded by the state through the Medicaid program lack a financial incentive to sue a negligent provider. Many states would exert a right to be repaid for their Medicaid expenditures on the patient's behalf out of any proceeds of a civil judgment, leaving the plaintiff with only the remainder. For all of these reasons, older patients usually make rather unattractive clients for plaintiffs' malpractice attorneys, who work on a contingency arrangement in which the attorney's compensation is tied directly to the size of the plaintiff's legal recovery (Saks, 1992).

Besides these systemic obstacles, the nature of geriatric practice and of older persons contribute also to the relative scarcity of geriatric malpractice lawsuits, compared with other medical specialties. Geriatric practice tends to emphasize conservative management and rehabilitative care, entailing fewer and less severe clinical—and hence legal—risks than practice specialties that rely more heavily on dramatic, curative, technologically oriented interventions that are calculated to produce more immediate and definitive results. In geriatrics, the objectives and expectations of the patient and family ordinarily are more realistic and limited than in other medical arenas, and thus the probability of serious patient or family dissatisfaction with unexpectedly bad outcomes is reduced.

Moreover, even though physicians working with older patients may confront a tremendous constellation of ethical issues, ranging from assessment of mental capacity to confidentiality considerations to limitation of life-sustaining treatment, these kinds of issues seldom actually erupt into malpractice claims. The fear of malpractice litigation inspired by these issues is disproportionate to the factual risk (Kapp, 1991b).

Finally, it has been suggested that older patients as a group are likely to impose less stringent demands and expectations on their physicians than do younger patients and to be more satisfied with the quality of medical attention that they receive (President's Commission, 1982). The elderly tend to show greater deference to authority figures generally, including physicians, than do the rest of the population.

DEFENSIVE MEDICINE

Although, as explained above, as a general matter the potential liability exposure for physicians treating older patients is less than for practitioners serving younger persons, the fear of medical malpractice litigation is still a very real and substantial factor in geriatric practice (Dubler & Nimmons, 1992) and attention to the topic of defensive medicine must still be paid. There is a consensus among participants in and observers of the contemporary health care industry that the practice of defensive medicine is now widespread across medical specialties, entailing extensive misuse and overuse of scarce and sometimes risky diagnostic and therapeutic resources (Institute of Medicine, 1990b).

As one national health policy leader has put it, "There can be no doubt that fear of litigation drives many physicians to wasteful styles of practice which, when added to the ever-increasing premiums for liability insurance, contribute to the rising costs of health care" (Relman, 1989). Beyond that general notion, though, there exists broad and strongly felt disagreement over a precise working definition of the defensive medicine phenomenon and the magnitude and distribution of its actual clinical and economic ramifications (Weiler, 1991).

For example, there certainly is a dispute about the extent to which the ordering of extra tests and procedures that are widely attributed to the physician's felt need to engage in defensive medicine are more accurately an artifact of the traditional fee-for-service payment system, in which the physician's compensation is directly related to the expenses the physician can induce the patient to incur. Similarly, are extra tests and procedures driven less by defensive medicine than by the prevalent technological imperative philosophy that more is always better and that, once invented and purchased, no machine should ever sit idle? The depth of feeling on this point is reflected in the recent statement by an official of the federal Department of Health and Human Services Inspector General's Office:

> If a doctor is running unsound tests, not for the beneficiary [patient] but for his or her own benefit, then the doctor should pay for it, not [the government's Medicare or Medicaid programs]. Health practitioners hold themselves out as experts and are highly paid for that expertise. They should be using their judgment to provide services as efficiently and cost-effectively as possible. (Patton, 1992)

Considerations of necessity and efficiency aside, there is even a total lack of consensus about how effective extra tests and procedures are in accomplishing their supposed objective of lawsuit avoidance or mitigation for the physician (Harris, 1987). Performing tests and procedures that are not part of the standard of good practice, as defined by the physician's professional peers in similar circumstances, adds nothing to the physician's legal prophylaxis and may actually expose the patient—and therefore the physician whose legal fate rides in large part on the patient's clinical outcome—to unnecessary and unjustifiable risk of negative side effects. At the same time, refraining from performing medical tests or procedures in circumstances where the physician's prudent peers also would not have performed them obviously does not expose the physician to a liability risk for deviation from acceptable medical standards.

Instead of reflexively ordering the maximum feasible number of tests and procedures, regardless of anticipated benefit for the patient, in every situation in which the theoretical possibility of malpractice litigation is remotely sensed, the physician ordinarily would be much better advised to utilize the medical technological arsenal thoughtfully and cautiously, weighing relative risks and benefits for the patient informed by available data and also to undertake several strategies that are more likely to bear meaningful risk management results in daily practice (Kapp, 1985, 1987). Physicians can realistically evaluate the sorts of legal risks that are likely to arise in their professional activities and work toward implementing effective risk management programs to anticipate those risks, prevent them from occurring, and minimize the damage if they do materialize. While legal risks will never be eliminated completely for the physician (nor for anyone else in our complicated modern society), risks may be managed in a way that makes a difference.

Within their private offices, physicians who treat elderly patients should pursue such tested risk management strategies as drafting of written policies and procedures for office staff; special attention to informed consent for risky and/or intrusive interventions and confidentiality of sensitive patient information; full, timely, accurate, legible, and objective documentation of patient care, including open lines of communication with the patient or surrogate; and appropriate procedures for selecting, training, and supervising support staff. If the physician practices within a health care facility, he or she should exert influence to ensure that these same strategies are instituted on the institutional level and should participate enthusiastically in making those strategies work within the facility. Special sensitivity to particular characteristics of older patients (such as sensory deficits or memory impairments) and their care needs to be exhibited in devising and carrying out risk management initiatives in geriatric medicine.

Physicians may also work collectively to address the defensive medicine issue by supporting and participating in activities of professional associations and governmental agencies that are developing and promulgating clinical practice parameters for various medical problems. These practice parameters, or guidelines, may be cited by physicians as their basis for handling certain medical situations in a particular way and specifically may be relied on to justify a decision not to order a certain test or procedure for a patient, given the clinical scenario (Hall, 1991; Havighurst, 1991).

CONCLUSION

Anxiety concerning potential malpractice litigation and liability exposure may encourage physicians caring for older persons to sometimes order medical tests and procedures that are not clinically indicated in terms of likely risks and benefits for the patient. This type of so-called defensive medicine is wasteful and often even counterproductive in achieving its purported goal. Physicians would be better advised to devise a plan for the older patient's care, in conjunction with the informed patient or surrogate decision maker, on the basis of relevant clinical factors, with an emphasis on rendering and documenting high-quality professional services and fostering a positive professional/patient/family dynamic consistent with the values and aims of the patient. The physician's legal welfare is fully consistent with taking a rational approach, based on facts rather than mythology, to the use of advanced diagnostic and therapeutic technology in elderly patients.

References

Brennan, T. A., Leape, L. L., & Laird N. M., et al. Incidence of adverse events and negligence in hospitalized patients: Results of the Harvard medical practice study I. *N Engl J Med, 324*: 370–376. 1991.

Dubler, N. N., & Nimmons, D. *Ethics on call.* New York: Harmony Books. 1992.

Fiscina, S., Doumil, M. M., Sharpe, D. J., & Head, M. *Medical Liability, American Casebook Series.* St. Paul, MN: West Publishing Co. 1991.

Hall, M. A. The defensive effect of medical practice policies in malpractice litigation. *L & Contemp Prob, 54*: 119–145. 1991.

Harris, J. E. Defensive medicine: It costs, but does it work? *JAMA, 257*: 2801–2802. 1987.

Havighurst, C. C. Practice guidelines as legal standards governing physician liability. *L & Contemp Prob, 54*: 87–117. 1991.

Institute of Medicine. (1990a). *Medicare: A strategy for quality assurance, Vol. 1*. Washington, DC: National Academy Press.

Institute of Medicine. (1990b). *Medicare: A strategy for quality assurance, Vol. II, sources and methods*. Washington, DC: National Academy Press.

Kapp, M. B. The malpractice crisis: Relevance for geriatrics. *J Am Geriatr Soc, 37*: 364–368. 1989.

Kapp, M. B. Malpractice liability in long-term care: A changing environment. *Creighton L Rev, 24*: 1235–1260. 1991a.

Kapp, M. B. Our hands are tied. Legally induced moral tensions in health care delivery. *J Gen Intern Med, 6*: 345–348. 1991b.

Kapp, M. B. Preventing malpractice in long-term care: Strategies for risk management. New York: Springer. 1987.

Kapp, M. B. Legal guide for medical office managers. Chicago: Pluribus Press. 1985.

Patton, J. Dir of Health Care Administrative Sanctions, Office of Inspections, Office of Inspector General, U.S. Dept of Health and Human Services; Quoted in Amer Med News 27; January 13, 1992.

President's Commission for the Study of Ethical Problems in Medicine and Biomedical and Behavioral Research. Making health care decisions: The Ethical and Legal Implications of Informed Consent in the Patient–Practitioner Relationship. Washington, DC: Government Printing Office. 1982.

Relman, A. S. The national leadership commission's health care plan. *N Engl J Med, 320*: 314–315. 1989.

Rozovsky, F. A. Consent to treatment: A practical guide. (2nd ed.). Boston: Little, Brown. 1991.

Sager, M., Voeks, S., Drinka, P., Langer, E., Grimstad, P. Do the elderly sue physicians? *Arch Intern Med, 150*: 1091–1093. 1990.

Saks, M. J. Do we really know anything about the behavior of the tort litigation system—and why not? *U Penn Law Rev, 140*: 1147–1292. 1992.

Weiler, P. C. Medical malpractice on trial. Cambridge, MA: Harvard University Press. 1991.

Chapter Five

The Role of the Physician in Decisions to Use or Forgo Life-Sustaining Technologies

Lydia O'Donnell and Mildred Z. Solomon

Over the past several decades, the number and types of medical treatments available to prolong life in the elderly patient have markedly increased. Through advances in the field of gerontology, we know more about how to manage the complex medical needs of older men and women who present with a variety of acute and chronic illnesses. At the same time, advances in medical specialty areas have improved our ability to diagnose problems and prescribe interventions that help sustain older hearts, kidneys, and other organ systems. While undoubtedly offering benefits to millions of people, these advances also bring with them serious physical, psychological, and financial burdens.

Today, many Americans worry that they will get too much treatment at the end of life and too little medication to ease their pain. They are concerned that their values and wishes about care will not be respected, especially in the event they become unable to make their own decisions. Discontent with the status quo is evident in the popular appeal of Dr. Kevorkian and his "suicide machine," as well as in the heated debate over whether physician-assisted suicide is ethically and legally permissible. As a *New York Times* reporter has expressed it, "There is a wide gulf between rapidly changing societal beliefs about appropriate treatment and the practice of medicine on the firing line" (Brody, 1993).

Research with physicians and nurses indicates that the public's fears may indeed be well-founded. A recent national survey that we conducted as part of our ongoing work in clinical ethics education has documented that health professionals are themselves concerned that patients are not adequately provided with the information they need to make decisions about their own care and that, in many cases, patients near the end of life receive inappropriate, overly burdensome treatment. Two-thirds of the physicians and nurses surveyed expressed concern that mechanical ventilation and cardiopulmonary resuscitation were used inappropriately. More than half expressed concerns about the inappropriate use of artificial nutrition and hydration and dialysis. Four times as many respondents were concerned about overtreatment than undertreatment, with more than half of those surveyed reporting that they sometimes offer treatments that are "overly burdensome" to their patients. Furthermore, 81% agreed that "the most common form of narcotic abuse in the care of the dying is undertreatment of pain" (Solomon, O'Donnell, Jennings et al., 1993). Many others have also recognized this problem (e.g., Foley, 1985; McGiveney & Crooks, 1984; Melzack, 1990; Wanzer, Adelstein, Cranford et al., 1984). Indeed, there is widespread acknowledgment that in the United States dying patients receive inadequate pain control.

Moreover, it is impossible to ignore the fact that concerns about care, and particularly the provision of overly burdensome treatments near the end of life, are occurring within the context of rapidly escalating health-care costs. As a nation, we now devote more economic resources to the last few years of adults' lives than to any other portion of the life span. About one-third of all Medicare expenses are spent on the last year of life (Goodman, 1993).

Over the past decade, a number of strategies have emerged to address the problem of unwanted treatment. Advance directives, including both Living Wills and health care proxies are now legal in most states (e.g. Emanuel, Barley, Stoeckle, Ettelson, & Emanuel, 1980; Omnibus Act 1990). Yet even as these tools for planning are more widely available, doubts have been raised about whether they can solve the myriad problems associated with the use of life supports (Jackson & Carlos, 1991; Schneiderman, Pearlman, Kaplan, Anderson, & Rosenberg, 1992).

Although these planning tools can be helpful in many circumstances, they alone cannot resolve the ethical dilemmas physicians and patients now face. Consider these examples:

- Should a man in his 70s with severe chronic pulmonary disease and pneumonia necessarily be placed on a ventilator to treat respiratory failure, given that there is a significant chance that he could not be weaned from the ventilator after the pneumonia is successfully treated? Should he even be offered the option of ventilation? In the event weaning fails, how long should he remain ventilated? Under what circumstances should the ventilator be removed?

- Should a 68-year-old diabetic in cardiogenic shock and kidney failure necessarily be a candidate for coronary artery bypass surgery? On the basis of what criteria?

- Should a 70-year-old woman with a newly diagnosed and treatable skin cancer and a history of depression be allowed to leave the hospital without treatment? Under what circumstances, if any, should her physician override her desire to forgo treatment? What if she were 50 years old, or 85, instead of 70? Would this make a difference?

These cases are difficult because medical facts alone cannot resolve them. Their resolutions must be based not only on what is medically possible but also on patients' values about how they want to spend their final months and years. To arrive at adequate solutions, physicians must shepherd patients and their families through what can be a difficult and ambiguous decision-making process. Guiding patients through this territory requires knowledge of what is ethically and legally permissible, yet misinformation about ethics and the law often seriously limits what treatment options are considered (Meisel, 1991). In addition to knowing what is medically possible, it is important for physicians to reflect on their own personal values and the ways in which these values may influence their discussions with patients and their families. Most important, physicians must be comfortable dealing with dying patients.

Given their relatively frequent exposure to death, one might assume that health care providers who work with the elderly would be adequately prepared to help patients and their families cope with dying. In fact, this often is not the case. Medical education prepares physicians well for treating illness and preserving life but offers less preparation for handling the death process. Just as the study of medical ethics frequently has been assigned to the periphery of medical training, scant attention has been devoted to the skills required to provide care and comfort to patients who are dying. In addition, in American culture there is reluctance to enter into discussions about dying and what it may entail. As a result, physicians may provide their older patients with insufficient information about the treatment and nontreatment alternatives available to them, as well as with inadequate support during the dying process. This state of affairs bears consequences not just for patients and families but for physicians too, who end up quietly shouldering responsibility for life and death treatment decisions that are not really theirs to make.

In an essay entitled "The Seductive Beauty of Physiology," Botkin (1992) argues that:

> For better or worse, human values often lie well within the realm of uncertainty. Even our own personal values may be frequently uncertain—at least in the context of illness, where complex choices may be layered by pain and fear. The values of our patients are all the more remote from our grasp. It is little wonder that physicians may seek refuge in the science of the organism, and that our patients are often eager followers of our firm—but perhaps misguided—lead on technical adventure. (p. 277)

Resorting to the use of technology to maintain physiologic function is simpler than addressing the inevitability of death and sorting through the complex human values and emotions that such discussions entail. Stabilizing blood pressure and maintaining adequate kidney function and normal blood gases are all undeniably important. Yet, as Botkin argues, the practice of medicine is more than keeping an organism alive. Within that practice, there must be recognition of the central role task should play in defining treatment goals and decisions.

The often underacknowledged burden of medical uncertainty further complicates decisions about whether to use available treatments. As Gerrity et al. (Gerrity, Earps, DeVellis, & Light, 1992) point out, "The rapid growth of technology and scientific knowledge has brought with it, paradoxically, a rapid increase in uncertainty. Uncertainty borders the edges of knowledge, so that the larger the territory known, the more extensive are the settings in which uncertainty is experienced" (p. 1022). The more we know about maintaining health and controlling disease in the elderly, the more questions arise about the costs and benefits of extending life near its natural limits.

Several distinct types of uncertainty complicate medical decision making. First is the uncertainty posed by gaps and deficiencies in our individual and collective knowledge about the causes and treatment of many terminal illnesses. The field of geriatric medicine is growing but still incomplete. Second is the lack of prognostic certainty: What exactly does this knowledge mean for any given patient? How should statistics on medical success and failure be used to guide this particular patient's course of action? Third is the difficulty of ascertaining the patient's values and preferences. Decision making is hard enough when competent patients are able to make their views known, but the choices become even more difficult if the patient is incapacitated and has left no indication of his or her values and preferences.

Finally, there is the uncertainty that arises when it is necessary to seek resolution between two incompatible but perhaps equally compelling goals. For example, some of the most morally distressing cases arise when physicians are called upon to reconcile their desire to protect a patient's well-being with their respect for a patient's right to make his or her own decisions. Good examples of such beneficence–autonomy conflicts are cases in which patients wish to forgo treatments that physicians believe are relatively simple yet likely to yield clear benefits.

Other rival claims, such as those between autonomy and distributive justice, also give rise to great uncertainty. In so-called futile cases, are physicians under an obligation to provide care that patients (or their families) insist upon? In such cases, physicians may not only worry that treatment poses undue, perhaps even injurious, burdens on their patients. They may also feel that the costs of that care are unjustified.

While our society has not resolved how to deal with all of these issues, particularly when they pertain to cost and equity in care, there *is* growing consensus about fundamental principles that are helpful for guiding decisions at the bedside. The field of clinical ethics provides support for physicians who must face such dilemmas in their practice and offers guidelines for closing the gap between what patients want and what medical science can do.

DECISION MAKING, CLINICAL ETHICS, AND THE CARE OF THE ELDERLY

As described by Pellegrino (1993), clinical ethics "focuses on the realities of moral choices as they are confronted in day-by-day health and medical care" (p. 1162). According to this formulation, the emphasis of clinical ethics is not on an abstract set of principles or philosophy. Rather, it is on the context in which choices occur and the process through which decisions are made and implemented.

Over the past few decades, as the field of clinical ethics has become established, there have been significant shifts in both the context and process of medical decision making. A number of interacting factors have contributed to these changes, including advances in science and medical treatment; shifts in philosophical opinion, the law, and public sentiment; and an evolving social context of health care, including changes in the nature of patient–provider relationship and health care institutions.

For example, little over a generation ago, most physicians did not feel it was necessary to inform patients that they had a terminal condition; indeed, such knowledge was even viewed as detrimental to patients' well-being (Beauchamp & Childress, 1983). Bearing the burden as well as the power of withheld information, physicians were relied upon to make decisions and control the dying process. In contrast, patients today are seen as entitled to know what is happening to them. In both ethics and law, a respect for individuals and their right to self-determination underlies the principle of autonomy in which the patient, not the physician, is assigned the role of central decision maker (Hastings Center 1987; Haug & Lavin, 1981; President's Commission, 1983). Now physicians not only must collect and interpret information; they also are expected to share their findings in ways that enable patients to make decisions for themselves.

In addition, physicians increasingly share decision-making authority with an expanding number of providers at their institutions. As nurses, administrators, lawyers, and others have become more involved in patient management, they are more likely to challenge physicians' orders (Ku & Fisher, 1990). As Vladeck (1993) notes,

> Indeed, in hospitals decision-making processes, even about more mundane clinical matters, have become so complex and involve so many different participants that it may not be unfair to say that

often decisions are made by no one. . . . [P]rofessionals work—perhaps increasingly—in large, complex systems that frustrate their ability to be as sensitive and compassionate as they would like. (p. 13)

Thus, it is not only the larger array of medical devices we now have available to sustain life that may cause problems; the structure of our health care delivery system adds a layer of complexity to the decision-making task.

Since the landmark Karen Quinlan case almost two decades ago *In re Quinlan* (1976), there has been extensive discussion in both law and ethics on issues pertaining to the withdrawal of life-sustaining treatments. It is now clearly recognized that competent patients have the right to refuse or terminate life supports, even if that refusal leads to death. Moreover, it is well established, both in existing ethical guidelines and in the law, that patients do not lose that right when they become incapacitated. A large number of court cases have upheld the rights of competent patients to refuse unwanted treatment *and* the authority of family members or other appropriate surrogates to refuse on behalf of those who can no longer speak for themselves. In 1990, the Supreme Court noted in the *Cruzan* decision that Constitutional protection for the right to refuse treatment could be inferred from the Court's earlier decisions (Cruzan v. Director, 1990). In addition, nearly all states have recognized the force of advance directives—so-called Living Wills and proxy appointment documents or both—through legislation, court decisions, or both. In 1990, the U.S. Congress passed the federal Patient Self-Determination Act, which ties Medicaid and Medicare reimbursement for hospitals and other health care facilities to the requirement that patients be informed of their right to accept or refuse medical and surgical treatment and the right to formulate advance directives (Omnibus Reconciliation Act, 1990; Patient's Rights, Accreditation Manual for Hospitals, 1992).

For the most part, there is consensus that what happens to a patient's body is a matter of self-determination. This emphasis on autonomy casts the physician in the role of facilitator, not decision maker. The physician's responsibility is to make sure that the patient has the information and support necessary to reach a good decision. To uphold this responsibility, before the determination is made to use or not use a given treatment, it is important for physicians to address two basic questions:

- How can I help my patient weigh the benefits and burdens associated with each treatment (and nontreatment) option?
- What does the patient want?

In the following two sections we take up each of these questions in turn.

Assessing Benefits and Burdens

In addition to acknowledging the right of patients and surrogates to refuse or terminate treatment, national guidelines and landmark court decisions are in agreement that there is no *ethical* difference between withholding and withdrawing treatment. The acknowledgment that these two acts are ethically equivalent affords providers, patients and families the option of initiating a treatment, such as mechanical ventilation, and later withdrawing it—if the patient or surrogate decision maker assesses that its burdens outweigh its benefits. Providing such a "trial of treatment" is viewed as ethically preferable to the alternative of withholding life support because of the fear that, once initiated, therapy cannot be later withdrawn (Silvestri & O'Donnell, 1989).

Further, most guidelines agree that when considering withholding or withdrawing life supports, the often relied upon distinction between "extraordinary" or "heroic" treatments and ordinary or nonheroic treatments is not ethically relevant. A decision to use a treatment should be based on its potential benefits and burdens to a patient, as *the patient* perceives them, not on the technological complexity of the treatment. Thus, most commentators feel there is no ethically relevant distinction between making the decision to withdraw a ventilator or to withdraw dialysis, antibiotic therapy, or artificial nutrition and hydration.

Assuming there is no ethical difference, however, does not eliminate inherent differences between technologies and their implications for patients and providers. There can be emotional, psychological, and even technical differences among life-support modalities that influence decision making. Unplugging the ventilator may be a greater emotional burden than not starting it in the first place; deciding to disconnect a feeding tube may be more laden with symbolic meaning for patients, families, and providers than choosing to forgo a course of antibiotics; withdrawing dialysis may cause less staff and patient distress than removing ventilatory support (Lynn & Childress, 1983). Obviously, these differences are relevant when formulating treatment plans with patients. They do not, however, negate the patient's right to initiate, forgo, or stop any given therapy.

Guidelines also address the ethical quandary physicians and nurses confront concerning the provision of adequate pain medication. Nearly all published guidelines hold that "providing large quantities of narcotic analgesics does not constitute wrongful killing when the purpose is not to shorten [patients' lives] but to alleviate their pain and suffering, and the alternatives have been carefully evaluated and this course found to serve the patient's best interest" (Hastings Center, 1987, p. 73).

Finally, existing guidelines recognize that providers who are ethically opposed to a course of action chosen by a patient have the right to withdraw from that case. Withdrawal from a case may be advisable not only when there is an ethical disagreement but also when a provider has become so close to a patient that he or she is unable to consider treatment alternatives or a course of action that the patient or surrogate thinks is best (Belkin, 1993).

The existence of these guidelines does not in itself ensure good practice. Indeed, research has documented a pervasive gap between existing ethical and legal recommendations and clinical practice (Solomon et al., 1993). While the knowledge base is established and public policy quite advanced, there needs to be far more attention to these concerns, both in medical education and in the hospitals and nursing homes where these decisions get made.

In this regard, there are some promising developments. For example, some changes in medical education and clinical training are taking place—changes that emphasize the importance of supporting dying patients and easing their pain (e.g., Botkin, 1992; Randall, 1992). In addition, one major national program now in use in nearly 100 hospitals and nursing homes brings together multidisciplinary teams of physicians, nurses, social workers, pastoral counselors, and hospital lawyers to examine how decisions near the end of life are made in their institutions. Participants are encouraged to compare their views about the use of life-sustaining treatments with their colleagues' views and with those promulgated in national guidelines (Solomon et al., 1991).

Yet even with these shifts, helping elderly patients make decisions about the use of life-sustaining treatments and ensuring that they receive adequate pain control and palliative support will not be easy. There is no substitute for the centrally important role physicians play.

What Does the Patient Want? The Physician's Role

Physicians frequently assume they know what patients want, but as research has shown, they are often incorrect in this assessment (Danis, Gerrity, Southerland & Patrick, 1988; Danis, Karr, & Southerland 1987; Uhlmann, Pearlman, & Cain, 1983). A significant minority of physicians still feel that many patients do not want to know that they are dying, despite growing evidence to the contrary ("Medical News & Perspectives," 1993). If patients are going to have as much say as possible in how they live and how they die, physicians need to raise the possibility of death with their elderly patients. When physicians do not initiate these conversations, they may limit patients' options and constrain their ability to plan and prepare for what is, ultimately, inevitable.

Research on aging indicates that most adults need time to consider what they want near the end of life; they do not come to such discussions with clearly articulated preferences. But they *are* prepared to face the future: "As one geriatrician put it, 'Most of my older patients don't view death as optional' " (Deutsch, 1989, p. 12). Indeed, even more than death itself, many patients fear the pain and suffering they associate with dying (Wanzer et al., 1989). This is a concern that providers, with currently available knowledge about palliation, can and should help alleviate.

As noted above, in 1991 the federal Patient Self-Determination Act (PSDA) became the first federal legislation that required hospitals and nursing homes to provide patients with information about their right to specify what treatment they wish if they become incapacitated (Omnibus Act, 1990). However, one of the authors of this legislation admits, "It is difficult to require the delicate skills necessary to talk to people about death and dying" (McCloskey 1991, p. 167). These skills are too often overlooked and unrewarded in general medical practice. In addition, it can take considerable time and effort to ensure that such conversations are done correctly. What's more, these discussions must be repeated as patients' conditions change.

Despite the PSDA and other efforts to expand the use of advance directives, physicians have expressed doubts about whether patients are sufficiently informed to assess the implications of different treatment alternatives and whether any form can contain sufficient information to guide treatment (e.g., Brett, 1991; Jackson & Carlos, 1991). There are also concerns that written documents become outdated, overridden, or lost as patients move from one setting to another (Miles, 1987). Acknowledgment of these limitations places even more importance on the physician's role in assuring that patients get what they want. Physicians are in an ideal position to ensure that death and dying is discussed with patients *before* medical emergencies dictate and limit what options can be chosen.

Perhaps the best way to learn the requisite skills is by observing other physicians engaging their patients in such conversations. While this form of mentoring is a commonly accepted practice for transferring other medical practices (e.g., learning how to do physical exams, surgical techniques, medical testing procedures), a training priority has not been assigned to modeling the important communication skills that come with experience. Indeed, in teaching hospitals, physicians-in-training often are not sufficiently informed by staff physicians about the nonmedical background, values, and preferences of a patient to be comfortable with treatments that are made or recommended. This lack of opportunity to share information about patients and their wishes is probably one reason house officers are more likely than staff physicians to report that treatments are overly burdensome and that they have acted against their conscience in providing care (Solomon, O'Donnell et al., 1993).

Some of the most complex situations arise when patients are not able to make decisions on their own or when there is doubt about their capacity to do so. Especially in the care of the elderly who have some cognitive impairment, it is too easy to assume that patients are unable to make decisions about what they do and do not want. Even older patients with diminished or fluctuating capacity may be able to communicate, verbally or nonverbally, what their desires are when provided with adequate opportunities to do so.

Patients who cannot remember what day it is or who are not able to choose what to have for breakfast from the hospital menu may be able to participate in decisions about their care if approached correctly. A number of techniques can be used to support the older patients' capacity to make decisions. Some examples include avoiding medical jargon and making sure to use words that patients understand; taking care not to overwhelm the patient with too much information or too many decisions at any one time; allowing patients time to absorb information, especially bad news about their health, before they have to make any decisions; choosing for conversation a time of day when patients are most alert and the side effects of medication least evident; making multiple assessments, on different days, assuming that patients will not always be at their best; having a family member, nurse, or someone else present to help the patient focus and to provide support; being creative in overcoming barriers to physical impairments, such as hearing loss or aphasia; and being aware of factors that may impair cognitive abilities (Deutsch, 1989).

Older patients may take longer to process information and to respond to questions, so their timing needs to be honored. Touching the patient, maintaining eye contact, reaching out and holding hands can be crucial. These small efforts help keep cognitively impaired patients focused and, above all, show that they are people whose wishes and values will be respected. The negative effects of hospitalization must also be considered. Older men and women can become disoriented, upset, and uncooperative due to the stresses entailed in altering their routines, sleep patterns, medications, and so on. The more they are allowed to follow their own schedules and body rhythms, the more they may be empowered to participate in decisions about their own care.

It can be especially difficult for a physician new to a case to determine the sources of patients' confusion and the extent to which they can be supported to make their own decisions. By working together, medical and nursing staff can often address these problems. Discussions with those who have known the patient longer—family, staff at a nursing home, etc.—can provide a more accurate portrait of the patient. In difficult cases, rather than assuming a lack of capacity, it is at times necessary to call in a gerontologist or psychologist trained in communicating with the elderly and cognitively impaired to help make an assessment of the patient's capacity.

Moreover, it is important that such assessments be made periodically. Not only may patients be more able to participate at a later date, but their opinions may change over time. What was once not an acceptable form of therapy—dialysis or a feeding tube, for example—may seem less burdensome as time passes, psychological and physical adjustments are made, and options become more limited.

There are, of course, many elderly patients who are unable to participate in decision making, and from an ethical as well as legal standpoint, these can be some of the most difficult cases. Again, recommendations from national guidelines are in agreement: patients who are incapacitated must be assigned a surrogate decision maker, hopefully someone who can provide information about *what the patient would have wanted* in such circumstances. Only when there is not enough information to make this assessment is it appropriate to fall back on a "best interest" standard, choosing what a reasonable person is likely to consider is in the patient's best interests.

To date, there is less agreement about whether physicians are appropriate surrogate decision makers for their patients or whether this assignment poses a conflict of interest (Clark & Duffy, 1989). Physicians themselves are split on the issue, although they are almost twice as likely as nurses to feel they can serve as appropriate surrogates (Solomon et al., 1993). However, most guidelines recommend that physicians should not just assume they can make decisions for their patients. A process of selecting an appropriate surrogate must be followed, and the same standards of surrogate decision making should guide treatment, regardless of who plays the surrogate role (Hastings Center, 1987).

RESOLVING DIFFICULT CASES

Given the issues raised in the above sections, it is evident that the two basic questions posed—what do patients want and how do they assess the benefits and burdens of treatment—really are composed of a host of related questions. Table 5.1 expands upon these two questions and provides a brief checklist of related questions that can be used to guide and evaluate the decision-making process. Case examples are then used to illustrate how these questions apply to particular clinical situations.

• CASE 1: CARL MERKIN* •

Carl Merkin is a 65-year-old man with a history of chronic obstructive pulmonary disease (COPD) due to emphysema. His breathing capacity is only one-third of what would normally be expected for a man of his age. He experiences shortness of breath when performing minimal activities, such as dressing himself or walking to the

TABLE 5.1 Decisions About Life Supports in the Care of the Elderly: A Physician Self-Assessment

When working with the elderly, do I:
1. Fully explain treatment and nontreatment options, using language my patients understand?
2. Help my patients assess the likely burdens and benefits associated with each of these options?
3. Consider how my own values and feelings may influence the way I present different options?
4. Take care not to assume I know what the patient wants?
5. Talk with patients (and their families) about the possibility of death, and help them deal with their fears and concerns about dying?
6. Initiate conversations in advance of a crisis—when patients are most able to make their wishes known?
7. Engage in an ongoing dialogue, listening to how patients' wishes and concerns change over time?
8. Devote the time and care necessary to assess whether patients are able to participate in decisions about their treatment, even if they are functionally or cognitively impaired?
9. Share information about what my patients want with other staff, so that if I'm not available in a time of crisis, patients' wishes will be known?
10. Encourage patients to share this information with their loved ones, to reduce the possibility of future conflict?
11. Record my patients' wishes in the medical record.
12. Assure patients and their families that comfort care measures, including adequate palliation of pain, will be provided, even if life supports are discontinued?
13. Encourage patients to complete an advance directive or assign a proxy decision maker, in the event they become unable to make decisions?
14. Make sure an appropriate surrogate decision maker is assigned to guide the course of treatment, if a thorough assessment indicates a patient does not have the capacity to make decisions?
15. Take steps to keep current on laws and guidelines regarding the use of life-sustaining treatments?

bathroom, and he often must lie still in bed. Several days ago, Mr. Merkin caught the flu. His breathing became even more difficult than usual, and his wife brought him to the emergency room, where he was met by his regular physician, Dr. Phillips, a pulmonary specialist. Dr. Phillips diagnosed acute decompensation of lung function due to the respiratory infection.

Since his diagnosis of emphysema several years ago, Mr. Merkin has repeatedly stated that he would not want to be maintained on a respirator. As he put it to his wife, "I've been independent all my life; I don't want to be tethered to a machine." When Mrs. Merkin reminds Dr. Phillips of her husband's feelings, Dr. Phillips responds by explaining that without immediate ventilatory support,

Mr. Merkin will almost certainly go into respiratory failure. With support, his deterioration could be slowed and he might be able to live for years. "I don't know if he would have to stay on the ventilator or not," Dr. Phillips explains, "but in either case he could live a long time."

• *CASE 2: ROSE KANTOR* •

Rose Kantor entered the Bedford Hills Nursing Home after her 76th birthday. She was alert, ambulatory, and able to manage most activities of daily living with minimal assistance. Approximately 5 years later, she began to experience increased weakness. A complete blood count, taken as part of a routine exam, showed that Ms. Kantor had a nonaggressive leukemia. Dr. Myers prescribed oral steroid therapy. Several months later, however, her platelet count remained low. She was referred to a hematologist, who recommended a relatively benign course of chemotherapy.

To the surprise of the staff who care for her, Ms. Kantor refuses the recommended treatment. She explains that although Bedford Hills is a first-rate facility and she is cared for in every way, she still feels that she has lived long enough and that the quality of her life in the nursing home is not worth prolonging. Dr. Myers disagrees, feeling the benefits of prolonged life outweigh the burdens of the proposed treatment.

These cases illustrate the importance and difficulty of using our knowledge and technology wisely, so that patients can be cared for in the ways they themselves want. They also highlight the physician's responsibility to make clear to the patient (or surrogate decision maker) the full range of available treatment and nontreatment options and what the benefits and burdens of each choice are likely to be. More detailed analysis of each case reveals the subtleties involved in carrying out these responsibilities.

In Carl Merkin's case, the physician's immediate focus is on the treatment options and alternative futures that the patient faces, with and without ventilation. Rather than simply insisting that ventilation be implemented in this life-threatening situation, she advises the patient and his wife that, if the decision is made to initiate lifesaving treatment, it will be possible to withdraw such treatment at a subsequent date if the patient assesses that its benefits do not outweigh its burdens. By suggesting a trial of treatment, she provides her patient with the opportunity to sustain his life and a chance to see what life on the machine is like. Beyond presenting these options, the physician could take further steps to assure Mr. Merkin that she will treat any pain and discomfort he experiences. During this conversation, or soon after, it would also be necessary to discuss treatment options in the event of complications (e.g., DNR status, antibiotics for infection).

Mr. Merkin is competent to make his own decision about what treatment he wants and has the right to refuse treatment even though he could live for years with ventilatory support. In the past, he has expressed strong preferences about his wishes not to be hooked to a machine but is willing, at his physician's suggestions, to try it for a while.

The difficulty of this situation does not end, however, with the initiation of treatment. In fact, this may be the easiest step for the physician to take. In addition, Dr. Phillips will want to be sure that her patient understands what kind of life is possible on long-term ventilator support: Has the patient seen or talked to any other ventilator-dependent patients or their caregivers? Autonomous action must be premised on being truly informed of all options. It is quite possible that Mr. Merkin was unaware of the portability of modern respirators or held some incorrect beliefs or exaggerated fears that might be corrected or assuaged through information, dialogue, and psychological support. However, there is a fine line between persuasion and coercion. And even when there is no overt coercion, patients may go along with a caregiver's wishes for fear they will be abandoned if they actively disagree.

Now assume that the agreed-upon 2-week trial of treatment has ended and unsuccessful attempts at weaning have been carried out, yet Mr. Merkin remains firm in his decision to be removed from ventilator. Dr. Phillips has made the promise that it can indeed be removed. What then? Is there anything for the physician to do other than withdraw treatment?

Clearly, Dr. Phillips still has a very important role to play in Mr. Merkin's care. Before going ahead, she may ask the patient some additional questions—Is there a will? Are there any good-byes to make?—that help the patient and his family prepare themselves for impending death or cause them to reevaluate their preference.

Finally, if Mr. Merkin is firm in his decision, she still has an important role in supporting the patient and his loved ones once a decision is made. This includes psychological comfort as well as attention to pain medication and other symptom relief. Too often, patients fear they will be abandoned by their physician if they decide to stop aggressive treatment. Dr Phillips, through her continued attention, can show that this fear is unfounded and that she cares about her patient's overall well-being, not only his lung function.

The case of Rose Kantor is similar in that the patient also does not want to make use of available treatment. In this case, however, there is substantial disagreement between the patient and the physician, as well as other staff at the nursing home where she has lived for many years. Unlike Ms. Kantor, they assess the burden of chemotherapy as relatively light compared with the benefit of extending her life. The patient disagrees, saying she has lived long enough. Her assessment is a shock to those around her: they see her as someone who would want this chance to "fight."

One question that arises is why Ms. Kantor's determined refusal of life-sustaining treatment is so surprising. Are staff projecting their values and assumptions onto her, surprised she does not react as they would have—or at least the way they thought she would have—under the same circumstances. This illustrates how important it is for health care professionals not to use their own values, hopes, fears, and expectations as the basis for reacting to patients' wishes.

An additional question is whether Dr. Myers fulfills his responsibility to Ms. Kantor by agreeing to forgo treatment. From the evidence provided, this is not clear. He assesses the patient as not incompetent just because she chooses to forgo chemotherapy, so he respects her right to decide for herself. However, he may be remiss if he does not try to uncover the underlying reasons for her desire to refuse treatment and if he does not offer her the chance to reassess her feelings at a later date, once her symptoms worsen.

For example, why does the nursing home think she is doing fine, while Ms. Kantor seems to believe her life is no longer worth living? Are there ways to improve her life in the nursing home and make it more meaningful? Is depression a contributing factor in her decision? What if treatment had been initiated 5 years ago, when the leukemia was first diagnosed? Finding the answers to these questions would not necessarily change Ms. Kantor's decision not to prolong her life. However, without additional evidence and without informing the patient about her options to change her mind, the dialogue between patient and physician is not complete.

In sum, working with the elderly presents special challenges. Physicians with a commitment to providing appropriate care to patients near the end of life attend to many issues. They sort through the complex medical histories that accrue as one grows old, assess the interactions of chronic and acute conditions and treatments, strive to maximize the patient's participation in the decision-making process despite limited or fluctuating capacity, deal with the needs and sometimes conflicting demands of emotionally vulnerable spouses and adult children, and so on. Working within a context of uncertainty, physicians have to explain what treatments are and are not reasonable alternatives and what the likely benefits and burdens of different options are in terms that the patient (or surrogate) can understand. In addition to medical and technical expertise, this requires excellent communication skills and a willingness to comfort patients and support family members through their grief. Physicians who possess these skills see their patients as whole persons with long histories behind them and a continuing stake in directing, to as great an extent as possible, their own futures.

In the not too distant past, there was relatively little we could do to extend the lives of elderly men and women. Now there is an arsenal of tools we can use to extend biological functioning, but a growing number of questions arises about how these tools should be employed.

In this chapter, we have focused on areas of growing consensus regarding how decisions about the use of life supports for patients near the end of life should be made. In recent years, the focus in clinical ethics has been on questions of patient autonomy and conflicts between autonomy and beneficence. In the decades to come, the study of clinical ethics is likely to turn its attention to different dilemmas, such as those related to the allocation of scarce resources. In addition, the development of new technologies and treatments, as well as other changes in the context of medical decision making, will bring new ethical and legal questions to center stage (Meisel, 1993; Pellegrino, 1993). Some of these are already plain: Do patients have the right to life-sustaining treatment that, in their physicians' view, is futile? Do they have they right to be informed of the availability of such treatment? Can physicians decide on what treatments are appropriate based on economic grounds? Is physician-assisted suicide ethical? Should it be legalized? What effect would its widespread practice have on physicians, patients, and society? As we proceed to the next century, these and other questions will emerge. Then, as now, physicians will be on the front line, called upon to utilize and harness life-sustaining technologies.

ACKNOWLEDGMENTS

Funding was provided to the authors by a grant from the W. K. Kellogg Foundation to the Decisions Near the End of Life Program. The authors thank Vivian Guilfoy, Rebecca Jackson, and Dieter Koch-Weser, MD, for their contributions to this chapter. Additional thanks are extended to Ms. Jackson, Ellen Olson, MD, and Carl O'Donnell, ScD for their preparation of the case study materials we discuss in this chapter.

References

Beauchamp, T. L., & Childress, J. F. *Principles of biomedical ethics.* (2d ed.). New York: Oxford University Press. 1983.

Belkin, L. *First do no harm.* New York: Simon & Schuster. 1993.

Botkin, J. R. The seductive beauty of physiology. *Journal of Clinical Ethics,* (Winter), 274–77. 1992.

Brett, A. S. Limitations of listing specific medical interventions in advance directives. *Journal of the American Medical Association, 266*: 825–28.1991.

Brody, J. E. Doctors admit ignoring dying patients' wishes. *New York Times,* A18m January 14, 1993.

Clark, H. W., & Duffy, T. P. *Is a surrogate always necessary, decisions near the end of life.* Newton: MA: Education Development Center. 1989.

Current Opinions of the Council on Ethical and Judicial Affairs of the American Medical Association: Withholding or withdrawing life prolonging treatment. Chicago: American Medical Association. 1992.

Danis, M., Gerrity, M. S., Southerland, L.I., & Patrick, D. L. A comparison of patient, family and physician assessments of the value of medical intensive care. *Critical Care Medicine, 16*: 594–600. 1988.

Danis, M., Karr, J. L., & Southerland, L. I. A comparison of patient, family , and nurse evaluations of usefulness of intensive care. *Critical Care Medicine, 15*: 138–43. 1987.

Deutsch, C. *Living with dying in nursing homes. Decisions near the end of life.* Newton, MA: Education Development Center. 1989.

Emanuel, L. L., Barley, M. J., Stoeckle, J. D., Ettelson, L. M., Emanuel, E. J. Advance directives for medical care—a case for greater use. *N Engl J Med, 92*: 832–36. 1980.

Gerrity, M. S., Earp, L. L., DeVellis, R. F., & Light, D. W. Uncertainty and professional work: Perceptions of physicians in clinical practice. *American Journal of Sociology, 97*: 1022–51. 1992.

Goetzler, R. M., & Moskowitz, M. A. Changes in physician attitudes toward limiting care of critically ill patients. *Arch Inter Med, 151*: 1537–40. 1991.

Goodman, E. Medicine and money. *Boston Globe, 71*, January 31, 1993.

The Hastings Center: *Guidelines on the termination of life sustaining treatment and the care of the dying.* Bloomington, IN: Indiana University Press. 1987.

Haug, M. R., & Lavin, B. Practitioner or patient: Who's in charge? *Journal of Health and Social Behavior, 22*: 2122–219. 1981.

Jackson, R., & Carlos, A. Getting ready for the PSDA: What are hospitals and nursing homes doing? *Journal of Clinical Ethics, 2*: 177–80. 1991.

Ku, L., & Fisher, D. The attitudes of physicians toward health cost containment policies. *Health Services Research, 25*: 25–42. 1990.

Lynn, J., & Childress, J. F. Must patients always be given food and water? *Hastings Center Report, 10*: 17–21. 1983.

McCloskey, E. L. The patient self-determination act. *Kennedy Institute of Ethics Journal*, 163–64. June 1991.

Miles, S. H. Advanced directives to limit treatment: The Need for Portability. *Journal of the American Geriatric Society, 35*: 74–76. 1987.

Miles, S. H. Commentary: Listening for the healing story. *Second Opinion, 18*: 87–89. 1992.

Medical News & Perspectives: Talk to people about dying—they can handle it, say geriatricians and patients. *Journal of the American Medical Association, 269*: 321–2. 1993.

Meisel, A. The consensus about forgoing life-sustaining treatment: Its status and prospects. *Kennedy Institute of Ethics Journal, 2*: 309–345. 1993.

Meisel, A. Legal myths about terminating life support. *Archives of Internal Medicine, 151*: 1497–1502. 1991.

Omnibus Budget Reconciliation Act of 1990, Pub L. No. 101–508, 4206, 4751.

Patients Rights. In: Accreditation manual for hospitals, 1992. Chicago: Joint Commission on Accreditation of Healthcare Organizations: 103–05. 1992.

Pellegrino, E. Metamorphosis of medical ethics. *Journal of the American Medical Association, 269*: 1159–62. 1993.

Randall, T. Students challenged to make ethics part of their habit of thought. *Journal of the American Medical Association, 268*: 2349–50. 1992.

President's Commission for the Study of Ethical Problems in Medicine and Biomedical and Behavioral Research. *Deciding to forego life-sustaining treatment: Ethical, medical, and legal issues in treatment decisions.* Washington, DC: US Government Printing Office. 1983.

In re Quinlan, 70 NJ 20, 355x A2nd 647, *cert denied sub nom Garger v New Jersey*, 429 US 922 (1976).

Schneiderman, L. J., Pearlman, R. A., Kaplan, R. M., Anderson, J. P., & Rosenberg, E.M. Relationship of general advance directive instructions to specific life-sustaining treatment preferences in patients with serious illness. *Archives of Internal Medicine, 1152*: 2114–18. 1992.

Silvestri, R., & O'Donnell, C. *The benefits of time-limited treatments. Decisions Near the End of Life.* Newton, MA: Education Development Center. 1989.

Solomon, M. Z., Jennings, B., Guilfoy, V., Jackson, R., O'Donnell, L., Wolf, S.M., Nolan, K., Koch-Weser D., & Donnelley, S. Toward an expanded vision of clinical ethics education: From the individual to the institution. *Kennedy Institute of Ethics Journal, 1*: 225–45. 1991.

Solomon, M. Z., O'Donnell, L., Jennings, B., Guilfoy, B., Wolf, S. M., Nolan, K. Jackson, R., Koch-Weser, D., & Donnelley, S. Decisions near the end of life: Professional views on life-sustaining treatments. *American Journal of Public Health, 83*: 14–23. 1993.

Uhlmann, R. F., Pearlman, R. A., & Cain, K. A. Physicians and spouses' predictions of elderly patients' resuscitation preferences. *Journal of Gerontology, 43*: 112–21. 1983.

Vladek, B., Editorial: Beliefs vs behaviors in healthcare decision making. *American Journal of Public Health, 83*: 13–14. 1993.

Wanzer, S. H., Federman, D. D., & Adelstein, S. J., et al. The physician's responsibility toward hopelessly ill patients. *New England Journal of Medicine, 320*: 844–49. 1989.

Chapter Six

The Rational Use of Tube Feeding in Elderly Long-Term Patients

Roberta M. Meyers and Michael A. Grodin

BACKGROUND AND DEFINITION OF THE PROBLEM

In 1790 a patient with paralysis of the muscles of deglutition was successfully fed using a tube made of a whalebone probe covered with an eelskin and attached to a bladderlike container that delivered "jellies, eggs beaten up with a little water, sugar and milk or wine" to the patient. In the 1940s and 1950s a variety of case reports were published in which patients were fed by means of fine polyethylene tubes. The ailments treated included anorexia resulting from trauma, burns, cardiovascular accidents, tuberculosis, depression, coma, and terminal cancer, as well as mechanical impediments to eating (Randall, 1990).

Nasogastric and gastrostomy ("appliance") feedings for both acute and chronic medical conditions have become commonplace. As the population ages and the prevalence of chronic diseases that affect the ability to aliment increases, questions regarding the use of and the decision-making processes surrounding the application of appliance feeding technologies are under closer scrutiny.

Feeding "failure" or disability in long-term care patients is not well understood. Forty-seven percent to 67% of skilled nursing facility residents have been described as requiring eating assistance, whether verbal supervision or actual physical assistance (Siebens et al., 1986; Zimmer, 1975). It has been estimated that the cost of

managing eating dependency is 25% of the cost of caring for a totally dependent individual (Kottkee, 1974).

Multiple reasons may exist for feeding disability in long-term
care patients. These include physical illness, cognitive loss, neurologic disability, and psychiatric and emotional disorders. Some of
these, such as physical and psychiatric illness, may be treatable
and reversible. For these patients, the goal of appliance feedings—
to support them through a potentially reversible period—enables a
straightforward decision-making process in which the feedings are
postulated as short-term and beneficial. The goal is to sustain the
patient until other treatments, and time, correct the underlying
condition. Other causes of feeding disability are irreversible. There
are multiple possible neurologic contributors to swallowing dysfunction that may be thought of as manifesting themselves
through a "final common pathway" of oral-pharyngeal dysfunction. Included are any phenomena that change muscle control or
coordination of the swallowing mechanism. Stroke syndromes may
have obvious neurologic sequelae leading to swallowing dysfunction, although the anatomic lesion does not necessarily predict the
type or severity of the swallowing disability (Robbins & Leverne,
1988; Veis & Logemann, 1985). The same is true for Parkinson's
disease; the severity of the disease and the severity of the swallowing dysfunction are not clearly correlated (Lieberman et al., 1980).
Dementing illness of any type may lead to swallowing dysfunction
through a variety of mechanisms, including damage to the neurologic control of the muscles of mastication and swallowing, as well
as the loss of integrative control, leading to "swallowing apraxia."
In a group of nursing home residents with eating dependency, abnormal oral-motor function, as identified either by the observation
of nurses or by the physical examination of a speech-language pathologist, was the characteristic most likely to be present (Siebens
et al, 1986).

Clinical examinations by speech pathologists are used to charac-
terize swallowing dysfunction and to develop treatment options.
More recently, videofluoroscopy swallowing studies have been used
to evaluate the nature of swallowing dysfunction. Videofluoroscopic
examinations delineate specific anatomic characteristics of the patient's swallow and also enable the measurement of specific functional components, such as transit time. Aspiration of swallowed
substances into the trachea can also be documented (Dodds, Stewart, & Logemann, 1990; Sorin, Somers, Austin, & Bester, 1988).

Aspiration can be broadly defined as the misdirection of oropharyngeal contents into the larynx, but it can also refer to the reflux of stomach contents into the bronchial tree. Patients with swallowing dysfunction may aspirate from the oropharynx; they may also aspirate from the stomach.

The relationship between swallowing dysfunction, aspiration, and the development of pneumonia is not clear. It is likely variable and influenced by other factors besides aspiration, including the failure of immunologic and pulmonary defense mechanisms of the patient. Whether or not the course is affected by placement of a feeding tube is also unclear. In long-term care populations the percentage of nasogastric-, gastrostomy-, or jejeunostomy-fed patients developing aspiration pneumonia ranges from 39% to 57% (Ciocon, Silverstone, Graver, & Foley, 1988; Cogen & Weinryb, 1989; Hassett, Sunby, & Flint, 1988; Peck, Cohen & Mulvihill, 1990; Pritchard, 1988). These studies are problematic because there is no comparably impaired control group to follow regarding the incidence of aspiration pneumonia in patients who receive spoon feedings instead of appliance feedings. Patients who require appliance feedings are often so impaired that adequate intake with spoon feedings is not possible. It has been contended that, for debilitated, noncommunicative, bed-bound patients, the risk of aspiration pneumonia may be increased when appliance feedings, rather than careful spoon feedings, are supplied (Campbell-Taylor & Fisher, 1987). Of note is that studies in acute care hospitals have primarily been done in intensive care units in patients with tracheostomies or endotracheal tubes. Complication rates, including aspiration and the incidence of pneumonia, are markedly fewer, 0% to 5.7% (Cataldi-Betcher, Seltzer, Slocum, & Jones, 1983; Metheny, Eisenberg, & Spies, 1986; Treolar & Stechmiller, 1984; Winterbauer, Durning, Barron, & McFadden, 1981).

TUBE FEEDINGS AS MEDICAL TREATMENTS

Tube feedings may or may not result in fewer episodes of aspiration pneumonia than do oral feedings. For those elderly patients whose swallowing dysfunction is irreversible and who become malnourished despite conscientious attempts at spoon feeding, the initiation of appliance feedings on a long-term basis may, however, be the only alternative for reliably supplying nutrition. Episodes of dehydration may be prevented, nutritional integrity restored, and life sustained. All of these may be viewed as benefits.

The prolongation of life by appliance feedings may, however, also potentially be viewed as a burden. This depends on the views of the patient and his or her valuation of the life circumstances that include feeding disability of a severity that requires appliance feedings to sustain life. There are other burdens to appliance feeding. The patients may need to be restrained or sedated if they repeatedly remove the feeding tube. This may increase the risk of pressure sores and pneumonia (Lo & Dornbrand, 1984). If the decision is made to place a gastrostomy tube, endoscopic or surgical placement is required, with its attendant risks, including operative hemorrhage and peritoneal leakage of tube feedings and gastric contents around the stoma (Ho, Yee, & McPherson, 1988; Steffes, Weaver, & Bouwman, 1989; Stiegmann et al., 1990).

Benefits and burdens of supplying long-term appliance feedings for elderly patients with feeding disability exist, and therefore a benefits/burdens assessment must be made. There is extensive commentary regarding the similarity of appliance feedings to other medical treatments and whether or not both require a decision-making process that balances benefits. Callahan (1988) has noted that the provision of nutrition may have symbolic significance and be important in and of itself; the method, whether simple or not, technological or not, is irrelevant. More typically, tube feedings have been equated with medical treatments, as in the U.S. Supreme Court concurring decision regarding *Cruzan v. Director, State of Missouri* (1990) written by Justice O'Connor: "Artificial feeding cannot readily be distinguished from other forms of medical treatment. . . Whether or not the techniques used to pass food and water into the patient's alimentary tract are termed 'medical treatment' it is clear they all involve some degree of intrusiveness and restraint."

Appliance feedings are also like medical treatments in that their use is subject to ongoing assessment. The benefit/burden ratio may change as the clinical circumstances change. Appliance feedings that were supplied and viewed as being beneficial may later be viewed as burdensome enough to warrant their withdrawal. There is no moral reason that appliance feedings, once begun, cannot be stopped if the feedings are judged as no longer benefiting the patient. There is a recognized psychological distinction for physicians and nurses, although not well characterized, between withdrawing feedings that have begun and not beginning them at all (Smith & Veatch, 1987). It seems more difficult for some caregivers to stop feedings that are in place than to withhold them initially. One difference may be that withholding appliance feedings requires no action and thus appears to be less explicit than withdrawing them. There is no moral prohibition against withdrawing feedings that are in place, and there are often many medical reasons for doing so.

COMPARISONS AND CONTRASTS WITH PATIENTS IN PERSISTENT VEGETATIVE STATE

Most of the commentary regarding the ethical dilemmas of appliance feedings relates to the withdrawal of feedings in patients in persistent vegetative states (PVS). Similarities and contrasts exist between the withdrawal of appliance feedings in patients with PVS and the initiation of feedings in the elderly with irreversible feeding disability.

The diagnosis of PVS is specific. These patients breathe without assistance, but their degree of neurologic disability essentially precludes their ability to swallow. Their only realistic option for feeding is via nasogastric or gastrostomy tube. Appliance feedings are typically initiated during a period when the prognosis is uncertain. As the prognosis becomes clearer, the benefits of continued nutritional support require review.

In contrast, elderly patients with feeding disability initially have the ability to be maintained by spoon feedings. They often fail spoon feedings in an uneven fashion, taking in variable amounts of oral food and fluids and usually maintaining some semblance of being able to aliment. It is possible to forestall, and even ignore, decisions surrounding the initiation of appliance feedings.

A second contrast between PVS patients and elderly patients with irreversible dementia is the perception of discomfort. Because of the severity of their neurologic condition, PVS patients cannot perceive discomfort; it has been argued that, in fact, they can neither be benefited nor harmed by appliance feedings (Lynn & Childress, 1986).

Elderly patients with feeding disability are fundamentally different from PVS patients; they can perceive discomfort. They can potentially be burdened by appliance feedings. They can feel the tube and may try to pull it out, necessitating keeping their hands physically restrained. Furthermore, depending on their mental status, they may retain their awareness of themselves and of their condition. This awareness may be burdensome if they would not have wished to continue life in the circumstances in which the feeding disability has arisen.

Many elderly patients with feeding disability are similar to PVS patients in that neither group is considered "terminally ill," since both types of patients can be expected to live years if appliance feedings are supplied.

THE VALUE OF AN EXPLICIT DECISION-MAKING PROCESS

Spoon-feeding failure can be uneven and unpredictable. Some elderly patients with feeding disability may never totally lose a semblance of being able to eat. Nutritional decline in these patients may be ignored and explicit decision making forestalled. The number of times malnutrition in these patients goes unrecognized versus the number of times it is recognized but either not acknowledged or left untreated is unknown.

An explicit diagnosis of nutritional deficiency and underlying feeding disability is preferable, because a deliberate decision-making process about the subsequent treatment can then occur. A deliberate decision-making process necessitates an articulation of the principles underlying the decision, as well as the patient's diagnoses, treatment options, and goals. Clear articulation facilitates communication between physicians, other caregivers, and patients' families. Unilateral decision making that potentially isolates physicians, families, and other caregivers from the support of others is avoided. Furthermore, these patients, who are often incapacitated, are safeguarded from care that occurs by default. They are often vulnerable and need some protection from decisions in which respect for their best interests might be diminished.

Some would argue there is value in not being explicit, especially in terms of avoiding the emotional or psychological stress that may accompany active decision making. Being inexplicit may be justified when there are no effective options although, even then, some would argue that it is not justified. As long as options exist, however, decision making must be explicit. Options do exist with the use of appliance feedings. They may be effective for some treatment goals and ineffective for other goals. Decision making must, therefore, be explicit.

THE LIMITS OF AUTONOMY AND BENEFICENCE

Two principles are important to the decision-making process regarding the initiation of appliance feedings in the elderly with irreversible feeding disability: respect for autonomy and beneficence. Autonomy is limited when a patient becomes incapacitated. Once capacity has been lost, patients should no longer be viewed as autonomous, and a different mechanism for assuring respect for them as persons and for respecting their interest in self-determination must be in place (Ellman, 1990). The ability to respect the personhood and autonomy of incapacitated patients is limited because, short of a clear written or oral advance directive, certainty about what they would have wanted for themselves is imperfect.

Beneficence, as a principle, also has limits in that it is not always possible to ascertain which treatment course is most beneficent. There is a general consensus that certain aspects of care are clearly beneficent: keeping patients clean and dry, offering feedings by spoon and cup, providing a comfortable room temperature, treating pain with analgesics, keeping bed-bound patients turned and positioned to prevent skin breakdown. The provision of this level of care is not inconsequential. But extending life by providing appliance feedings may be viewed as a benefit or a burden, depending on each individual's values and perceptions about his or her life in the circumstances in which the feeding disability arises.

Determining which treatment choices are beneficent is further obscured by the emotional issues surrounding the withholding of feeding. Deciding to forgo placement of a feeding appliance in a patient who still has some semblance of orally alimenting does not immediately result in death. Forgoing a ventilator for respiratory failure will, in contrast, usually result in death within a relatively short period of time. Death from dehydration may not occur as quickly; the deterioration that accompanies that process may be difficult for caregivers to observe.

THE LIMITS OF SURROGACY

The goal of decision making is to choose for the patient what the patient would have chosen if he or she had the capacity to make an informed decision. Who should make these decisions, based on either what a patient would have wanted (substituted judgment) or on an analysis of the patient's best interests? The assumption has been, and should continue to be, that families and loved ones best represent the values and interests of the patient. Rhoden (1988) has argued that the rebuttable presumption should be in favor of families (or loved ones) as the appropriate surrogates. Those who challenge this assumption must show, in a given case, why the family is not the best decision maker. Historically, families and loved ones have acted as surrogates. There is no evidence that others—for example, courts—represent patients more effectively. It is reasonable to believe that the family, as the context within which a person first develops his or her values, can best represent those values (Rhoden, 1988). Cases in which there is disagreement among the family or reason to suspect the good will of the family should have the arena of surrogate decision makers broadened. The purpose of including other decision makers in these cases is to protect inherently vulnerable patients from decisions that are not representative of their wishes nor based on their best interests.

A fundamental dilemma surrounding surrogacy is that, short of clearly expressed advance directives, surrogate decision makers can never truly know what an incapacitated person would have wanted. Respect for the principle of autonomy requires that surrogates try to determine, as accurately as possible, what an incapacitated patient would have wanted in a given situation. The inherent potential of inaccuracy when exercising substituted judgment must, however, be recognized.

Additionally, advance directives may have limitations. An elderly, incapacitated person may be "discontinuous" with his past. Though severely demented, for example, he may be contented. Hypothetically, he may not wish to be bound by a prior perception of an incapacitated state that led him to complete an advance directive explicitly shortening the duration of that state.

Surrogates struggle to respect the principle of autonomy and to act beneficently. The issue is complicated because, among the outcomes of the decision making process is extending life in a state in which irreversible feeding disability has arisen. This may be seen as either desired or hated by the patient. Neither the level of self-awareness of the patient nor the discomfort he or she is experiencing is certain. Surrogates cannot perfectly know what he or she would have wanted. Furthermore, safeguards are needed to protect these vulnerable patients from hastily made decisions or those that would devalue the quality of their lives.

ARGUMENTS AT THE EXTREMES

Some would contend that withholding appliance feedings from patients whose intake is suboptimal is always unacceptable. Proponents of this position argue that appliance feedings are substantially different from medical treatments, and a benefit/burden analysis cannot be applied. Appliance feedings are viewed as equivalent to food and fluids, which can never be withheld because they are beneficent without qualification. There are professional and societal proscriptions, for example, against giving a patient a lethal injection. Similarly, it may be argued that failure to supply appliance feedings is prohibited.

In response to these claims, others would assert that the extension of life that may result from the use of appliance feedings can be analyzed as a benefit or burden, much the same way in which the extension of life with the use of antibiotics is analyzed. Furthermore, appliance feedings can be viewed as potentially intrusive and burdensome regardless of the outcome.

Although a benefit/burden analysis can be applied to appliance feedings, we do not believe it can be similarly applied to feeding a patient orally with a spoon and cup. The level of intrusiveness of supplying oral feedings is not that of appliance feedings. Offering food and fluids to patients and feeding them by hand can be viewed as one of the aspects of care that, except in unusual circumstances, is an unqualified beneficent act.

At the other extreme of the spectrum is the stance that elderly patients with irreversible feeding disability should never be fed. Otherwise healthy but incapacitated elders who are failing spoon feeding are experiencing a natural progression of the aging process. Withholding appliance feeding is simply allowing a fatal pathology to take its course (Volicer, Rheaume, Brown, Fabiszewski, & Brady, 1986).

This argument, however, fails to recognize the plurality of belief systems that exist. For some patients and their families, life is viewed as having intrinsic quality; food and fluids are seen as natural resources, which, regardless of the method, should always be supplied. For these patients, appliance feedings may not be viewed as particularly burdensome in relation to the valued life. To assert that no failing elder with feeding disability should ever be provided appliance feedings is to ignore the patient-centered principle of respect for autonomy. Many patients may, in fact, elect appliance feedings. Supplying appliance feedings in some cases may restore nutritional integrity and improve the quality of life of a patient. Clearly, where it is unknown whether or not supplying appliance feedings will be beneficial, a trial of them is indicated. Initiation and then withdrawal after reevaluation of the treatment objectives is a better option than withholding feedings.

The value premise that follows rejecting either end of the spectrum recognizes the desirability of respecting a variety of outcomes of the decision-making process. If either absolute position is accepted, there is no respect for individuals as persons. If the extension of life that results from appliance feeding may be viewed as either a benefit or a burden, a tolerance for a plurality of belief systems regarding appliance feedings will result. The difficulties that arise are practical ones, such as the decision-making process itself, facilitating communication, and determining appropriate surrogate decision makers for patients lacking autonomy.

THE DECISION-MAKING PROCESS

The underlying ethical principles that guide this decision making are beneficence and the principle of respect for patient autonomy. The provision of appliance feedings in elderly patients with irreversible feeding disability can be subjected to a benefit/burden analysis in much the same way that other medical treatments are analyzed. Variability exists in the way different persons view the extension of life in the circumstances in which their feeding disability has arisen. Whether or not appliance feedings are viewed as beneficial may depend, most importantly, on personal values. A variety of outcomes of the decision-making process may thus result. Decisions for these incapacitated patients will most often be made by surrogates. Safeguards to protect patients against poor decision making are necessary. Respect for a plurality of values does not imply there is no ethic at all. Physicians who defer decision making solely to the family, without providing any guidance and support, and physicians who simply do what they personally feel is correct have equally abrogated their responsibility.

The challenge for the decision-making process is to facilitate communication, respect the ethical principles of autonomy and beneficence, tolerate a plurality of belief systems, and yet safeguard vulnerable patients. Within this framework, physicians and other health care workers must maintain their own professional and personal ethic. Who will participate in this process and what will it consist of?

One place to look for information regarding the development of an ethic to clarify these dilemmas is the caregivers themselves. Physicians and nurses, as professionals, need both to convey information based on their training and clinical experience and to develop a sense of themselves as moral agents (Hauerwas, 1986). To be a professional is to profess; to be involved in a creative process that lays a foundation for one's work that evolves with experience, and from which others, including patients and their families, can learn (Churchill, 1989). Caregivers can express this moral creativity through direct involvement in the policy-making of the institutions in which they work.

A second place to look for useful information in developing an ethical process for resolving feeding dilemmas is the caregiving institution. In much the same way "Do Not Resuscitate" policies are in place in institutions (a requirement for those that are accredited by the Joint Commission of Accreditation of Health Care Organizations), feeding "policies" could be developed. An unknown but probably small number of nursing homes have formal policies for decisions about the use of nutritional support and hydration (Miles & Ryden, 1985; Office of Technology Assessment, 1987). Institutions should develop guidelines for the initiation of appliance feedings whenever the feedings can be expected to be chronic. These guidelines should be oriented toward treatment goals (S. H. Miles, personal communication, April 1991). For example, in the case of a nursing home resident who is malnourished, if the goal is supportive care, for comfort, the reversal of the undernutrition is moot. If the goal is to improve nutrition for whatever reason, including maintaining weight or promoting healing of a pressure sore, this may require appliance feeding, and this should be explicit.

Institutions with certain religious affiliations may seek to promulgate a certain stance toward appliance feedings. Policies should reflect this. It should be explicit to the patients prior to entering the institution, to their families, and to the caregivers employed by and affiliated with the institution.

Guidelines for decision making regarding the initiation of tube feedings need these elements: an elucidation of the patient's prognosis, an assessment of the patient's decision making capacity regarding the issue of appliance feeding, a discussion with the patient's surrogates (if the patient lacks capacity to make the decision) about what the patient would have wanted, and, most important, an elucidation of the overall treatment goals. Acknowledgment of the policies of the institution in which the patient resides should be included. Discussions among the patient, family, physician, and nursing staff should also be included as part of the process.

A third place to look for input in these decisions is the larger community, including the religious institutions that exist within it. It has been argued that modern medicine has created a paradox for itself. The power of its technology has created a problem (i.e., the termination of life support) so fundamental that solving it has moved beyond the boundaries of medicine (Carton, 1990). Problems concerning termination of life support are societal in that the community sets the limits within which patient autonomy can operate. The argument that, in a pluralistic society, debate about such value-laden issues cannot be useful because a clear consensus is not possible ignores the potential benefits of the debate itself. These benefits include eliciting the values that may be shared: autonomy, beneficence, respect for basic care and hygiene, and affirmation of the value of emotional support for patients, families, and caregivers. Eliciting these values can only help strengthen them and lead to a community-based framework for meeting the need these values imply.

Jennings (1989) reminds us, "to say that a society is ethically pluralistic is not to say that it is ethically fragmented." To fail to involve communities in these decision making processes is to ignore a vital resource for problem solving and to isolate medicine from the community of which it is an integral part.

There are several valuable potential outcomes to this open and explicit decisionmaking process. Decisions are not made unilaterally by physicians. Families are not stranded struggling to represent a patient's best interests, in relative isolation. They can draw on the expertise of medicine, nursing, and institutions, as well as the commonly derived values of the larger community, for information and support. Likewise, caregivers, especially physicians, are not isolated in a vacuum of speculation and second guessing. When explicit discussions occur, the potential exists for planning in advance what other treatment modalities may or may not be appropriate.

Additionally, it is hoped that policy making would reflect the need to accommodate individual decisions. Humane hospice and home care may be seen as valuable alternatives to continued feeding and institutionalization. A society that works to provide the flexibility to support patients and their families in these end-of-life decisions will be a richer, more thoughtful one.

The process of deliberate decision making applied to a patient such as this would include the following important aspects. First, a discussion would be held with the patient's family, the caregivers on the hospital or nursing home ward, and the physician. Risks and benefits of feeding tube placement would be discussed by the doctors and nurses. The family would be asked to imagine what the patient would have wanted. The policy of that particular institution would be used as a resource.

A trial of appliance feeding might be the outcome. Alternatively, a hospice level of care may be chosen, either in a formal setting or at home, with support services, during which food and fluids would be offered, fevers and discomfort treated with antipyretics and analgesics, and basic hygiene and nursing care provided. (In this hypothetical community, accustomed to involvement in such decisions, such alternatives for care would be readily available.) Each hypothetical outcome has its own integrity derived from a process that is deliberate and informed.

The price of informed deliberation in feeding dilemmas is time, energy, and tolerance. The price of failing to deliberate carefully in these practical dilemmas is continued isolation of medicine from the very people it professes to serve: patients, their families, and their communities. These deliberations require more than a calculation of risks and benefits. They require a fundamental respect for individual values. Without this respect, medicine loses the quality that illumines all of its technology—compassion.

References

Callahan, D. Commentary. In C. B. Cohen (Ed.). *Casebook on the termination of life-sustaining treatment and care of the dying*, (pp. 56–58). Bloomington: Indiana University Press. 1988.

Campbell-Taylor, I., & Fisher, R. H. The clinical case against tube feeding in palliative care of the elderly. *Journal of the American Geriatrics Society*, 35: 1100–1104. 1987.

Carton, R. W. The road to euthanasia. *Journal of the American Medical Association, 263*: 2221. 1990.

Cataldi-Betcher, E. L., Seltzer, M. H., Slocum, B. A., & Jones, K. W. Complications occurring during enteral nutrition support: A prospective study. *Journal of Parental and Enteral Nutrition, 7*(6): 546–552. 1983.

Churchill, L. R. Reviving a distinctive medical ethic. *Hastings Center Report,* May/June: 28–34. 1989.

Ciocon, J. O., Silverstone, F. A., Graver, M., & Foley, C. J. Tube feedings in elderly patients: Indications, benefits, and complications. *Archives of Internal Medicine, 148*: 429–433. 1988.

Cogen, R., & Weinryb, J. Aspiration pneumonia in nursing home patients fed via gastrostomy tube. *Am J Gastroenterol, 84*(12): 1509–1512. 1989.

Cruzan v. Director, Missouri Department of Health, 110 S. Ct. 2841 (1990).

Dodds, W. J., Stewart, E. T., & Logemann, J. A. Physiology and radiology of the normal oral and pharyngeal phases of swallowing. *Am J Roentgenol, 154*: 953–963. 1990.

Ellman, I. M. Can others exercise an incapacitated patient's right to die? *Hastings Center Report,* January/February: 47–50. 1990.

Hassett, J., Sunby, C., & Flint, L. M. No elimination of aspiration pneumonia in neurologically disabled patients with feeding gastrostomy. *Surgery, Obstetrics and Gynecology, 167*: 383–388. 1988.

Hauerwas, S. *Suffering Presence: Theological reflections on medicine, the mentally handicapped, and the church.* Notre Dame, IN: University of Notre Dame Press. 1986.

Ho, C., Yee, A. C. H., & McPherson, R. Complications of surgical and percutaneous non-endoscopic gastrostomy: Review of 233 patients. *Gastroenterology, 95*: 1206–1210. 1988.

Jennings, B. Bioethics as civic discourse. *Hastings Center Report,* September/October: 34–35. 1989.

Kottkee, F. J. Historia obscura hemiplegiae. *Archives of Physical Medicine and Rehabilitation, 55*: 4–13. 1974.

Lieberman, A. N., Horowitz, L., Redman, P., Pachter, L., Lieberman, I., & Leibowitz, M. Dysphagia in Parkinson's disease. *American Journal of Gastroenterol, 74*: 157–160. 1980.

Lo, B., & Dornbrand, L. Guiding the hand that feeds: Caring for the demented elderly. *N Engl J Med, 311*: 402–404. 1984.

Lynn, J., & Childress, J. F. Must patients always be given food and water? In J. Lynn (Ed.), *By no extraordinary means: The choice to forego life-sustaining food and water* (pp. 48–60). Bloomington: Indiana University Press. 1986.

Metheny, N.A., Eisenberg, P., & Spies, M. Aspiration pneumonia in patients fed through nasoenteral tubes. *Heart & Lung, 15*(3): 256–261. 1986.

Miles, S. H., & Ryden, M. B. Limited-treatment policies in long-term care facilities. *Journal of the American Geriatrics Society, 33*: 707–711. 1985.

Office of Technology Assessment. Nutritional support and hydration. In: *Life-sustaining Technologies and the Elderly* (OTA Publication No. OTA-BA-306, pp. 274–329). Washington, DC: U.S. Government Printing Office. 1987.

Peck, A., Cohen, C. E., & Mulvihill, M. N. Long-term feeding of aged demented nursing home patients. *Journal of the American Geriatrics Society, 38*: 1195–1198. 1990.

Pritchard, V. Tube feeding-related pneumonias. *Journal of Gerontological Nursing, 14*(7): 32–36. 1988.

Randall, H. T. The history of enteral nutrition. In J. L. Rombeau & M. D. Caldwell (Eds.), *Clinical nutrition: Enteral and tube feeding* (pp. 1–9). Philadelphia: Saunders. 1990.

Rhoden, N. K. Litigating life and death. *Harvard Law Review, 102*: 375–446. 1988.

Robbins, J., & Leverne, R. L. Swallowing after unilateral stroke of the cerebral cortex: Preliminary experience. *Dysphagia, 3*: 11–17. 1988.

Siebens, H., Trupe, E., Siebens, A., Cook, F., Anshen, S., Hanauer, R., & Oster, G. Correlates and consequences of eating dependency in institutionalized elderly. *Journal of the American Geriatrics Society, 32*: 192–198. 1986.

Smith, D. H., & Veatch, R. M. (Eds.) Introduction In *Guidelines on the termination of life-sustaining treatment and the care of the dying* (pp. 1–14). Bloomington: Indiana University Press. 1987.

Sorin, R., Somers, S., Austin, W., & Bester, S. The influence of videofluoroscopy on the management of the dysphagic patient. *Dysphagia, 2*: 127–135. 1988.

Steffes, C., Weaver, D. W., & Bouwman, D. L. Percutaneous endoscopic gastrostomy: New technique—old complications. *American Surgery, 55*: 273–277. 1989.

Stiegmann, G. V., Goff, J. S., Silas, D., Pearlman, N., Sun, J., & Norton, L. Endoscopic versus operative gastrostomy: Final results of a prospective randomized trial. *Gastrointestinal Endoscopy, 36*: 1–5. 1990.

Treolar, D. M., & Stechmiller, J. Pulmonary aspiration in tube-fed patients with artificial airways. *Heart & Lung, 13*(6): 667–671. 1984.

Veis, S. L., & Logemann, J. A. Swallowing disorders in persons with cerebrovascular accident. *Archives of Physical Medicine and Rehabilitation, 66*: 372–375. 1985.

Volicer, L., Rheaume, V., Brown, J., Fabiszewski, K., Brady, R. Hospice approach to the treatment of patients with advanced dementia of the Alzheimer type. *J Am Med Association, 256*: 2210–2213. 1986.

Winterbauer, R. H., Durning, R. B., Barron, E., & McFadden, M. C. Aspirated nasogastric feeding solution detected by glucose strips. *An Inter Med, 95*(1): 67–68. 1981.

Zimmer, J. G. Characteristics of patients and care provided in health-related and skilled nursing facilities. *Medical Care, 13*: 992–1010. 1975.

Chapter Seven

Advanced Diagnostic Technology in Cardiovascular Disease of the Aged

Kirsten E. Fleischmann and Richard T. Lee

Recent advances in imaging and other technologies have led to an explosion in the number of diagnostic tests, both invasive and noninvasive, available to the clinician to assess the cardiovascular system. Choosing the appropriate diagnostic modality requires knowledge of the potential and limitations of each test, as well as a sense of what information it may provide above and beyond history, physical examination, and electrocardiographic data. This is particularly crucial in the elderly patient in whom cardiovascular disease ranks as the leading cause of death in both men and women (National Center for Health Statistics, 1991) and in whom the history and physical examination may be less specific or difficult to interpret (Cobb, Higginbotham, & Mark, 1986). Factors that may influence suitability of each test in the aged include the following:

1. A rising incidence of comorbidities that can affect the logistics of testing.
2. Changing physician and patient preferences with advancing age.
3. Different prevalence of disease when compared to a younger population.
4. Changes in standards or normal values with "normal" aging.

Thus, age may directly affect the desire or ability to perform a given diagnostic test or alter the sensitivity (probability that the test is positive in the presence of disease) or specificity (probability that the test is negative in the absence of disease)(Henneken & Buring, 1987) of an adequate study in the elderly population. While information regarding direct comparison of diagnostic and imaging modalities is relatively sparse, this chapter will provide an overview of the commonly utilized diagnostic techniques, along with a discussion of special considerations applicable to the elderly.

STRESS TESTING

Stress testing assesses the heart's response to physiologic (e.g., exercise, pacing) or pharmacologic (e.g., dipyridamole, adenosine, dobutamine) stimulation and is a mainstay of cardiac diagnostic testing, particularly in known or suspected coronary artery disease but also in valvular heart disease and arrhythmias. It can be coupled with imaging modalities such as two-dimensional echocardiography or radionuclide scintigraphy to yield additional information in some patients (Brown, 1991; Coyne, Belvedere, Vande Streek, et al., 1991; Marwick, Nemec, Pashkow, Stewart, & Salcedo, 1992; Picano, 1992).

In treadmill exercise testing, the most widely used form, the patient is asked to walk at increasing speed and against increasing incline according to a predetermined protocol (Naughton, Bruce, protocols etc.). Endpoints include development of symptoms, abnormal hemodynamic response to exercise and diagnostic ST changes, all of which can signal significant stenosis in the coronary circulation. In addition, treadmill testing provides valuable information on exercise capacity and, in conjunction with measurement of maximal oxygen uptake, is often used to gauge functional status in evaluation of cardiomyopathy or in patients being considered for transplantation. Contraindications to exercise testing include an unstable ischemic syndrome, critical aortic stenosis, severe hypertrophic obstructive cardiomyopathy, uncompensated heart failure, acute systemic illness or inflammatory disease such as myocarditis or pericarditis, uncontrolled hypertension, untreated life-threatening arrythmias, or high-degree atrioventricular block (Chaitman, 1992).

In the elderly, exercise testing may be complicated by several factors. First, decline in exercise tolerance or increased incidence of comorbidities such as pulmonary disease, peripheral vascular disease, or musculoskeletal disorders can limit technical adequacy of the study. Careful clinical assessment of the patient's exercise tolerance and use of a protocol that increases work more gradually, such as the modified Bruce or Naughton protocols, help maximize the probability of a successful test (Vasilomanolakis, Licht, & Ellestad, 1985). Should a patient still be unable to exercise adequately, consideration should be given to a pharmacologic stress test. The incidence of resting ECG abnormalities such as left bundle branch block or ST and T wave abnormalities, with or without digitalis use, rises in the aged (Fisch, 1981), diminishing the utility of ECG criteria in these patients. Addition of echocardiographic imaging during exercise to look for development of regional wall motion abnormalities, left ventricular dysfunction, or mitral regurgitation may be helpful here (Picano, 1992; Marwick et al., 1992). Alternatively, perfusion imaging with stress and at rest using injections of radioactive tracers such as thallium-201 or technicium-99 MIBI can help identify defects corresponding to areas of altered perfusion (Brown, 1991; Parodi et al., 1991).

The predictive value of any screening test is dependent on the pretest likelihood of disease (Bayes' theorem) as well as the sensitivity and specificity of the test (Cobb et al., 1986; Henneken & Buring, 1987). While overall sensitivity for treadmill testing is usually in the range of 70% in a mixed population, the work of Hlatky et al.(1984) has identified age as an important independent factor influencing the sensitivity of exercise testing in multivariate analysis. In this study, sensitivity rose from 65% in the 40–49-year-old age range to 84% in the group over 60 years of age. The authors also reported slightly decreased specificity in patients over 60 years of age (from 85% in the younger group to 70% in patients over 60), However, specificity did not show a clear downward trend with increasing age. Thus, exercise testing can be expected to maintain or even increase sensitivity in the older population.

ECHOCARDIOGRAPHY

Doppler echocardiography utilizes reflected sound waves and differences in acoustic impedance among tissues to create images providing both structural and functional information regarding the heart and great vessels. Modalities currently in widespread use include M-mode (time-motion) one-dimensional scanning, two-dimensional real-time imaging, and Doppler and color Doppler flow mapping. Doppler ultrasound provides flow and velocity information; color Doppler flow mapping uses color coding of the Doppler signal to display visually both flow direction and velocity (Feigenbaum, 1992).

Due to its noninvasive nature, safety, reproducibility, portability, and applicability to a wide range of clinical situations, transthoracic echocardiography, in which the ultrasound transducer is applied to the chest wall in the parasternal, apical, subcostal, and suprasternal areas, is widely performed in patients suspected of having cardiovascular disease at any age. More recently, it has been joined by transesophageal echocardiography (TEE), in which the ultrasound probe is actually inserted via an endoscopic probe into the esophagus and stomach, under sedation and local anesthesia (Matsuzaki, Toma, & Kusakawa, 1990). This approach provides an alternative "window" to the heart, as well as high-quality, high-resolution images. The following discussion will focus first on the more commonly used transthoracic approach and its use in the elderly and then describe situations in which TEE may be particularly helpful.

The indications for transthoracic echocardiography are varied and include most of the major classes of cardiac disease. There is general agreement that echocardiography can provide valuable diagnostic and prognostic information in valvular disease, ischemic heart disease (especially after myocardial infarction), pericardial disease, cardiomyopathies, cardiac masses, diseases of the great vessels and congenital heart disease ("Guidelines for the Clinical Application of Echocardiography," 1990). In addition, it may provide helpful information in some clinical scenarios in patients with pulmonary disease or hypertension or those with evidence of peripheral embolic events.

Echocardiography can assess the presence and severity of both stenotic and regurgitant valvular lesions, though, in general, accuracy in evaluation of severity of regurgitant lesions is more limited ("Guidelines for the Clinical Application of Echocardiography," 1990). It can identify lesions consistent with vegetation in endocarditis, though it is important to remember that this is a clinical diagnosis, not to be based solely on the presence or absence of echocardiographic abnormalities. It can also help assess the function of mechanical and bioprosthetic valves. In patients with ischemic heart disease, the presence of regional wall motion abnormalities at rest can serve as a marker of current or past infarction, while the development of hypokinetic segments with exercise is often indicative of ischemia in the area. Assessment of global left ventricular function can have important implications for therapy and prognosis, particularly after myocardial infarction, where echocardiography remains invaluable for identifying complications of infarction such as thrombus, ventricular rupture, aneurysm, infarct expansion, or mitral regurgitation. Determination of wall thickness, ventricular function, chamber sizes, and diastolic flow parameters are useful in distinguishing hypertrophic, dilated, and restrictive cardiomyopathies. While assessment of pericardial disease remains imperfect, echocardiography reliably detects the presence of pericardial effusion and, by identifying evidence of right ventricular collapse in diastole or excess variation in valvular flow velocities, can help assess its hemodynamic significance. In all of these applications, however, transthoracic echocardiography may be limited by the quality of the images obtainable in a given patient and is operator- and reader-dependent.

The minimal discomfort and risk associated with transthoracic echocardiography make it extremely valuable for evaluation of the aged patient. However, several pitfalls deserve mention. First, adequate ultrasound images may be difficult to obtain in the elderly secondary to changes in body habitus (e.g., kyphosis), difficulty in positioning, or increasing incidence of concomitant lung disease (Coodley, 1988). Second, ultrasonographic studies, even in the absence of disease, have documented changes in the appearance of the heart with age. For example, the ratio of early diastolic mitral inflow to peak atrial mitral inflow, or E: A ratio, is markedly decreased in elderly patients, and peak ventricular filling is diminished (Gerstenblith et al., 1977; Kitzman, Sheikh, Beere, Philips, & Higginbotham, 1991). Changes in these parameters, traditionally related to left ventricular filling patterns and thus to diastolic function imply a "stiffening" of the left ventricle with age, even in the absence of overt cardiac disease. This is also supported by a mild increase in diastolic left ventricular wall thickness on M-mode study with age (Gerstenblith et al., 1977). Mild aortic root dilatation with age has also been reported (Gerstenblith et al., 1977). In contrast, resting ejection fraction and fractional shortening are well-preserved in aged normals (Gerstenblith et al., 1977; Kitzman, et al, 1991).

While the transthoracic approach remains the mainstay for ul-

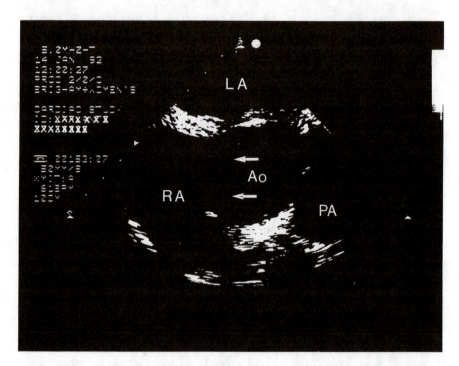

FIGURE 7.1 Transesophageal echocardiogram showing an intimal flap (arrows) in the ascending aorta (Ao), suggestive of aortic dissection. Surrounding structures include the right atrium (RA), left atrium (LA), and pulmonary artery (PA).

trasound evaluation, it is being increasingly supplemented by TEE. Indeed, for some indications, such as suspected aortic dissection (Figure 7.1), TEE is an important modality due to its speed of acquisition, safety, portability, and high diagnostic accuracy (sensitivity of 97%–100% and specificity of 68%–100%) (Ballal et al., 1991; Erbel et al., 1989; Nienaber et al., 1992). TEE is also particularly useful in the evaluation of atrial masses and thrombi, evaluation of the atrial septum, assessment of prosthetic valves (particularly in the mitral position), and detection of vegetations in endocarditis (Fisher, Stahl, Budd, & Goldman, 1991; Matsuzaki et al., 1990). While this technique is clearly more invasive than the transthoracic approach, it is generally well tolerated, with a less than 1% incidence of complications such as bradycardia, nonsustained arrhythmia, or transient ischemia (Matsuzaki et al., 1990). Damage to or perforation of the esophagus remains a possibility but can be minimized by avoiding TEE in patients with known or suspected esophageal disease. As always, care in the use of and potential reduction in the total dosage of sedative agents, such as midazolam or morphine, are appropriate in elderly patients.

NUCLEAR CARDIAC IMAGING

The use of radioactive tracers in noninvasive evaluation of the cardiovascular system has burgeoned with the development of both new tracer substances and improved imaging techniques. In general, the available studies serve three major purposes:

1. Measurement of global left ventricular function as well as regional wall motion.
2. Assessment of myocardial perfusion.
3. Determination of myocardial viability, both in terms of identifying infarction and in terms of localizing reversibly injured myocardium that may respond to therapeutic or revascularizing interventions.

The first purpose is often served by standard radionuclide ventriculography (RVG), traditionally using a technetium-99-based tracer, which outlines the intracardiac blood pool throughout the cardiac cycle either at rest or with concomitant exercise. By gating to the ECG and then comparing diastolic and systolic images, quantitative, relatively reproducible assessment of ejection fraction is possible, using either the initial cardiac cycles (first-pass technique) or the summation of many cardiac cycles (equilibrium technique) (Rocco, Dilsizian, Fischman, & Strauss, 1989). The first-pass technique allows assessment of both left and right ventricular function, while equilibrium images, in general, provide higher count totals and thus better resolution. While RVG is most often used for assessment of systolic function in coronary artery disease or valvular lesions, it has also been used to identify diastolic abnormalities (Rocco et al., 1989). As a technique for detection of coronary disease, it has been largely supplanted by perfusion studies using radioactive tracers that distribute in proportion to cardiac blood flow.

The best known and most widely used of these agents is thallium-201, in conjunction with either planar imaging or the newer single photon emission computed tomography (SPECT). Thallium, which acts as a potassium analog, is quickly and efficiently extracted by the myocardium in relation to blood flow but can also redistribute in relationship to changes in blood flow (Zaret, Wackers, & Soufer, 1992). In conjunction with exercise testing, images are usually obtained at peak exercise and then 3–4 hours later, after redistribution. The appearance of a reversible defect generally indicates an area of ischemia with viable myocardium (Zaret et al., 1992). The significance of a "fixed" defect present on both stress and rest images is less clear, however. Traditionally, such defects were considered evidence of infarction or scar, but recent data suggest some of these areas are still viable and may show improved function after revascularization (Brunken et al., 1989; Cloninger et al., 1988; Tamaki et al., 1988). Overall sensitivity and specificity for the detection of coronary artery disease from pooled data is reported as approximately 85% (Detrano et al., 1988). However, it is important to remember that sensitivity also increases with severity of disease. Thallium imaging after dipyridamole injection has also been used in preoperative assessment of patients with peripheral vascular disease (Boucher et al., 1985), although a recent study casts doubt on its routine use (Mangano et al., 1991).

Currently, technetium-99 MIBI has generated great interest as a perfusion tracer. Its favorable imaging characteristics result in higher count rates with better resolution as well as the option of performing first pass ventricular function studies (Wackers et al., 1989). Of note is that it undergoes minimal redistribution, necessitating separate rest and stress injections (Wackers et al., 1989). This technetium compound also shows promise in myocardial viability assessment, as does metabolic imaging with positron emission tomography (PET).

In the PET technique, positron-emitting isotopes such as rubidium-82 chloride, nitrogen-13 ammonia, and oxygen-15 water are injected and imaged to assess perfusion (Zaret et al., 1992). Shortly thereafter, a metabolic marker, usually fluorine-18 fluorodeoxyglucose, is injected and after about 30–50 minutes a second set of images is obtained (Zaret et al., 1992). Uptake of the labeled glucose compound reflects glucose utilization and is used as a marker of metabolic activity. Mismatch between perfusion and metabolic images is interpreted as ischemic yet viable myocardium (Zaret et al., 1992). Limitations include high cost, limited availability, imaging resolution, and the need for on-site generation of tracers given the short half-life of many isotopes.

Finally, studies with infarct-avid tracers are available (Willerson et al., 1991). These accumulate in irreversibly damaged myocardium and have been used for detection, sizing, and localization of acute infarcts. While the largest experience is with technetium-99 pyrophosphate, studies with indium-labeled monoclonal antibodies to cardiac myosin appear promising as well (Beller, Khaw, Haber, & Smith, 1977; Johnson et al., 1989; Khaw et al., 1986).

Few data are available specifically concerning the use of radionuclide imaging in the elderly. However, recent studies do suggest that thallium-201 imaging, coupled with either exercise or dipyridamole, may be used effectively to assess and risk-stratify elderly patients with known or suspected coronary artery disease (Hilton et al., 1992; Iskandrian, Joekyeong, Decoskey, Askenase, Segal, 1988; Shaw et al., 1992). Moreover, as noninvasive techniques, radionuclide studies remain attractive alternatives in cardiac evaluation.

HOLTER MONITORING

Continuous ambulatory heart monitoring, or "Holter monitoring," is a useful noninvasive method of assessing cardiac rhythm, heart rate variability, and ST changes during normal activity, often on an outpatient basis. In its most common form, the technique involves continuous recording of two ECG channels by a monitor worn on the patient's belt or slung across the chest, usually for a 24- or 48-hour period (Kennedy, 1988). Any symptoms experienced during the monitoring period are recorded in a diary and then correlated with the corresponding area of tape. Holter monitors are most often used in noninvasive assessment of known or suspected cardiac arrhythmias and can help document the type and frequency of spontaneous arrhythmia as well as any correlation with symptoms. As an alternative, transtelephonic monitoring, in which monitoring signals are transmitted by phone line to the interpreting physician at the time of symptoms, or patient-activated recorders are available. However, these methods are obviously limited to symptomatic arrhythmia and are also difficult in cases where syncope or significant hemodynamic compromise occurs. More recently, Holter monitoring has been used to assess heart rate variability, as data suggest that decreased variability correlates with a higher mortality after myocardial infarction (Kleiger, Miller, Bigger, & Moss, 1987).

Another active area of research involves episodes of asymptomatic ST shifts documented by Holter and felt to represent "silent" ischemia. Recent data suggest that the majority of electrocardiographically detected ischemic episodes are asymptomatic in unstable angina patients and that such episodes occur in over half of patients admitted to the coronary care unit with this diagnosis (Gottlieb et al., 1986). Moreover, the presence of silent ischemia in patients with angina or myocardial infarction or in those who have undergone bypass surgery appears to correlate with poor prognosis, though its significance in the asymptomatic population is not yet well defined (Gottlieb et al., 1986, 1988; Rocco et al., 1988; Weiner et al., 1991). In addition, the detection of ST segment changes on Holter has proved useful in assessing cardiac risk in patients with peripheral vascular disease undergoing revascularization (Raby et al., 1989).

Given the increased prevalence of arrhythmias and coronary artery disease in the elderly, Holter monitoring is particularly valuable in this age group, though one must remember that arrhythmias such as bradycardia, sinoatrial or high atrioventricular block, or frequent atrial and ventricular premature beats are more common in the aged and not necessarily pathologically important (Fleg, 1988). In the patient with documented arrhythmia, Holter monitoring may be useful in assessing suppression of ambient arrhythmia, though its utility in comparison to more invasive electrophysiologic studies in assessing efficacy of pharmacologic therapy is still debated. Age-stratified data concerning the utility of silent ischemia detection by continuous ambulatory monitoring are lacking.

CARDIAC MAGNETIC RESONANCE IMAGING

Magnetic resonance imaging (MRI) is another modality that shows great promise for noninvasive evaluation of the cardiovascular system, and it is in a phase of rapid growth in interest and applications. The basic magnetic resonance signal is based on perturbation of nuclei in a strong magnetic field by radiofrequency pulses in a smaller magnetic field applied at an angle to the first. Information on the return of these nuclei to their equilibrium or baseline state is then encoded on a frequency spectrum and used to generate an image (Higgins, 1992). A variety of pulse sequences are available, including spin-echo; gradient reversal, or GRASS, images, which can be displayed in rapid succession, like a movie, to simulate motion (cine-MRI); and phase shift or phase velocity images, which can provide information regarding velocity and flow in cardiac structures and large vessels (Bryant, Payne, Firmin, & Longmore, 1984; Higgins, 1992). Potential advantages of MRI scanning include the absence of ionizing radiation, excellent structural resolution (Figure 7.2), flexibility in terms of image orientation, and ability to obtain flow information without contrast agents. However, the technique may also be limited by relatively high cost, prolonged acquisition times, incompatibility with metallic devices such as pacemakers and aneurysm clips, and artifact related to blood flow or to cardiac or respiratory motion (Wozney, Prorok, & Petcheny, 1991). Some of these limitations may be addressed by new fast-imaging or gating techniques now under development.

Currently, areas of active applications research include determination of cardiac dimensions and mass, assessment of global and regional function, cardiac masses, pericardial disease, and questions related to flow, such as shunt calculations, cardiac output, evaluation of valvular lesions, and even myocardial perfusion. While direct visualization of the coronary anatomy is still limited (Manning, Lei, Boyle, & Edelman, 1993), the use of paramagnetic contrast agents that distribute in proportion to blood flow shows promise as an alternative method for assessing regional blood flow to the myocardium (Manning, Atkinson, Grossman, Paulin, & Edelman, 1991; Schaefer et al., 1989). As might be expected given the recent emergence of the technique, extensive data on the use of MRI in the aged are lacking.

CARDIAC CATHETERIZATION

While noninvasive imaging and evaluation of the heart can provide definitive diagnostic information in many cardiac diseases, more invasive techniques, such as cardiac catheterization, remain invaluable in some cases. Catheterization is usually performed by passing catheters through the great vessels and into the heart, either by a percutaneous (usually femoral) approach or by direct visualization of peripheral vessels by means of a 'cutdown' approach (often brachial). Manometer-tipped or, more commonly, fluid-filled catheters measure pressures in the cardiac chambers and great vessels and provide hemodynamic information throughout the car-

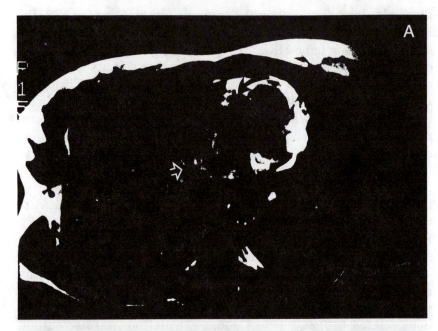

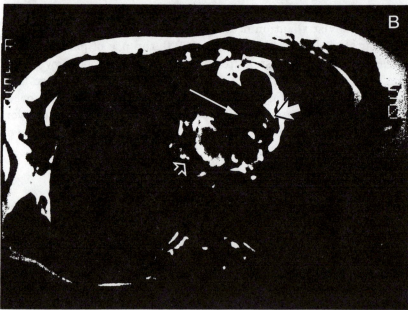

FIGURE 7.2A/B EKG-gated spin-echo (SE) magnetic resonance images of a sinus of Valsalva aneurysm. (A and B) Axial SE T1-weighted images of the thorax at the level of the aortic root. There is an encapsulated lobular mass located posterior to the aortic root (open arrow heads). Note the dilated left sinus of Valsalva (straight arrow) and extrinsic compression of the left main coronary artery (closed arrow head) as well as roof of the left atrium. Origin of the normal right coronary artery is visualized (curved arrow).

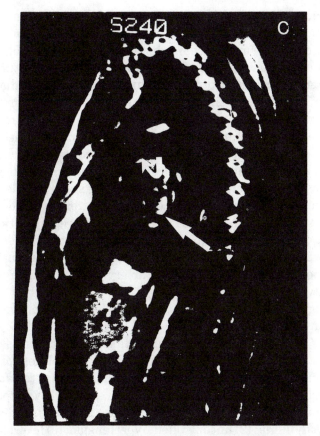

FIGURE 7.2C EKG-gated spin-echo (SE) magnetic resonance images of a sinus of Valsalva aneurysm. (C) Sagittal SE T1-weighted images through the mid thorax. The thrombus-filled aneurysm is visualized posterior to the aortic root (arrow head), displacing the pulmonary artery superiorly (curved arrow). (Courtesy of D. Piwnica-Worms, Department of Radiology, Brigham and Women's Hospital, Boston, MA.)

diac cycle helpful in detecting and assessing a variety of cardiac conditions (Grossman &Barry, 1992). For example, evidence of a significant pressure gradient across the mitral valve in diastole by comparison of pulmonary wedge and left ventricular pressures is a hallmark of mitral stenosis, while cardiac tamponade often results in equalization of end diastolic pressures in both right- and left-sided chambers.

Cardiac output may be measured by the Fick method, which relies on the ratio of oxygen consumption to arteriovenous oxygen difference, or by the thermodilution method, in which an indicator substance of known temperature is injected and subsequently sensed by a thermistor some distance away in the bloodstream (Grossman & Barry, 1992). The magnitude of temperature change is related to cardiac output. Information concerning cardiac output, in turn, can allow estimation of valve areas or determination of vascular resistances when used in conjunction with intracardiac pressures. Concomitantly, angiography is often performed by injection of contrast material, or "dye" into the coronary arteries, great vessels, and left ventricle. Films of these structures as they are outlined by dye can detect stenoses in the coronary arteries, provide information on left ventricular ejection fraction, and aid in the assessment of valvular disease such as aortic regurgitation. Thus, cardiac catheterization can provide diagnostic information, help assess severity of disease, or be used as a guide for interventions such as angioplasty (PTCA), coronary artery bypass grafting (CABG), and valve replacement.

Though cardiac catheterization is, in general, considered safe, with an overall mortality rate of 0.14% (0.25% in those over 60 years of age), it should not be undertaken without careful assessment of the risks and benefits involved ("Guidelines for Cardiac Catheterization," 1991). Relative contraindications to catheterization include (1) uncontrolled ventricular irritability, hypokalemia or digitalis toxicity, as these may increase the likelihood of significant arrhythmia; (2) uncontrolled hypertension; (3) fever; (4) decompensated heart failure; (5) anticoagulated state (though emergency catheterization in patients on heparin is often performed); (6) significant contrast allergy; and (7) severe renal insufficiency (unless dialysis can be used to remove fluid and dye postprocedure) (Grossman, 1991). In addition, mortality risk is felt to increase with severe coronary disease, mitral valve disease, acute myocardial infarction, unstable angina, and congenital heart disease ("Guidelines for Cardiac Catheterization," 1991), though the information obtained from catheterization is often also of most benefit in these patient subgroups.

Catheterization in the elderly is generally well tolerated, though the higher prevalence of comorbidities and conditions listed above obviously increase both morbidity and mortality. In addition, special care is appropriate in choice and dosage of sedation (tolerance to and metabolism of drugs is often reduced in the aged) (Roberts, Goldberg, & Woldow, 1985) and in fluid management after a dye load to avoid large-scale shifts in intravascular volume, which may be poorly tolerated in the aged, generally less compliant heart. Ambulatory cardiac catheterization, for which the patient is admitted and discharged on the day of the procedure, is growing increasingly popular. However, due to the considerations above, the Joint Task Force of the American College of Cardiology and the American Heart Association has recommended against its routine use in patients over 75 years of age ("Guidelines for Cardiac Catheterization," 1991).

INTRACARDIAC ELECTROPHYSIOLOGIC STUDIES

Invasive intracardiac electrophysiologic studies have become a widely used tool in the diagnosis and management of patients with significant arrhythmia or conduction system disease. These studies routinely employ multipolar catheters positioned via the peripheral vasculature to both record and stimulate a variety of locations in the heart, most commonly the atria, ventricles, and coronary sinus (Zipes, 1992). Generally accepted indications include (1) symptomatic patients (most often syncope or near-syncope) in whom sinus node dysfunction, A-V block, or intraventricular conduction delay with ventricular arrhythmia is the suspected etiology but in whom a causal relationship cannot be documented by other means (e.g., electrocardiography or Holter); (2) patients with frequent or poorly tolerated narrow-complex tachyarrhythmias or patients with sustained or symptomatic wide-complex tachyarrhythmias for which additional information is needed to help guide care; (3) patients with unexplained syncope and known or suspected underlying structural heart disease; (4) survivors of cardiac arrest, except within the first 48 hours of an acute myocardial infarction or when a clearly identifiable cause is present (e.g., reversible ischemia); (5) patients with palpitations and documented inappropriate tachycardia not explicable by other means; (6) as a guide in selecting drug therapy for refractory AV nodal reentrant tachycardia, some Wolff-Parkinson-White patients and patients with sustained ventricular tachycardia or ventricular fibrillation not associated with a long QT syndrome or within 48 hours of a myocardial infarction; (7) patients in whom antiarrhythmic surgery or ablative therapy or implantation of an electrical device to control arrhythmias is being considered or in selected instances for follow-up of such patients ("Guidelines for Clinical Intracardiac Electrophysiologic Studies",

TABLE 7.1   Comparison of Diagnostic Imaging Modalities in Cardiac Disease

	Echo	Angio	RVG	Spect Perfusion Imaging	MRI	PET
Cardiac Anatomy						
Chamber size	+ + +	+ + +	+ +	0	+ + + +	+ +
Intracardiac masses	+ + +	+ +	+	0	+ + +	0
Valve anatomy	+ + + +	+ +	0	0	+ + +	0
Pericardial disease	+ +	+	0	0	+ + + +	0
Coronary anatomy	+	+ + +	0	0	+ +	0
Graft patency	0	+ + + +	0	+	+	+ +
Cardiac Physiology						
Diastolic filling	+	+ +	+ + +	0	+	0
Stenosis/insufficiency	+ + +	+ + + +	+	0	+ +	0
Intracardiac shunt	+ + +	+ + + +	+ +	0	+ +	0
Myocardial function	+ +	+ + +	+ + + +	0	+ + + +	+
Myocardial blood flow	+	0	0	+ +	+	+ + +

Scale: 0 = no information to + + + + = maximal information
Definitions: ECHO = transthoracic echocardiography with Doppler flow assessment; ANGIO = cardiac catheterization with angiography; RVG = radionuclide ventriculography SPECT PERFUSION = single photon emission computed tomography perfusion imaging MRI = magnetic resonance imaging; PET = positron emission tomography

Source: Modified, with permission, from Grover-McKay M., & Skorton D. Comparative aspects of modern imaging techniques. In D. P. Zipes, D. J. Rowlands, Eds. (1990). Progress in cardiology. 3/1 Philadelphia: Lea and Febiger.

1989). The risks of such studies are similar to those associated with catheterization, and an overall mortality rate of 0.12% has been reported (Horrowitz, 1986). Though data specific to the elderly are limited, a report from the Mayo Clinic suggests that intracardiac electrophysiologic study may be particularly helpful in evaluation of the elderly patient with as yet unexplained syncope after noninvasive evaluation, identifying potential causes in 68% of these cases (Sugrue et al., 1987).

CONCLUSION

A variety of diagnostic modalities are available for evaluation of the cardiovascular system (Table 7.1). Although all may be applied in the elderly population, their optimal utilization requires understanding of the special characteristics of each test in the elderly and a careful consideration of the risks and benefits involved.

Hopefully, future research will help to clarify these issues in one of our fastest-growing patient populations.

• Editor's Comment •

The complexity of factors that, especially in aged patients, will determine which of many modern diagnostic methods to employ in any given case is well illustrated in this chapter. Only a well-informed specialist will be able to arrive at a truly rational choice.

As information on the risks and effectiveness of new diagnostic procedures in this field increases, the criteria of what constitutes their rational use change. This is indicated, for example, for coronary angiography regarding which Graboys et al. (Graboys, Biegelsen, Lampert, Blatt, & Lown, 1992) estimated that "50% of coronary angiography currently being undertaken in the United States is unnecessary, or at least could be postponed."

Reference for Editor's Comment

Graboys, B., Biegelsen, B., Lampert, S., Blatt, M., Lown, B. Results of a Second Opinion Trial Among Patients Recommended for Coronary Angiography. *JAMA*, Vol. 268, No. 18 p. 2537–40. 1992.

References

Cobb, F., Higginbotham, M., & Mark, D. Diagnosis of coronary disease in the elderly. In N. Wenger, C. Furberg, E. Pitt, (Eds.), Coronary heart disease in the elderly. New York: Elsevier. 1986.

Ballal, R., Nanda, N., & Gatewood, R., et al. Usefulness of transesophageal echocardiography in assessment of aortic dissection. *Circulation*, *84*(5): 1903–14. 1991.

Beller, G., Khaw, B., Haber, E., & Smith, T. Localization of radiolabeled cardiac myosin-specific antibody in myocardial infarcts: Comparison with technetium-99m stannous pyrophosphate. *Circulation*, *55*(1): 74–78. 1977.

Boucher, C. A., Brewster, D. C., & Darling, R. C., et al. Determination of cardiac risk by dipyridamole thallium imaging before peripheral vascular surgery. *N Engl J Med*, *312*(7): 389–94. 1985.

Brown, K. Prognostic value of thallium-201 myocardial perfusion imaging: A diagnostic tool comes of age. *Circulation*, *83*(2): 363–81. 1991.

Brunken, R., Kottou, S., & Nienaber, C., et al. PET detection of viable tissue in myocardial segments with persistent defects in T1–201 SPECT. *Radiology*, *172*(1): 65–73. 1989.

Bryant, D. J., Payne, J. A., Firmin, D. N., & Longmore D. B. Measurement of flow with NMR imaging using a gradient pulse and phase difference technique. *Journal of Computer Assisted Tomography*, *8*(4): 588–593. 1984.

Chaitman, B. Exercise stress testing. In E. Braunwald (Ed.), *Heart Disease: A Textbook of Cardiovascular Medicine*. Philadelphia: Saunders. 1992.

Cloninger, K., DePuey, G., Garcia, E., & Roubin, G., et al. Incomplete redistribution in delayed thallium-201 single photon emission computed tomographic (SPECT) images: An overestimation of myocardial scarring. *JACC, 12*(4): 955–63. 1988.

Cobb, F., Higginbotham, M., & Mark, D. Diagnosis of coronary disease in the elderly. In N. Wenger, C. Furberg, E. Pitt, (Eds.), *Coronary heart disease in the elderly*. New York: Elsevier. 1986.

Coodley, E. Clinical spectrum and diagnostic techniques of coronary heart disease in the elderly. *Journal of the American Geriatrics Society, 36*(5): 447–456. 1988.

Coyne E., Belvedere D., Vande Streek P. R., et al.: Thallium-201 scintigraphy after intravenous infusion of adenosine compared with exercise thallium testing in the diagnosis of coronary artery disease. JACC 17(6): 1289–94. 1991.

Detrano, R., Janosi, A., & Lyons, K. P., et al. Factors affecting sensitivity and specificity of a diagnostic test: The exercise thallium scintigram. *American Journal of Medicine, 84*: 699–710. 1988.

Erbel, R., Engberding, R., Daniel, W., & Roelandt, J., et al. Echocardiography in diagnosis of aortic dissection. *Lancet, 1*: 457–61. 1989.

Feigenbaum, H. Echocardiography. In E. Braunwald, (Ed.), *Heart Disease: A Textbook of Cardiovascular Medicine*. Philadelphia: Saunders. 1992.

Fisch, C. Electrocardiogram in the aged: An independent marker of heart disease? *Am J Med, 70*: 4–6. 1981.

Fisher, E., Stahl, J., Budd, J., & Goldman, M. Transesophageal Schocardiography: Procedures and clinical practices. *JACC, 18*(5): 1333–48. 1991.

Fleg, J. L. Ventricular arrhythmias in the elderly: Prevalence, mechanisms and therapeutic implications. *Geriatrics, 43*(12): 23–9. 1988.

Gerstenblith, G., Frederiksen, J., Yin, F. C. P., Fortuin, N. J., Lakatta, E. G., & Weisfeldt, M. L. Echocardiographic assessment of a normal adult aging population. *Circulation, 56*(2): 273–8. 1977.

Gottlieb, S. O., Gottlieb, S. H., & Achuff, S. C., et al. Silent ischemia on Holter monitoring predicts mortality in high-risk postinfarction patients. *JAMA, 259*(7): 1030–5. 1988.

Gottlieb, S. O., Weisfeldt, M. L., & Ouyang P., et al. Silent ischemia as a marker for early unfavorable outcomes in patients with unstable angina. *New England Journal of Medicine, 314*(19): 1214–1219. 1986.

Grossman, W. Cardiac catheterization: Historical perspective and present practice. In W. Grossman, D. S. Baim, (Eds.), *Cardiac Catheterization, Angiography and Intervention*. Philadelphia: Lea and Febiger. 1991.

Grossman, W., & Barry, W. Cardiac catheterization. In E. Braunwald, (Ed.). *Heart Disease: A Textbook of Cardiovascular Medicine*. Philadelphia: Saunders. 1992.

Guidelines for cardiac catheterization and cardiac catheterization laboratories: A report of the American College of Cardiology/American Heart Association. *Circulation*, 84 (5): 2213–47. 1991.

Guidelines for clinical application of echocardiography: A report of the American College of Cardiology/American Heart Association Task Force on Assessment of Diagnostic and Therapeutic Cardiovascular Procedures. *Circulation, 82*(6): 2323–45. 1990.

Guidelines for clinical intracardiac electrophysiologic studies: A report of the American College of Cardiology/American Heart Association Task Force on Assessment of Diagnostic and Therapeutic Cardiovascular Procedures. *Circulation, 80*(6): 1925–1939. 1989.

Hennekens, C., & Buring, J. Screening. In Epidemiology in Medicine. Boston/ Toronto: Little, Brown and Co. 1987.

Higgins, C. Newer cardiac imaging techniques (computed tomography, magnetic resonance). In E. Braunwald, (Ed.), *Heart Disease: A Textbook of Cardiovascular Medicine.* Philadelphia: Saunders. 1992.

Hilton, T. C., Shaw, L. J., & Chaitman, B. R., et al. Prognostic significance of exercise thallium-201 testing in patients aged greater than or equal to 70 years with known or suspected coronary artery disease. *Am J Cardiol, 69*: 45–50. 1992.

Hlatky, M. A., Pryor, D. B., Harrell, F. E., Califf, R. M., Mark, D. B., & Rosati, R. A. Factors affecting sensitivity and specificity of exercise electrocardiography: Multivariable analysis. *Am J Med, 77*: 64–71. 1984.

Horowitz, L. N. Safety of electrophysiologic studies. *Circulation, 73* (Suppl II) 28–31. 1986.

Iskandrian, A. S., Joekyeong, H., Decoskey, D., Askenase, A., & Segal B. L. Use of exercise thallium-201 imaging for risk stratification of elderly patients with coronary artery disease. *Am J Cardiol, 61*: 269–72. 1988.

Johnson, L. L., Seldin, D. W., & Becker, L. C., et al. Antimyosin imaging in acute transmural myocardial infarction: Results of a multicenter clinical trial. *JACC, 13*: 27–35. 1989.

Kennedy, H. L. Long-term electrocardiographic recordings. In D. Zipes, D. J. Rowlands, (Eds.), *Progress in cardiology.* Philadelphia: Lea and Febiger. 1988.

Khaw, B. A., Gold, H. K., & Yasuda, T. et al. Scintigraphic quantification of myocardial necrosis in patients after intravenous injection of myosin-specific antibody. *Circulation, 74*: 501–8. 1986.

Kitzman, D., Sheikh, K., Beere, P., Philips, J., & Higginbotham, M. Age-related alterations of Doppler left ventricular filling indices in normal subjects are independent of left ventricular mass, heart rate, contractility and loading conditions. *JACC, 18*(5): 1243–1250. 1991.

Kleiger, R. E., Miller, J. P., Bigger, J. T., & Moss, A. J. Decreased heart rate variability and its association with increased mortality after acute myocardial infarction. *Am J Cardiol, 59*(4): 256–262. 1987.

Mangano, D. T., London, M. J., Tubau, J. F., & Browner, W. S., et al. Dipyridamole thallium-201 scintigraphy as a preoperative screening test: A reexamination of its predictive potential. *Circulation, 84*(2): 493–502. 1991.

Manning, W. J., Lei, W., Boyle, N. G., & Edelman, R. R. Fat-suppressed breath-hold magnetic resonance coronary angiography. *Circulation, 87*(1): 94–104, 1993.

Manning, W. J., Atkinson, D. J., Grossman, W., Paulin, S., & Edelman, R. R. First-pass nuclear magnetic resonance imaging studies using gadolinium

DTPA in patients with coronary artery disease. *JACC, 18*(4): 959–65. 1991.

Marwick, T., Nemec, J., Pashkow, F., Stewart, W., & Salcedo, E. Accuracy and limitations of exercise echocardiography in a routine clinical setting. *JACC, 19*(1): 74–81. 1992.

Matsuzaki, M., Toma, Y., & Kusakawa, R. Clinical applications of transesophageal echocardiography. *Circulation, 82*(3): 709–722. 1990.

National Center for Health Statistics. Death rates for 72 selected causes (1988). In *Vital Statistics of the United States.* Washington, DC: Public Health Service. 1991.

Nienaber, C., Spielmann, R., & Kodolitsch, Y., et al. Diagnosis of thoracic aortic dissection: Magnetic resonance imaging versus transesophageal echocardiography. *Circulation, 85*(2): 434–447. 1992.

Parodi, O., Marcassa, C., & Casucci, R., et al. Accuracy and safety of technetium-99m hexakis 2–methoxy-2–isobutyl isonitrile(sestamibi) myocardial scintigraphy with high dose dipyridamole test in patients with effort angina pectoris: A multicenter study. *JACC, 18*(6): 1439–44. 1991.

Picano, E. Stress echocardiography: From pathophysiologic toy to diagnostic tool. *Circulation, 85*(4): 1604–12. 1992.

Raby, K. E., Goldman, L., & Creager, M. A., et al. Correlation between preoperative ischemia and major cardiac events after peripheral vascular surgery. *N Engl J Med, 321*(19): 1296–1300. 1989.

Roberts, J., Goldberg, P., & Woldow, A. Pharmacologic basis for the response to cardiac drugs in the elderly. In E. Coodley, (Ed.), *Geriatric Heart Disease.* St. Louis, MO: Mosby Year Book, Inc. 1985.

Rocco, M. B., Nabel, E. G., & Campbell, S., et al. Prognostic importance of myocardial ischemia detected by ambulatory monitoring in patients with stable coronary disease. *Circulation, 78*(4): 877–84. 1988.

Rocco, T. P., Dilsizian, V., Fischman, A. J., & Strauss, H.W. Evaluation of ventricular function in patients with coronary artery disease. *Journal of Nuclear Medicine, 30*(7): 1149–65. 1989.

Schaefer, S., Lange, R., & Kulkarni, P., et al. In vivo nuclear magnetic resonance imaging of myocardial perfusion using the paramagnetic contrast agent manganese gluconate. *JACC, 14*(2): 472–80. 1989.

Shaw, L., Chaitman, B., & Hilton, T., et al. Prognostic value of dipyridamole thallium-201 imaging in elderly patients. *JACC, 19*(7): 1390–8. 1992.

Sugrue, D. D., Holmes, D. R., & Gersh, B. J., et al. Impact of intracardiac electrophysiologic testing on the management of elderly patients with recurrent syncope or near syncope. *Journal of the American Geriatrics Society, 35*(12): 1079–83. 1987.

Tamaki N., Yonekura Y., Senda M., et al.: Value and limitation of stress thallium-201 single photon emission computed tomography: comparison with nitrogen-13 ammonia positron tomography. Journal of Nuclear Medicine 29(7): 1181–8. 1988.

Task Force on assessment of Diagnostic and Therapeutic Cardiovascular Procedures. *Circulation, 84*(5): 2213–47. 1991.

Vasilomanolakis, E., Licht, J., & Ellestad, M. Exercise physiology, testing, and training in the geriatric population. In E. Coodley, (Ed.), *Geriatric Heart Disease.* St. Louis: Mosby Year Book, Inc. 1985.

Wackers, F., Berman, D., Maddahi, J., & Watson, D., et al. Technetium-99m hexakis 2–methoxyisobutyl isonitrile: human biodistribution, dosimetry, safety and preliminary comparison to thallium-201 for myocardial perfusion imaging. *Journal of Nuclear Medicine, 30*(3): 301–11. 1989.

Weiner, D., Ryan, T., & Parsons, L., et al. Prevalence and prognostic significance of silent and symptomatic ischemia after coronary artery bypass surgery: A report from the Coronary Artery Surgery Study (CASS) randomized population. *JACC, 18*(2): 343–348. 1991.

Willerson, J., McGhie, I., Parkey, R., Bonte, F., Buja, L. M., & Corbett, J. Infarct avid imaging. In Marcus, Schelbert, Skorton, & Wolf (Eds.), *Cardiac imaging: A companion to Braunwald's heart disease.* Philadelphia: Saunders. 1991.

Wozney, P., Prorok, R., & Petcheny, R. Optimizing MR image quality: artifact causes and cures. In: Marcus, Schelbert, Skorton, & Wolf (Eds.), *Cardiac imaging: A companion to Braunwald's heart disease.* Philadelphia: Saunders. 1991.

Zaret, B., Wackers, F., & Soufer, R. Nuclear cardiology. In E. Braunwald, (Ed.), *Heart disease: A textbook of cardiovascular medicine.* Philadelphia: Saunders. 1992.

Zipes, D. Genesis of cardiac arrhythmias: electrophysiological considerations. In E. Braunwald, (Ed.), *Heart disease: A textbook of cardiovascular medicine.* Philadelphia: Saunders. 1992.

Chapter Eight

Cardiovascular Surgery in the Elderly

Sary F. Aranki

The number of the elderly continues to rise steadily. There are 31 million people over the age of 65 in the United States, comprising 12.5% of the population (U.S. Bureau of the Census, 1991). By the year 2010, it is estimated that 40 million people will be over the age of 65, and 30 million will be over the age 70 (National Center for Health Statistics, 1990; U.S. Bureau of the Census, 1991).

Heart disease is currently the leading cause of death among the elderly, with a prevalence of almost 50%, accounting for more than 40% of deaths in people over the age of 65 (Siegal, 1980; Wei, 1984). Elderly patients with heart disease tend to present at an advanced stage of the disease, are usually in congestive heart failure, and may have other comorbid conditions such as diabetes or renal insufficiency. They also have diminished multisystem, reserve, which functions appropriately under resting physiologic conditions but decompensates rapidly under stressful conditions such as cardiopulmonary bypass (CPB), with its multisystem nonphysiologic effects, and global myocardial ischemia during the procedure of aortic cross-clamping. All of these factors combine to influence mortality and morbidity after cardiac surgery in this group of patients. However, the recent improvement in surgical techniques, especially in the field of myocardial protection, modern cardiac anesthesia, and intensive care, coupled with proper selection of patients, resulted in improved short- and long-term survival. If elderly patients survive the operation and suffer no major permanent morbidity such as a stroke or renal failure, they tend to bounce back within a few weeks after surgery and lead a normal and independent life (Butler, 1991).

CARDIOPULMONARY BYPASS (CPB)

The recent practice of cardiac surgery, with its varied and complex procedures, would have been impossible without CPB. As a result of the continued evolution and development of CPB that occurred during the past 30 years, the reliability and safety of such devices are well established. This has led to a dramatic reduction in the mortality and morbidity rates of cardiac surgical procedures and to a continuous increase in the number of high risk procedures being performed. Continuous improvement in CPB will undoubtedly lead to further lowering of risk in the elderly. Further development in this regard will be biocompatible materials and heparin-coated devices that will abolish the harmful effects of complement activation, blood cellular destruction, and bleeding complications. Pulsatile perfusion (Jacobs et al., 1969; Taylor, 1981), for which the technology is already available but needs further refinement, will probably allow a more physiologic CPB—especially in the elderly, in whom the preservation of organ function will contribute to a more favorable outcome.

MYOCARDIAL PROTECTION

Modern cardiac surgery, whether for congenital or acquired lesions, is performed on a motionless heart and a bloodless field. To achieve this objective, an effective form of myocardial protection has to be applied. The interruption of coronary blood flow and oxygen during the period of aortic cross-clamping can initiate serious metabolic, structural, and functional changes that can result in severe myocardial necrosis and failure. This can be avoided by manipulating the myocardial supply–demand balance whereby the minimum myocardial energy demand is met by an equally adequate minimum supply that exists under ischemic anoxic conditions (Buckberg, 1979; Silverman & Del Nido, 1988). Anaerobic energy supply, if continued uninterrupted, can maintain prolonged myocardial viability. Cardioplegia, which is the cornerstone of myocardial protection, is designed to meet this challenge. It is a pharmacologic solution with a high potassium concentration that allows rapid depolarization of the cell membrane and sustained diastolic arrest (Follette, Mulder, Maloney, & Buckberg, 1978; Hearse, Stewart, & Braimbridge, 1975). It is delivered cold (4°c), which, along with moderate systemic and local hypothermia, reduces the metabolic rate and prevents the return of electromechanical activity (Follette, Steed, Foglia, Fey, & Buckberg, 1978). In addition, cardioplegia should provide a substrate for continued energy production during aortic cross-clamping, such as glucose (Hewitt et al., 1974) and a buffer (sodium bicarbonate or blood), to counteract extensive lactate production.

CARDIAC SURGERY IN THE ELDERLY

Although advanced age in itself is a risk factor for operative mortality and morbidity (Goldman et al., 1987; Kennedy et al., 1981; Scott et al., 1985; Stephenson, McVaugh, & Edmunds, 1978), identification of other independent incremental risk factors permits estimates of probability of death or serious morbidity for individual elderly patients (Parsonnet, Dean, & Bernstein, 1989). Emergency operation, cachexia, New York Heart Association Class IV, and previous myocardial infarction have been identified as independent risk factors for early death after cardiac surgery (Edmunds, Stephenson, Edie, & Ratcliffe, 1988). These factors are quite common in the elderly (Rowe, 1985). As a result, preoperative selection of elderly patients becomes the most important determinant of operative mortality (Buckley, Cheitlin, Goldman, Kaplan, & Kouchoukos, 1987). With this knowledge, selection bias toward continued medical management (O'Keefe, Vliestra, Bailey, & Holmes, 1987) or alternative therapies (Letac, Bribiera, Koning, & Lefebre, 1989) becomes obvious in light of the increased probabilities of undesirable results. Paradoxically, high-risk patients are often the ones that benefit most from surgery (Jones, 1989).

With the increasing realization that chronological age in itself is not a valid basis for treatment decisions and that every elderly patient is individually characterized from others in his or her age group (Wetle, 1987), it becomes obvious why guidelines for operating on the elderly do not exist. The decision to operate becomes a complex one involving the patient, family, and physician (Edmunds, 1990). Presenting in detail the odds of a bad result and assessing the willingness of the patient's family to go all the way following a prolonged course of intensive postoperative treatment and rehabilitation make the decision of whether or not to proceed with surgery both valid and ethical.

CORONARY ARTERY BYPASS IN THE ELDERLY (CABG)

Atherosclerotic coronary artery disease (CAD) in the elderly accounts for 85% of all deaths due to heart disease (Wei, 1984). Occult significant CAD is present during life in the majority of elderly individuals (Elveback & Lie, 1984). Coronary artery bypass graft (CABG) surgery is performed on a rapidly increasing number of older patients (Feinleib et al., 1989; Gersh et al., 1981). Preoperatively, older patients are sicker, have more unstable angina, congestive heart failure, and a higher prevalence of comorbid conditions such as hypertension, diabetes, cerebrovascular disease, peripheral vascular disease, and chronic lung disease. They also have a higher incidence of severe triple vessel disease, left main disease, and depressed left ventricle function (Rahimtoola et al., 1981).

Perioperative mortality

In the coronary artery surgery registry study (CASS), perioperative mortality of 1,087 patients > 65 years of age was 8.2%, (vs. 1.9% in 7,827 younger patients) undergoing isolated CABG. Mortality increased with advancing age, with a 4.6% mortality for the 65–69-year-old age group, which increased to 9.5% in patients > 75 years of age (Gersh et al., 1981). A review of the literature shows a varied perioperative mortality for the elderly, widely ranging from 0% to as high as 21% (Wei & Gersh, 1987). This trend has significantly declined; more recent perioperative mortality ranges from 1% to 12%, with the higher mortalities in octogenarian patients (Edwards et al., 1991; Ko et al., 1991). Surgical mortality was increased in the presence of left ventricular dysfunction and/or cardiomegaly and significant left main coronary artery disease (Rahimtoola et al., 1981). Recent reports demonstrated the significant impact of emergency surgery on perioperative mortality, which ranged from 17%–33% to 1%–8.6% for elective cases (Horvath et al., 1990; Ko et al., 1991).

Perioperative morbidity

Perioperative morbidity is increased in the elderly, ranging from 0.17 to 2.31 complications per patient (Cohn & Horvath, 1991). Frequent serious complications include perioperative myocardial infarction, strokes, deep vein thrombosis, pulmonary embolism, pneumonia, respiratory failure, sepsis, acute respiratory distress syndrome, deep sternal wound infections, and renal failure requiring dialysis. Other complications include superficial cellulitis and wound infections, urinary tract infections, and mild renal insufficiency (Edwards et al., 1991). Atrial fibrillation and flutter occurs in nearly 30% of older patients and is directly related to age (Leitch, Thompson, Band, & Harris, 1990). Again, emergency surgery was significantly associated with a higher rate of complications; 92% versus 17% for elective surgery (Edwards et al., 1991). The CASS Registry study showed that age was an independent risk factor but not the most powerful predictor of perioperative mortality and morbidity compared to left ventricular dysfunction, severe left main coronary artery disease, female sex, and unstable angina, which are more frequently present (Gersh et al., 1981).

Long-Term Results

The 5-year survival in the CASS Registry was 83%, compared with 91% in younger patients. The long-term survival, as expected, declines with age. The 5-year survival was 84% for the 65–69 year age group, 80% for the 70–74 year age group, and 70% for those > 75 years old. The corresponding figures for hospital survival were 88%, 85%, and 77% respectively, for the three age groups (Gersh et al., 1981). Similar results were reported from other large studies (Horvath et al., 1990; Rhimtoola, Grunkemeier, & Starr, 1986). Major predictors of long-term mortality were indices of left ventricular dysfunction and the number of associated comorbid conditions. The 5-year survival in patients without myocardial dysfunction and without associated medical conditions was 90% in the CASS Registry (Gersh et al., 1981).

Symptomatic relief and the quality of life after coronary artery surgery was similar in older and younger patients. Freedom from angina was 70% at 5 years and 50% at 10 years. The rate of reoperation was 0.5%–1% per year (Guadagnoli, Ayanian, & Cleary, 1992).

USE OF THE INTERNAL MAMMARY ARTERY

Routine use of the internal mammary artery (IMA) in the elderly is controversial. It has proven long-term patency rates and has improved patient survival. However, its use in the elderly is unpopular. A recent study by Gardner and his group (1990), showed a significant reduction in perioperative mortality and morbidity as well as improved 4-year survival in IMA groups, compared with the vein grafts–only group. There is an increased risk (2.2%) of sternal wound dehiscence and infection after using the IMA (vs. 0.8% for vein grafts only) (Grossi et al., 1991). However, in the elderly group there is a qreater tendency to have poorer-quality veins and more calcified ascending aortas; under these circumstances the IMA might be the conduit of choice.

PERCUTANEOUS TRANSLUMINAL CORONARY ANGIOPLASTY

In comparing percutaneous transluminal coronary angioplasty (PTCA) to CABG it must be realized that they are not equivalent alternatives for the treatment of CAD. PTCA patients usually have single- or double-vessel disease and a preserved left ventricular function. CABG patients usually have multivessel disease and/or left main disease and depressed left ventricular function.

Recent published reports about PTCA in multivessel disease (Kahn et al., 1990; O'Keefe et al., 1990) should be analyzed carefully when comparing results with CABG, especially in the elderly subgroup. Elective versus emergency results, complete versus incomplete revascularization, the need for emergency CABG after unsuccessful PTCA, and the need for further PTCA and/or CABG during follow-up are all important factors in such analyses.

For multivessel disease surgery in elderly patients, whether elective or emergency, CABG offers complete revascularization and favorable immediate and late results in low- and high-risk patient. The role of angioplasty in the wide spectrum of multivessel disease remains undefined and in highly selected patients might safely postpone CABG for several years (Gersh, Phil, & Holmes, 1990).

VALVULAR SURGERY IN THE ELDERLY

Aortic Valve Stenosis

Calcific aortic valve stenosis (AS) in a trileaflet aortic valve is the commonest form in the elderly. The diagnosis of AS in the elderly can be difficult because symptoms associated with it could be attributed to CAD and cerebrovascular disease, and it is not uncommon for elderly people to have more than one of these problems (Roberts, Perloff, Costantino, 1971; Wei, 1984).

Aortic valve replacement (AVR) is the treatment of choice for symptomatic AS. Medical therapy carries a poor prognosis, with 1, 2, and 3-year survival of 57%, 37%, and 25%, respectively (Frank, Johnston, & Ross, 1973; O'Keefe et al., 1987). In asymptomatic patients with mild or moderate AS a careful follow-up with regular serial echocardiogram should monitor the progress of AS, left ventricular (LV) hypertrophy, and LV dysfunction to allow replacement of the valve in an optimal timely fashion before the onset of myocardial dysfunction and its potential operative risk (Hwang et al., 1989).

Aortic Valve Regurgitation

Chronic aortic valve regurgitation (AR) is the commonest form in the elderly, resulting from long-standing hypertension, atherosclerosis, valvular deformity (congenital, rheumatic, and following endocarditis), or aortic root dilatation. The hemodynamic effect of the volume overload results in increasing LV dilatation and hypertrophy. Symptomatic patients should undergo prompt AVR. Asymptomatic patients should have surgery as soon as signs of ventricular dysfunction or increased LV dimensions appear on echocardiogram (Bonow et al., 1984).

Acute AR results from infective endocarditis or aortic dissection. Hemodynamic compromise is acute because of absence of compensatory LV hypertrophy or dilatation following the sudden volume overload, and AVR is performed on an urgent basis (Wei & Gersh, 1987).

Mitral Valve Stenosis

Usually rheumatic in origin, acquired at a young age, and manifested many years later, silent mitral valve stenosis (MS) should be considered when dyspnea and/or atrial fibrillation are present. Surgical management in the form of open commissurotomy or valve replacement depend on the severity and rate of progression of the lesions and presence of pulmonary hypertension, atrial arrhythmias, or systemic embolism. Surgery can be postponed for a few years by maintenance of sinus rhythm alone. However, signs of LV dysfunction and progressive pulmonary hypertension should warrant earlier intervention (Ko et al., 1991).

Mitral Valve Regurgitation

Myxomatous degeneration, coronary artery disease, and mitral valve prolapse (Tresch et al., 1979) are the more common causes of mitral valave regurgitation (MR) in the elderly. Severe MR in the presence of normal leaflet motion is usually secondary to annular dilatation (LV dysfunction) or leaflet perforation (infective endocarditis). In the presence of leaflet prolapse MR is usually secondary to chordal dysfunction or papillary muscle dysfunction.

Surgery is indicated for MR when there is an increase in symptoms, increasing mechanical overload, and diminishing cardiac reserve. Mitral valve repair in the form of a ring annuloplasty, pericardial patch repair, or leaflet resection with or without an annuloplasty ring is preferred if feasible. Mitral valve replacement (MVR) is usually performed in cases of papillary muscle dysfunction and when repair is not possible or has failed. Acute postinfarction MR due to papillary muscle dysfunction usually requires an immediate MVR (Tresch, et al., 1979).

Tricuspid Valve Regurgitation

Left-sided valvular lesions account for the majority of tricuspid valve regurgitation (TR) (Cohn, 1991). TR should be surgically corrected when it is moderate to severe in the presence of preserved right ventricular function. However, if the right ventricle is severely dysfunctional, correction of TR could be harmful, especially in the presence of fixed pulmonary hypertension.

Tricuspid valve repair is more commonly used for treatment of TR, or alternatively a tricuspid valve replacement, usually with a bioprosthesis. Short- and long-term results are similar for both techniques (McGrath et al., 1990).

Results of Valvular Surgery in the Elderly

Elderly people undergoing valvular surgery have more advanced symptoms, decreased LV function, CAD in about 50% of the patients (Fremes et al., 1989), and other associated comorbid conditions. They are more likely to undergo urgent or emergent surgery. Each of these factors poses an elevated risk of mortality and morbidity in the elderly.

Perioperative Mortality

Significant predictors of perioperative mortality are urgent surgery, double-valve disease, grafted and nongrafted CAD, female gender, and depressed LV function. Fremes et al. (1989) reported a total operative mortality (OM) of 10% in 469 patients > 70 years of age undergoing valvular surgery: 6.11% for AVR, 15.1% for MVR, and 18.9% for double valve replacement (vs. 5.8%, 7.4%, and 11.3%, respectively, for younger patients. Urgent surgery was associated with a mortality of 21.9%, versus 7.8% for elective surgery. The presence of CAD increased the risk of valvular surgery (6.6% vs. 12.9%), and for patients undergoing CABG the OM was 11.5% (vs. 27.0% for patients with CAD who had no CABG). The OM for male patients was 5.6%, versus 14.4% for females. Similar results were reported by other studies (Jamieson et al., 1981). The range of OM for valvular surgery in the elderly ranged from 3% (Blakeman et al., 1987) to 37% (Tsai et al., 1986).

Perioperative Morbidity

There is a significant increase of perioperative morbidity following valvular surgery in the elderly. There is also a significant association between serious perioperative morbidity and increased mortality. Death occurred in half of the patients with perioperative myocardial infarction, intraaortic balloon, or deep sternal wound infections and in one third of the patients with low cardiac output or stroke. Nonfatal complications occurred in 28% of patients (Fremes et al., 1989).

Long-Term Results

Significant data concerning the long-term results of valve replacement with mechanical and porcine bioprosthesis are now available. The interrelationship between patient age and the choice of prosthesis is well documented (Cohn, 1991). Porcine bioprosthetic valves appear to be the valve of choice for the elderly because structural failure rates are markedly reduced. Also, the risk of thromboembolism and anticoagulation-related complications is reduced. Survival is significantly influenced by the presence of CAD and LV dysfunction. However, excellent survival rates with near-total freedom from reoperation for structural valve failure have been achieved (Jamieson et al., 1990; Jones et al., 1990). Although the MVR group has a lower but not significant survival rate compared to the AVR group, this might be explained by the increased perioperative mortality in the MVR group (Jones et al., 1990).

The AS group seems to be the only group that achieves a survival comparable to an age-matched population, which stresses the palliative nature of valvular surgery and the superiority of surgical treatment to other forms of therapy (Lindblom, Lindblom, Qvist, & Lundstrom, 1990). The earlier difference in survival between AS and aortic incompetence was most likely related to the degree of LV dysfunction associated with AR because of delayed referral for surgery. This has been recognized with more favorable results (Cohn, 1991).

The Role of Percutaneous Valvuloplasty

The interest in percutaneous balloon valvuloplasty that peaked in the 1980s has significantly diminished, especially for aortic valvuloplasty, which has proved to be an inadequate treatment for AS (Bernard et al., 1992). Mitral valvuloplasty in highly selected patients has a higher success rate and continues to play a supporting role to surgical treatment, postponing definite surgical treatment for variable periods of time (Legget et al., 1991). With the decreasing operative mortality and improved long-term survival, valvular surgery in the elderly continues to be the procedure of choice.

SUMMARY

Advances in surgical techniques, in CPB, myocardial protection, cardiac anesthesia, and intensive care have established modern cardiac surgery as the choice treatment for CAD and valvular heart disease. This has extended to the continually increasing elderly population with favorable short- and long-term results that outperform other forms of therapies. These results can only improve with future development and improvements in the technology of CPB, valvular prostheses, and bypass conduits. Cardiac surgery is costly, but in the long term it might prove to be cost-effective by reducing the number of hospital admissions, repeated nonsurgical procedures, and expensive medicines prescribed.

• Editor's Comments •

This chapter illustrates the complexity of factors that make it difficult for the physician to decide which therapeutic approach to suggest in any given case of an elderly cardiac patient. Age alone, while generally increasing the risk of most surgical procedures, is not an absolute guide to a rational decision. For all the cardiac, coronary, and valvular candidates for surgical intervention there are multiple and variable factors with effects on the outcome that can be evaluated adequately only by experienced specialized cardiac surgeons.

References

Bernard, Y., Etievent, J., & Mourand, J. L., et al. Long-term results of percutaneous aortic valvuloplasty compared with aortic valve replacement in patients more than 70 years old. *J Am Coll Cardiol, 20*: 796–801. 1992.

Blakeman, B. M., Pifarre, R., & Sullivan, H. J., et al. Aortic valve replacement in patients 75 years old and older. *Ann Thorac Surg, 44*: 637–639. 1987.

Bonow, R. O., Rosing, D. R., & Maron, B. J., et al. Reversal of left ventricular dysfunction after aortic valve replacement for chronic aortic regurgitation: Influence of duration of preoperative left ventricular dysfunction. *Circulation, 70*: 570–579. 1984.

Buckberg, G. G. A proposed "solution" to the cardioplegic controversy. *J Thorac Cardiovasc Surg, 77*: 803–15.

Buckley, M. J., Cheitlin, M. D., Goldman, L., Kaplan, J. A., & Kouchoukos, N. T. Cardiac surgery and noncardiac surgery in elderly patients with heart disease: *J Am Coll Cardiol, 10*: 35A-37A. 1987.

Butler, R. N. Harrision's principles of internal medicine, (12 ed.). In J. D. Wilson, G. Braunwald, K. J. Isselbacher, et al. (Eds.). *The challenge of geriatric medicine* (p. 16). New York: McGraw, Hill. 1991.

Cohn, L. H. Valvular surgery. *Current Opinion in Cardiology, 6*: 235–245. 1991.

Cohn, L. H., & Horvath, K. A. CABG in elderly patients: Risks vs. Benefits. *J Myocardial Ischemia, 3*: 1: 13–23. 1991.

Edmunds, L. H., Stephenson, L. W., Edie, R. N., & Ratcliffe, M. B.: Open heart surgery in octogenarians. *N Engl J Med, 319*: 131–136. 1988.

Edmunds, L. H., Jr. Uncomfortable issues. *Ann Thorac Surg, 50*: 173–4. 1990.

Edwards, F. H., Taylor, A. J., & Thompson, L., et al. Current status of coronary artery operations in Septuagenerians. *Ann Thorac Surg, 51*: 265–9. 1991.

Elveback, L., & Lie J. T. Combined high incidence of coronary artery disease at autopsy in Olmstead County, Minnesota, 1950–1979. *Circulation, 70*: 345–349. 1984.

Feinleib, J. M., Havlik, R. J., & Gillum, R. F., et al. Coronary heart disease and related procedures. *Circulation, 79*: 113–118. 1989.

Follette, D. M., Mulder, D. G., Maloney, J. V., Jr., & Buckberg, G. D. Advantages of blood cardioplegia over continuous coronary perfusion or intermittent ischemia. *J Thorac Cardiovasc Surg, 76*: 604. 1978.

Follette, D. M., Steed, D. L., Foglia, R. P., Fey, K., & Buckberg, G. D. Advantages in intermittent blood cardioplegia over intermittent ischemia during prolonged hypothermic aortic clamping. *Circulation, 58*(Suppl 3): 1–200. 1978.

Frank, S., Johnston, A., & Ross, J. Jr. Natural history of valvular aortic stenosis. *Br Heart J, 35*: 41. 1973.

Fremes, S. E., Goldman, B. S., Ivanov, J., Weisel, R. D., David, T. E., Salerno, T. & the Cardiovascular Surgeons at the University of Toronto Valvular surgery in the elderly. *Circulation, 80*(Suppl 1): I-77–I-99. 1989.

Gardner, T. J., Green, P. S., & Rykiel, M. F., et al. Routine use of the left internal mammary artery graft in the elderly. *Ann Thorac Surg, 49*: 188–94. 1990.

Gersh, B. J., Kronmal, R. A., & Frye, R. L., et al. Coronary arteriography and coronary artery bypass surgery: Morbidity and mortality in patients ages 65 years or older: A report from the Coronary Artery Surgery Study. *Circulation, 64*: 360–367. 1981.

Gersh, B. J., Phil, D., & Holmes, D. R. Coronary angioplasty as the preferred approach to treatment of multivessel: Promising, appealing but unproved. *Am Coll of Cardiol, 16*(5): 1104–1106. 1990.

Goldman, B. S., Scully, H. E., Tong, C. P., Weisel, R. D., Mickelborough, L. L., & Baird, R. J. Coronary artery bypass (CAB) in the elderly. *Circulation, 76*: (Suppl IV): IV-352 [Abstract]. 1987.

Grossi, E. A., Esposito, R., & Harris, L. J., et al. Sternal wound infections and use of internal mammary artery grafts. *J Thorac Cardiovasc Surg, 102*: 342–7. 1991.

Guadagnoli, E., Ayanian, J. Z., & Cleary, P. D. Comparison of patient reported outcomes after elective coronary artery bypass grafting in patients r65 and s65 years. *Am J Cardiol, 70*(1): 60–4. 1992.

Hearse, D. J., Stewart, D. A., & Braimbridge, M. V. Metabolic and myocardial protection during elective cardiac arrest. *Circ Res, 36*: 481. 1975.

Hewitt, R. L., Lolley, D. M., & Adrouny, G. A., et al. Protective effect of glycogen and glucose on the anoxic arrested heart. *Surgery, 75*: 1. 1974.

Horvath, K. A., Disesa, V. J., & Peigh, P. S., et al. Favorable results of coronary artery bypass grafting in patient older than 75 years. *J Thorac Cardiovasc Surg, 99*: 92–6. 1990.

Hwang, M. H., Hammermeister, K. E., Oprian, C., Henderson, W., Bousvaros, G., Wong, M., Miller, C. D., Folland, E., & Sethi, G Preoperative identification of patients likely to have left ventricular dysfunction after aortic valve replacement: Participants in the Veterans Administration Cooperative Study on Valvular Heart Disease. *Circulation, 80*(Supp 1, no 3): I65. 1989.

Jacobs, L. A., Vlopp, E. H., & Seamore, W., et al. Improved organ function during cardiopulmonary bypass with a roller pump modified to deliver pulsatile flow. *J Thorac Cardiovasc Surg, 58*: 703–712. 1969.

Jamieson, W. R. E., Allen, P., Miyagishima, R. T., Gerein, A. N., Munro, A. I., Burr, L. H., & Tyers, G. F. O. The carpentier-Edwards standard porcine bioprosthesis. *J Thorac Cardiovasc Surg, 99*: 543–561. 1990.

Jamieson, W. R. E., Dooner, J., & Muno, A. I., et al. Cardiac valve replacement in the elderly. A review of 320 consecutive cases. *Circulation, 64*(Suppl II): II-177–II-183. 1981.

Jones, E. L., Weintraub, W. S., Craver, J. M., Guyton, R. A., Cohen, C. L., Corrigan, V. E., & Hatcher, C. R. Ten-year experience with the porcine bioprosthetic valve: interrelationship of valve survival and patient survival in 1050 valve replacements. *Ann Thorac Surg, 49*: 370–384. 1990.

Jones, R. H. In search of the optimal surgical mortality. *Circulation, 79*(Suppl 1): 132–6. 1989.

Kahn, J. K., Rutherford, B. D., & McConahay, D. R., et al. Results of primary angioplasty for acute myocardial infarction in patients with multivessel coronary artery disease. *Am Coll of Cardiol, 16*(5): 1089–1096. 1990.

Kennedy, J. W., Kaiser, G. C., & Fisher, L. D., et al. Clinical and angiographic predictors of operative mortality from the Collaborative Study in Coronary Artery Surgery (CASS). *Circulation, 63*: 793–802. 1981.

Ko, W., Krieger, K., & Lazenby, et al. Isolated coronary artery bypass grafting in one hundred consecutive octogenarian patients. *J Thorac Cardiovasc Surg, 102*: 532–8. 1991.

Legget, M. E., Jaffe, W. M., & Ellis, C. J., Low mortality and morbidity with open mitral valvotomy: Implications for those performing balloon valvuloplasty [Abstract]. *Circulation, 84*(Suppl II): II-640. 1981.

Leitch, J. W., Thompson, D., Band, D. K., & Harris, P. J. The importance of age and prediction of atrial fibrillation and flutter after coronary artery bypass grafting. *J Thorac Cardiovasc Surg, 100*: 338–42. 1990.

Letac, B., Bribiera, A., Koning, R., & Lefebre, E. Aortic stenosis in elderly patients aged 80 or older. *Circulation, 80*: 1514–20. 1989.

Lindblom, D., Lindblom, U., Qvist, J., & Lundstrom, H. Long term relative survival rates after heart valve replacement. *J Am Coll Cardiol, 15*: 566–573. 1990.

McGrath, L. B., Gonzalez-Lavin, L., Bailey, B. M., Grunkemeier, G. L., Fernandez, J., & Laub, G. W.: Tricuspid valve operations in 530 patients. Twenty-five year assessment of early and late phase events. *J Thorac Cardiovasc Surg, 99*: 124–133. 1990.

National Center for Health Statistics. Vital Statistics of the United States, 1988, Vol. 11, Section 6, Washington DC. 1990.

O'Keefe, J. H., Jr, Vliestra, M. B., Bailey, K. R., & Holmes, D. R. Jr. Natural history of candidates for balloon aortic valvuloplasty. *Proc Mayo Clin, 62*: 986–91. 1987.

O'Keefe, J. H., Jr., Rutherford, B. D., & McConahay, D. R., et al. Multivessel coronary angioplasty from 1980 to 1989: Procedural results and long-term outcome. *Am Coll of Cardiol, 16*(5): 1097–1102. 1990.

Parsonnet V., Dean D., & Bernstein A. D. A method of uniform stratification of risk for evaluating the results of surgery in acquired adult heart disease. *Circulation, 79*(Suppl 1): 3–12. 1989.

Rahimtoola, S. H., Grunkemeier, G. L., & Teply, J. F., et al. Changes in coronary bypass surgery leading to improved survival. *JAMA, 246*: 1912–1916. 1981.

Rhimtoola, S. H., Grunkemeier, G. L., & Starr, A. Ten year survival after coronary artery bypass surgery for angina in patients aged 65 years and older. *Circulation, 74*: 3: 509–517. 1986.

Roberts, W. C., Perloff, J. K., & Costantino, T. Severe valvular aortic stenosis in patients over 65 years of age. *Am J Cardiol, 27*: 497–506. 1971.

Rowe, J. W. Health care of the elderly. *N Engl J Med, 312*: 827–35. 1985.

Scott, W. C., Miller, D. C., & Haverich, A., et al. Determinants of operative mortality for patients undergoing aortic valve replacement: Discriminant analysis of 1,479 operations. *J Thorac Cardiovasc Surg, 89*: 400–13. 1985.

Siegal, J. S. Recent and prospective demographic tends for the elderly population and some implications for health care. In Second Conference on the Epidemiology of Aging. bethesda, MD: National Institute of Health. 1980.

Silverman, N. A., Del Nido, P., Krukenkamp, I., & Levitsky, S. Biological rationale for formulation of antegrade cardioplegia solutions. In W. R. Clintwood, (Ed.), *Myocardial Preservation: Clinical Applications.* (pp. 181–95). Philadelphia: Hantey and Belfus.

Stephenson, L. W., McVaugh, H. M. III, & Edmunds, L. H., Jr. Surgery using cardiopulmonary bypass in the elderly. *Circulation, 58*: 250–4. 1978.

Taylor, K. M. Why pulsatile flow during cardiopulmonary bypass? In D. B. Longmoor (Ed.), *Towards safer cardiac surgery* (pp. 481–500). MTP. PRESS Lancaster, England; 1981.

Tresch, D. D., Siegel, R., & Keelan, M. H., et al. Mitral valve prolapse in the elderly. *J Am Geriatr Soc, 27*: 421–424. 1979.

Tsai, T. P., Matloff, J. M., & Chaux, A., et al. Combined valve and coronary artery bypass procedures in septuagenarians and octogenarians: Results in 120 patients. *Ann Thorac Surg, 43*: 681–684. 1986.

U.S. Bureau of the Census: Statistical abstract of the United States 1991 (111 edition). Washington, DC, 1991.

Wei, J. Y. Heart disease in the elderly. *Cardiovascular Med, 9*: 971–982. 1984.

Wei, J. Y., & Gersh B. J. Heart disease in the elderly. *Curr Probl Cardiol, 12*: 1–65. 1987.

Wetle, T. Age as a risk factor for inadequate treatment. *JAMA, 258*-4: 516. 1987.

Chapter Nine

Diagnostic Tests in the Elderly with Neurological Disorders

Pamela A. Cyrus, Janet Jankowiak, and Robert G. Feldman

The elderly patient with neurological disease is unique in many ways, and consequently, diagnostic and treatment approaches should be tailored to the patient's special circumstances. When considering diagnostic studies, the importance of weighing the risks versus benefits of each test must be even more seriously considered than in the younger patient. The discomfort of a test may be tolerated poorly by an elderly patient, and the caring physician should feel confident that the information gained from the study will justify the cost, time, inconvenience, and possible risks.

In this chapter, we will discuss some of the neurological changes that occur in the "normal" aging process, as understanding of such changes is essential when interpreting diagnostic tests. This will be followed by an overview of various diagnostic tools, both those currently used in the clinical setting and those still under investigation. We will give examples of some commonly encountered neurological disturbances where specific studies may be most valuable.

Our goal is to offer guidelines for ordering diagnostic studies that may be helpful in assessing an elderly patient with a neurological problem. However, each patient poses a unique challenge and merits consideration on an individual basis.

NEUROLOGICAL CHANGES IN "NORMAL" AGING

On neurological examination, the elderly patient has characteristics that would be considered pathological in a younger patient. As a person ages, a fine line develops between that which is considered normal aging and pathology. With the ever-increasing numbers of elderly persons in Western societies, the prevalence of neurological impairment in this group is notable. Neurologic disorders are the most common cause of disability in the aged, accounting for nearly 50% of morbidity (Drachman & Long, 1984).

One may question why the older population is so susceptible to neurological deterioration. One explanation may be that cell replication is finite; cell division ceases in the senescent cell despite a homeostatic environment (Hayflick, 1970). Neuronal elements undergo multiple and varied stresses during a lifetime. Eventually, the nervous system loses its reserve capacity, and neurologic deterioration ensues.

With the aging process, *morphologic and biochemical changes* occur in the nervous system. From young adult life to old age, there is a decrease in brain weight, the degree of decline accelerating during the sixth and seventh decades (Kemper, 1984). However, not all neuronal tissues appear to be equally susceptible. For example, the locus ceruleus and substantia nigra show a 35% reduction in cells. These anatomical and biochemical changes may contribute to the motoric slowing noted with normal aging and extending into pathological states such as parkinsonism. At autopsy, a 25% loss is seen in lumbosacral anterior horn cells, sensory ganglion cells, putaminal cells (part of the extrapyramidal motor system), and cerebellar Purkinje cells. On the other hand, the vestibular nuclei and inferior olivary nuclei (a relay station in the brainstem connecting to the cerebellum) maintain a fairly constant number of cells (Kemper, 1984). The elderly brain also undergoes metabolic changes. Cerebral metabolic rate of oxygen uptake decreases by 6% over the age of 50, while the cerebral metabolic rate of glucose utilization is reduced by 25% with normal aging (Duckett, 1991). These morphologic and biochemical changes may explain some of the clinical neurological changes seen in the elderly.

Clinically, the aging process seems to affect selective aspects of *cognitive function*. "Crystallized" intelligence (manipulation of previously learned material, which is dependent on education) is more resistant to the effects of aging than "fluid" intelligence (abstraction and cognitive flexibility, which are independent of educational and cultural experiences) (Gainotti, 1984). Tests of verbal abilities (vocabulary, auditory/written comprehension) appear to withstand the effects of aging better than visuospatial skills (Weintraub & Mesulam, 1985). Memory impairment, particularly retrieval of information, is considered part of the normal aging process (Crook, 1989). However, a fine line exists between that which is considered age-related memory impairment and early pathological memory impairments.

The elemental neurological examination reveals frequent changes associated with aging. On *cranial nerve* testing, diminished ability to identify odors is common (Jekyn, 1989). Pupils are small with restricted pupillary reflexes (Adams & Victor, 1989b). Ocular mobility tends to be slow, and upgaze is often limited (Drachman & Long, 1984), although the latter may represent early pathology. Progressive hearing loss is common. Sense of taste is also diminished (Drachman & Long, 1984).

Significant impairments in *motor function* are characteristic. Movements tend to be slowed; this may be multifactorial, including arthritic and other medical conditions. Muscle strength may be reduced by 20% to 40% in healthy 60–80-year-olds (Wolfson, 1992). Although increased muscle tone in the limbs has been reported in the elderly (Jekyn, 1989), some argue that this is not part of normal aging (Jankowiak, Knoefel, & Albert, 1991).

Reflexes also change with aging. Ankle jerks are commonly diminished or absent. Plantar reflexes may be neutral (no response) or extensor in 5% of the elderly (Drachman & Long, 1984), although the latter may represent underlying pathology (e.g., secondary to cervical spondylosis).

The *sensory exam* also shows changes with aging. Vibratory sensation is diminished in the lower extremities. These changes are most likely due to a 5%–8% dropout of peripheral nerve fibers per decade after the fourth decade. The largest fibers are most affected (Sabin, 1982).

One of the most common neurological changes in the healthy elderly patient is *gait* disturbance, sometimes termed senile gait. Approximately 13% of people over 65 exhibit this gait abnormality, which cannot be attributed to any specific disease (Greenspan, Knoefel, & Albert, 1990). The senile gait is characterized by its shuffling quality, slightly widened base, turning in stages, reduced arm swing, difficulty initiating the first step upon arising, and tendency to retropulsion (Jankowiak et al., 1991). This gait disturbance may be multifactorial, involving a combination of sensory, motor, visual, and vestibular disturbances (Manchester, Woollacott, Zederbauer-Hylton, & Marin, 1989).

Thus, a narrow margin seems to exist between findings of normal aging and early signs of pathology. When a pathological state is suspected, further evaluation is warranted. In the remainder of the chapter, the usefulness and limitations of diagnostic tools that may aid in the evaluation of the geriatric patient will be addressed.

COMPUTED TOMOGRAPHY SCAN

The computed tomography (CT) scan is one of the most widely used diagnostic tools for evaluating structural cerebral pathology. It is indicated in patients presenting with head trauma, cerebrovascular disease, new-onset seizures, or unexplained changes in mental status, including suspected tumors and dementia.

With normal aging, there is a loss of brain parenchyma volume and a relative increase in cerebrospinal fluid (CSF) spaces (Creasey & Rapoport, 1985). These changes are seen on the CT as widening of the sulci and enlargement of the ventricles, often called "cerebral atrophy, consistent with age." The perivascular spaces become more prominent (Rao, 1992). However, these changes do not seem to correlate well with clinical cognitive changes (Freedman, Knoefel, Naeser, & Levine, 1984).

An elderly patient presenting with a head injury, especially with loss of consciousness or altered mental status, merits a CT. The elderly are particularly susceptible to *subdural hematomas*, even with minor trauma, due to the increased incidence of cerebral atrophy and consequent vulnerability of the bridging dural veins. Subdural hematomas occur most commonly over the cerebral convexities or within the interhemispheric fissure and appear as crescent-shaped high-density masses adjacent to the calvarium (Austin, 1991). Within the brain parenchyma, trauma may result in hemorrhagic areas of necrosis (*contusions*). Contusions typically occur at the inferior frontal and anterior-inferior temporal poles, where the brain's surface is particularly vulnerable to the skull's bony prominences (Poirier, Gray, & Escourolle, 1990). On CT, contusions produce high-density (if hemorrhagic) or low-density (if nonhemorrhagic) areas of mass effect (Zimmerman, 1992). However,

CT may not detect a small contusion lying next to bone due to arti-fact created by bone. Generally, CTs are readily available and can provide much needed information in a timely fashion. The total exam time varies from 10 to 25 minutes. CT remains the most cost-effective means of evaluating cranial trauma.

A CT scan is also useful in the diagnosis and management of *cerebrovascular disease.* Cerebrovascular disease, the third leading cause of death in the United States, is particularly prevalent in the geriatric population. Although CT may show changes consistent with cerebral ischemia as early as 3 hours after the onset of symp-toms, generally the initial changes are only evident after 18–24 hours (Goldberg & Lee, 1992). The main reason for obtaining a CT in the early stages is to rule out hemorrhage, which may conse-quently influence treatment options such as anticoagulation. CT is preferable to MRI in this setting due to its ready availability and shorter imaging time. The main limitation of CT scans in cerebro-vascular disease is the poor sensitivity in infratentorial (cerebel-lum and brainstem) infarctions; only 31–44% are positive (Gold-berg & Lee, 1992). The posterior fossa is difficult to image on CT due to artifact created by the bones at the base of the skull; in this setting MRI is preferable.

Much debate exists regarding the correlation of CT findings and cognitive changes. Many authors believe that the degree of cortical atrophy does not correlate with cognitive function and specifically is not of predictive value in determining dementia. However, ven-tricular size may be increased in various types of dementia (Freed-man et al., 1984). In evaluating ventricular size, the ventricle–brain parenchyma ratio is considered. Various indices are used in determining this ratio. One is the *bicaudate index*, which measures the area of the lateral ventricle at its largest point above the cau-date, divided by the intracranial area (Brinkman, Sarwar, Levin, & Morris, 1981). Another index is the *bifrontal index*, which mea-sures the width of both frontal horns divided by the intracranial area (Kirkwood, 1990a). An increase in the ventricle–brain paren-chyma ratio is found to correlate well with severity of dementia (Brinkman, 1981). In Pick's disease, a cortical dementia character-ized by initial behavioral changes, there is prominent atrophy noted in the frontal and temporal lobes (Duara, 1992). Hun-tington's disease, an autosomal dominant movement disorder asso-ciated with a subcortical dementia, shows a marked increase in the bicaudate index due to prominent atrophy of the caudate nuclei (Sax & Vonsattel, 1992).

Another reason for obtaining a CT scan is to rule out treatable causes of cognitive dysfunction, such as *normal pressure hydrocephalus* (NPH). In the presence of the clinical triad of dementia, incontinence, and gait apraxia, characteristic of NPH, CT may be helpful. However, NPH must be differentiated from hydrocephalus *ex vacuo* (i.e., diffuse cortical atrophy). The finding of ventricular enlargement with absent sulci suggests NPH. Ventricular enlargement with large sulci is more consistent with hydrocephalus *ex vacuo*. In addition, "flattening" of the frontal horns is noted with NPH, while the angle formed by the frontal horns is more acute with diffuse atrophy (Rao, 1992). These findings are important as NPH is potentially treatable by CSF shunting. CT may help in the assessment of dementia due to small vessel disease (e.g., *multi-infarct dementia*), although it is not treatable per se. Other treatable causes of mental status change that can be diagnosed by CT are chronic subdural hematomas/hygromas and mass-occupying lesions such as *abscess* or tumor.

A patient with a suspected *neoplasm*, due to new-onset headache, seizures, mental status changes, or focal neurological findings should have a CT scan, preferably with contrast. Contraindications to contrast dye include hypersensitivity to iodine and renal failure, although hydration may help in the latter situation. CT has a 98% sensitivity in detecting intracranial tumors (Wolpert, 1991). Lesions in the posterior fossa are less well visualized by CT but are usually confirmed with MRI. Tumors may also be detected by mass effect, edema, or enhancement with contrast (Smirniotopoulos & Lee, 1992).

MAGNETIC RESONANCE IMAGING

MRI is another useful tool in the assessment of structural neurological lesions and, in many circumstances, surpasses the CT scan. In general, MRI is superior to CT in detecting posterior fossa, brainstem, and deep temporal lobe lesions due to bone artifact that occurs on CT. MRI is also preferred over CT for evaluation of white matter disease (especially demyelinating processes). MRI provides clearer contrast between gray and white matter and consequently is better for detecting edema and small amounts of blood (Goldberg & Lee, 1992). However, CT is superior to MRI in detecting calcium (e.g. in tumors) and in evaluating bone lesions (Smirniotopoulos & Lee, 1992).

With "normal" aging, MRI demonstrates increased frequency of small focal high T2 signal intensity, often called unidentified bright objects (UBOs). These occur predominantly in the periventricular white matter and are of unclear significance (Kirkwood, 1990e). Approximately 30% of healthy patients over age 60 show these lesions (Chi & Bello, 1992).

Because MRI is superior to CT for visualization of *white matter diseases*, it is used in diagnosing multiple sclerosis, progressive multifocal leukoencephalopathy (PML), Creutzfeldt-Jakob disease, central pontine myelinolysis (presumably secondary to overrapid correction of hyponatremia), postradiation necrosis and Binswanger's disease (subcortical arteriosclerotic encephalopathy). In addition, MRI better delineates lacunar infarcts in the deep white matter associated with "vascular" dementia and may aid in diagnosis. Vascular malformations, aneurysms, and tumors are better defined by MRI.

MRI is also very useful in evaluation of the *spinal cord*. Myelopathy, due to intrinsic or extrinsic compression of the cord, is relatively common in the geriatric patient. Spinal cord impingement is frequently due to osteophyte formation. Almost all patients over the age of 70 have significant osteophytic narrowing of the spinal canal, although most patients are asymptomatic (Wolfson & Katzman, 1992). Symptoms of myelopathy secondary to *cervical spondylosis* include a spastic gait, hyperreflexia, and extensor plantar reflexes; bladder symptoms may occur later. Other common causes of myelopathy in the elderly patient are disk herniation and malignancy (primary or metastatic). Intrinsic spinal cord pathology, intradural-extramedullary lesions, osteomyelitis, and vertebral metastasis are better seen on MRI than with CT or myelography. The use of gadolinium enhancement is particularly beneficial with cord tumors, transverse myelitis and multiple sclerosis (Kirkwood, 1990c). In cases of spinal trauma, the cord is best visualized by MRI while bone pathology is best viewed by CT (Kirkwood, 1990b).

The major limiting factors of MRI are cost, availability, and length of time required for testing. A study may take 45–75 minutes, during which time an elderly patient may find it very difficult to remain motionless, lying flat, in an enclosed space. Contraindications to MRI are pacemakers, claustrophobia, and any internal metal object (e.g., surgical clips, heart valves, shrapnel).

MYELOGRAPHY

A myelogram is a diagnostic study used to determine focal spinal cord/nerve root pathology. Although the use of aqueous contrast agents has reduced some of the serious risks of myelography, the incidence of postmyelographic reactions is about 33% (Kirkwood, 1990c). The most common problem is headache, although mental dysfunction and allergic reactions to iodine may occur. With the more recent availability of MRI imaging, myelography is used less often. However, myelography may be preferable in the case of acute cord compression if it can be obtained more expeditiously than MRI (Wolpert, 1991). Myelography may also be needed if the patient can not tolerate MRI.

SINGLE PHOTON EMISSION COMPUTED TOMOGRAPHY

Single photon emission computed tomography (SPECT) scanning provides a method for testing cerebral metabolic function. This technique, which uses iodine-containing isotopes and a rotating gamma camera, is becoming increasingly available for clinical use in many nuclear medicine departments. The isotope is injected intravenously and reflects regional blood flow. In cerebrovascular disease, SPECT demonstrates a decrease in uptake of the isotope in the area of infarction but not in areas of transient ischemia (Hill et al., 1984). SPECT scan may also prove beneficial in distinguishing various forms of dementia. In Alzheimer's disease there seems to be reduction of isotope uptake in the posterior temporal and parietal lobes early in the course of the disease; as the disease progresses, the anterior temporal lobes and frontal lobes become involved. In multi-infarct dementia, patchy and diffuse defects are noted (Holman & Devous, 1992). Patients with normal pressure hydrocephalus tend to have a symmetric reduction of isotope uptake in the periventricular white matter (Wolpert, 1991).

POSITRON EMISSION TOMOGRAPHY

Positron emission tomography (PET) scanning is an exciting tool to study cerebral metabolic function. It uses radioactive substances to measure cerebral blood flow, oxygen uptake, and glucose utilization (Wolpert, 1991). Although PET is currently limited to experimental protocols, it has received much publicity in its use in Alzheimer's disease research. PET scanning has demonstrated reduced cerebral blood flow, glucose metabolism, and oxygen utilization (with normal oxygen extraction) in the temporoparietal and frontal areas in Alzheimer's disease patients (Wolpert, 1991). In patients with Parkinson's disease, PET scanning with a radioisotope of L-dopa shows decreased accumulation in the striatum (part of the extrapyramidal motor system implicated in the pathology of Parkinson's disease) (Wolpert, 1991). PET scanning is also being used in cerebrovascular disease to differentiate transiently ischemic areas from permanently infarcted brain tissue, in hopes of predicting recuperation and prognosis. At this time, PET is not readily available clinically, but use of this technique is increasing our understanding of some of the unique changes in elderly brain function.

ELECTROENCEPHALOGRAPHY

The electroencephalogram (EEG) is the most commonly used diagnostic tool to assess brain electrical function. It records electrical current generated by the summation of excitatory and inhibitory synaptic potentials of cortical neurons (Pedley & Emerson, 1991). The normal waking EEG in adults with their eyes closed has a posterior rhythm of 8–13 cycles per second (Hz) alpha activity and anterior background rhythm consisting of a mixture of low-amplitude beta (>13 Hz) and theta (4–7 Hz) activity. Sleep produces characteristic changes, such as vertex sharp waves, sleep spindles, and slowing of background activity (4–7 Hz theta activity in lighter phases and <4 Hz delta activity in deeper phases of sleep). With aging, the posterior alpha frequency tends to slow but the rhythm should not fall below 8.0 Hz in a normal alert adult at any age (Katz & Harner, 1984). Intermittent focal slowing limited to the temporal lobes during wakefulness is often encountered in normal elderly subjects (Hughes & Cayaffa, 1977), predominantly on the left side (Arenas, Brenner, & Reynolds, 1986). This is generally considered to be a "normal variant of aging" unless greater than 0.6% of the recording shows delta (<4 Hz) or greater than 1.8% of the recording contains theta (4–7 Hz) activity (Arenas, et al., 1986).

A common indication for obtaining an EEG is a history of an unexplained loss of consciousness or other intermittent behavioral change raising a suspicion of *epilepsy*. The number of new cases of epilepsy in patients over 60 years of age varies from 7.5 to 15.5 per

100,000 (Hauser & Hessdorfer, 1990). Common causes of seizures in this age group include cerebrovascular disease, trauma, tumor, and degenerative disease. An EEG may localize a focus of abnormal activity and guide the choice of anticonvulsant therapy, depending on seizure type. However, a normal EEG can not exclude a diagnosis of epilepsy, given that recording electrodes are superficial and may not record a deep electrical abnormality (e.g., within the temporal lobe). To increase the chances of visualizing an epileptogenic focus, long-term ambulatory or video EEG monitoring may be beneficial.

An EEG may also be useful in *cerebrovascular disease*. The EEG may show slow-wave activity or suppression of normal background activity in the area of ischemia (Adams & Victor, 1989c). Rhythmic delta activity bifrontally may suggest severe cerebral edema (Katz & Harner, 1984).

The EEG may also be beneficial in evaluating fluctuating or altered levels of consciousness. The most common cause of *impaired consciousness* is diffuse encephalopathy due to metabolic disturbances, hypoxia, infection, postictal state, or drug intoxication (Plum & Posner, 1980). The EEG characteristically shows diffuse slowing in the delta or theta range. Bilaterally synchronous large, sharp triphasic waves are classically seen in hepatic encephalopathy but may also be found in uremia, various other metabolic abnormalities, vascular, degenerative, neoplastic, infectious, and traumatic brain lesions (Chatrian, 1990). A comatose patient with a midbrain lesion may show rhythmic slow activity with sleep spindles occurring in bursts (Katz & Harner, 1984). Another pattern noted in a comatose patient is "alpha coma." Although the EEG tracing resembles normal alpha activity, the patient is deeply comatose due to a lower brainstem lesion, and prognosis is generally very poor (Katz & Harner, 1984).

The EEG is also useful in the evaluation of *dementia*. In the early stages of a dementing process, it may be easy to mistake a change in behavior due to *depression* for dementia. The EEG will be normal in the case of depression (often termed pseudodementia) but may show various changes in a neurodegenerative disorder. In the early stages of Alzheimer's disease, the EEG may be normal or show diffuse, slightly slowed activity in the theta range (Markand, 1986). However, the severity of slowing on the EEG may not always predict the extent of cognitive dysfunction, and vice versa, especially in the early stages. As the dementia progresses, the EEG generally shows increased slowing. In patients with Huntington's disease, the EEG characteristically shows a very low amplitude (flat) background. Creutzfeldt-Jakob disease, a rare and rapidly progressive dementia, shows very characteristic features on the EEG that may help in the diagnosis. These are periodic sharp waves that are most prevalent in the second phase of the disease, though they may also be present in the terminal phase when the background amplitude diminishes (Markand, 1990). The EEG may also be useful in cases of multi-infarct "vascular" dementia, where 74% of patients show focal slow waves (Markand, 1990). Although these patterns are not pathognomonic, their presence may support a diagnosis of dementia and confirm the need to pursue the etiology.

SLEEP STUDIES

Normal aging is associated with marked changes in the daily sleep–wake cycle. These well-established changes include (1) decreased total time of nocturnal sleep, (2) decreased slow-wave sleep (Stages 3 and 4), (3) decreased amount of REM sleep, (4) increased awakenings, (5) increased daytime naps, and (6) disruption of circadian rhythms (Vitiello & Prinz, 1990). Studies suggest that 25%–40% of elderly patients complain of sleep disturbances (Vitiello & Prinz, 1990). The prevalence of these complaints explains the higher use of sedative-hypnotics (both prescription and over-the-counter) in this population (Moran, Thompson, & Nies, 1988). At the same time, it is well recognized that the elderly are particularly susceptible to the adverse effects of these medications. Consequently, an overnight sleep study may be advocated to further delineate the sleep disturbance and avoid unnecessary medication. Sleep studies are performed in many major electrophysiologic laboratories. The study entails basic EEG monitoring, with additional leads to measure nasal and oral air flow, and belts to monitor chest and abdominal wall movements.

Sleep studies are particularly useful in establishing the diagnosis of *sleep apnea*. Clinically, the patient with sleep apnea may complain of excessive daytime somnolence, while his/her sleeping partner may report profound snoring. Often these patients have concomitant obesity, chronic obstructive pulmonary disease (COPD), and/or hypertension. Sleep studies may reveal at least 10-second pauses in respiration, consistent with the diagnosis (Prinz,

Vitiello, Raskind, & Thorpy, 1990). Sleep apnea may be obstructive, central, or mixed in etiology. Obstructive sleep apnea, the most common type, may be treated with weight loss (if indicated), a trial of continuous positive airway pressure (CPAP), or surgery (removal of tonsils and adenoids or tracheostomy in severe cases) (Prinz et al., 1990). The central form of sleep apnea is due to medullary lesions of various etiologies (e.g., infarction, idiopathic "Ondine's curse" [breathing ceases with sleep]).

Another particularly common sleep disturbance in the elderly is nocturnal myoclonus or *restless leg syndrome*. This is characterized by stereotypic flexion of the hips and knees which last 0.5–10 seconds and may occur at 30-second intervals (Vitiello & Prinz, 1990). Restless leg syndrome may be diagnosed with a routine sleep study. Treatment may include clonazepam and other pharmacological agents (Prinz et al., 1990).

Other common causes of sleep disturbances in the elderly may be medical or psychological problems. *Nocturia*, which may be a symptom of an underlying medical condition (e.g., diabetes or benign prostatic hypertrophy) or secondary to medication effect (e.g., diuretics), may interfere with normal sleep. *Pain* from an underlying medical condition, especially arthritis or a painful peripheral neuropathy, frequently disrupts sleep in this age group. *Depression*, probably underdiagnosed in the elderly, is often associated with early morning awakenings and may aid in diagnosis. Many medications (both prescription and over-the-counter), particularly *alcohol*, commonly interfere with the sleep–wake cycle. Therefore, prior to undertaking a sleep study, each geriatric patient should be carefully questioned regarding potentially reversible causes of sleep disturbance which may profoundly effect his/her daily functioning and sense of well-being.

EVOKED POTENTIALS

Evoked potentials, or evoked responses, are primarily used in establishing the diagnosis of demyelinating disorders, the most common being multiple sclerosis. Since multiple sclerosis is rarely diagnosed de novo in the elderly patient, their clinical application in geriatric neurology is limited. However, ongoing research uses these studies to explore responses of the aging brain to various sensory stimuli. Brain potentials are generated by repetitive auditory, visual, or somatosensory stimuli and recorded from scalp electrodes. The earliest components of the sensory-evoked response represent the direct transmission of impulses from the periphery to sensory cortex while later components reflect central transmission to the corresponding association cortices (Katzman & Terry, 1992).

In normal aging, auditory evoked responses show prolonged latencies and decreased amplitudes in both the peripheral and central transmission rates (Polich & Starr, 1984). Latency for one of the later components seems to increase approximately 2 ms per year throughout life (Katzman & Terry, 1992). Visual evoked responses also show increased latencies in peripheral and central transmission but are more notable in later potentials. This is interpreted as a delay in central processing. However, researchers argue that some of the age-related evoked-response changes may be due to a reduction in the amount of light reaching the retina, caused by lens and pupil alterations (Katzman & Terry, 1992). Somatosensory evoked responses also demonstrate increased latencies with aging (Polich & Starr, 1984). In most of the sensory evoked studies, latencies tend to be more prolonged in the later components, supporting the hypothesis that speed of information processing decreases with normal aging (Katzman & Terry, 1992).

ELECTROMYOGRAPHY/NERVE CONDUCTION STUDIES

Electromyography (EMG)/nerve conduction velocities (NCV) should be considered when the history and neurological exam suggest a disturbance in the peripheral nervous system (i.e., spinal root, nerve plexus, peripheral nerve, neuromuscular junction, or muscle). These electrodiagnostic tests, although causing some discomfort, aid in diagnosis and also provide a means of monitoring disease progression and response to therapy.

With normal aging, there is a progressive slowing of sensory and motor nerve conduction velocities of about 16% and a 50% reduction in the amplitude of the action potentials from age 20 to 80 (Wolfson, 1992). On EMG, the mean motor unit potential increases with age (Lange, 1991).

Radiculopathies are frequently encountered in the elderly patient. With aging, the water content of the intervertebral disks decreases, contributing to herniation of the disk or a disk fragment into the spinal canal or neural foramina. However, it is the bony overgrowth of osteophytes that truly compromises the spinal canal and roots, producing a myelopathy or radiculopathy (Wolfson &

Katzman, 1992). When nerve root compression becomes sympto-matic, the patient may complain of back or neck pain that radiates down the leg or arm in a dermatomal fashion. The EMG reveals de-nervation (as evidenced by positive sharp waves and fibrillation po-tentials) in the paraspinal muscles and distal muscles supplied by the corresponding nerve root (Kimura, 1989b).

Peripheral neuropathy is common in patients over 55. The most frequent causes of peripheral neuropathy in this population are di-abetes, malignancy, alcohol, drugs, autoimmune disorders, and nu-tritional deficiencies (Vital & Vital, 1991). Patients may present with stocking-and-glove sensory changes, distal weakness, and hypo/areflexia, especially of ankle jerks. On electrophysiologic studies, nerve conduction velocities are slowed and have reduced amplitudes (Kimura, 1989e).

Disorders of *neuromuscular transmission* should be considered in patients with unexplained weakness. *Myasthenia gravis* is a disor-der of the postsynaptic acetylcholine receptor. When myasthenia gravis does present in the elderly, it usually occurs in men in the fifth and sixth decades and is sometimes associated with thymic tumors. Patients present with fluctuating weakness, especially of ocular, facial, and proximal limb muscles, worsened with exercise and improved with rest. Electrophysiologic studies support the clin-ical diagnosis. Repetitive stimulation of a peripheral nerve at 3–5/ second characteristically produces a "decrementing response" (de-crease in amplitude of compound muscle action potentials) which is reversed with neostigmine or edrophonium (Adams & Victor, 1989a). Single-fiber EMG, an even more sensitive test of neuromus-cular transmission, classically shows increased "jitter" (variability of interpotential intervals) (Kimura, 1989c). A less common disor-der of neuromuscular transmission is *Lambert-Eaton myasthenic syndrome*. It is due to decreased release of acetylcholine from the presynaptic motor nerve terminals. This disorder is usually associ-ated with oat-cell carcinoma of the lung, although in one-third of patients no associated malignancy is found (Sanders & Howard, 1991). Patients complain of weakness, especially involving the hip and shoulder girdles, but strength may often improve transiently during the first few muscle contractions. Electrodiagnostic studies classically show an incrementing response (increase in the ampli-tude of action potentials) with repetitive stimulation at high rates.

The most common *muscle diseases* in the elderly are polymyosi-tis, endocrine myopathies, and myopathies associated with carcinoma (Brooke, 1991). *Polymyositis* has a bimodal distribution, the majority occurring in the fifth and sixth decades, with a smaller peak in adolescence (Kimura, 1989d). Patients present with an insidious onset of proximal limb muscle weakness and vague pains and may occasionally experience muscle tenderness. Serum creatine phosphokinases are generally elevated. EMG demonstrates a typical myopathic pattern with abundant fibrillation potentials, complex repetitive discharges, and polyphasic brief action potentials of low amplitude (Kimura, 1989d). *Thyroid dysfunction* may also lead to neuromuscular problems, thyrotoxic myopathy being the most common. Although women have thyrotoxicosis more frequently, the myopathy is more common in men (Kimura, 1989d). Hypothyroidism may also cause proximal muscle weakness and spasms. *Steroids* used to treat medical problems (e.g., COPD, arthritis) may cause a myopathy in the elderly. However, there is a poor correlation between steroid dose and severity of myopathy (Adams & Victor, 1989a). With discontinuation of steroids the myopathy may improve. Other causes of myopathy in the elderly include *alcohol* and *carcinoma*.

Motor neuron disease is a degenerative disorder of the aging nervous system, the most common being *amyotrophic lateral sclerosis* (ALS). ALS is a disorder of both corticospinal tracts and anterior horn cells, thus producing signs of both upper and lower motor neuron disease. Classically, the disease manifests itself in middle or late life (Kim & Sung, 1991). Patients develop progressive weakness, atrophy, fasciculations, and hyperreflexia. EMG generally demonstrates findings consistent with diffuse denervation (i.e., widespread fibrillation potentials, positive sharp waves), and poor recruitment of motor units) (Kimura, 1989a).

RADIOISOTOPE CISTERNOGRAPHY

Radioisotope cisternography is a functional study of cerebrospinal flow and absorption, primarily used to assess possible normal pressure hydrocephalus (NPH). It is performed by injecting isotope-labeled tracer into the lumbar subarachnoid space via lumbar puncture. Normally, the isotope becomes concentrated over the cerebral convexities in approximately 12–24 hours and then reaches the parasagittal region in 36–48 hours (Wald, 1991). In some patients with NPH, the isotope tends to reflux into the ventricular system, where it may remain for over 72 hours (Kirkwood, 1990a). Interpretation of this test is controversial in terms of determining which patients may benefit from CSF shunting, the treatment of choice for NPH. Some studies have demonstrated benefit from shunting in patients with negative cisternograms, whereas other studies show no benefit from shunting despite positive cisternograms (Kaye, Grady, Haxby, Moore, & Friedland, 1990). Therefore, although cisternograms may aid in the diagnosis of NPH, their use in determining the prognosis of shunting remains controversial.

NONINVASIVE CAROTID STUDIES

Noninvasive carotid studies (NICS), including carotid ultrasound and carotid Doppler studies, provide an indirect measure of internal carotid artery disease. They are particularly useful in the geriatric population due to the high incidence of cerebrovascular disease and susceptibility of these patients to complications of invasive procedures. These studies should be obtained as part of the workup of suspected transient ischemic attacks (TIAs) or cerebrovascular accidents (CVAs) referable to the anterior cerebrovascular circulation. Recent studies suggest that symptomatic patients (i.e., CVA or TIA) with greater than 70% carotid stenosis benefit from carotid endarterectomy when compared with patients receiving only medical management (NASCET Collaborators, 1991). However, due to the relative limitation of this indirect technique, if NICs suggest >70% stenosis, a presurgical angiogram should be performed to better delineate the precise nature of the stenosis.

CEREBRAL ANGIOGRAPHY

Angiography is used to diagnose aneurysms, vascular malformations, mass lesions, and occluded/stenotic blood vessels. In patients with CT- or LP-proved subarachnoid hemorrhage, an angiogram may help in defining an aneurysm or vascular malformation as the etiology for the bleed. Often, neurosurgeons request an angiogram prior to surgical intervention for mass lesions to ascertain the vascular supply of the mass. Perhaps the most common use of angiogram is in assessing stenotic or occluded blood vessels. Angiography is usually performed after lesions have been suspected by noninvasive techniques as it carries certain risks. These include death (1: 5,000), stroke (1: 1,000), TIA (1: 500), contrast reaction (1: 100), and femoral hematoma (1: 50) (Kirkwood, 1990d).

MAGNETIC RESONANCE ANGIOGRAPHY

Magnetic resonance angiography (MRA) is a new and exciting noninvasive means of visualizing the extracranial and intracranial cerebral vasculature. However, there are limitations compared with conventional angiography. These include potential overestimation of the degree of stenosis, underestimation of occlusions, and inadequate visualization of the carotid siphon (Fine-Edelstein & Babikian, in press). At present, MRA is still limited as a noninvasive screening tool, and traditional angiography should be used prior to surgical intervention.

TRANSCRANIAL DOPPLER STUDIES

Transcranial Doppler ultrasonography (TCD) is another noninvasive means of imaging extracranial and intracranial cerebral blood supply. Using ultrasound technique, three natural bony windows in the skull are used to visualize specific vascular territories: (1) transtemporal (supraclinoid internal carotid artery, mainstem of the middle cerebral artery, A-1 segment of the anterior cerebral artery, and P-1 segment of the posterior cerebral artery); (2) transorbital (carotid siphon and the ophthalmic artery); and (3) suboccipital (distal vertebral and proximal basilar arteries) (Fine-Edelstein & Babikian, in press). This technique is being investigated in evaluating ischemic cerebrovascular disease and monitoring blood flow during carotid endarterectomy.

LUMBAR PUNCTURE

LP was historically the main diagnostic tool to assess neurological pathology. With the advent of CT and MRI, which are far superior in detecting and localizing lesions, the LP is less commonly used for diagnosing noninfectious processes. However, the use of LP should not be forgotten, especially in the elderly patient with a change in mental status. Very often the elderly do not show significant elevations of temperature or white cell counts in the presence of chronic or even acute meningoencephalitis. In addition, an LP may be diagnostic of a subarachnoid hemorrhage (SAH) even when a CT is negative, as occurs in 5% of cases (Adams & Victor, 1989c). Therefore, if an SAH is suspected (due to severe headache, nuchal rigidity, altered level of consciousness), an LP should be performed after the CT. Other reasons to perform an LP include evaluation of dementia, new-onset seizure, headache, and confusional states, especially to rule out a chronic inflammatory process. Although nonspecific, an elevated CSF protein may support a diagnosis of chronic inflammatory polyradiculoneuropathy.

An LP may be more difficult to obtain in an older patient because of bony changes of the lumbar spine, but if necessary it can be obtained with fluoroscopic guidance. Generally, a CT scan should be obtained prior to the procedure, as increased intracranial pressure is a relative contraindication. In this situation, the sudden release of elevated CSF pressure may allow herniation of swollen tissue with potentially fatal compression of the brainstem (Bradley, Daroff, Fenichel, & Marsden, 1991). When performing an LP, the opening pressure should always be recorded. CSF samples should be sent routinely for protein, glucose (with a simultaneous serum glucose), cell count, and Gram's stain. In addition, as much CSF as possible should be sent for bacterial and fungal cultures and cytology, if indicated. Immunoglobulins, VDRL, and other special studies may be requested.

CONCLUSION

The geriatric patient poses a challenging array of diagnostic and treatment problems due to the interaction of multiple medical/neurological pathologies as well as particular psychosocial, economic, and ethical issues. We hope that this chapter provides a reference for deciding which studies suit a particular patient with his/her unique clinical presentation.

ACKNOWLEDGMENT

We wish to thank Dr. Janice E. Knoefel, Chief of Geriatric Evaluation Unit, Boston VA Medical Center, for her suggestions and support in writing this chapter.

References

Adams, R. A., & Victor, M. Metabolic myopathies. In *Principles of neurology* (4th ed.). pp. 1133–1139. New York: McGraw-Hill. 1989a.

Adams, R. A., & Victor, M. The neurology of aging. In *Principles of neurology* (4th ed.) pp. 488–497. New York: McGraw-Hill. 1989b.

Adams, R. A., & Victor M. Special techniques for neurologic diagnosis. *Principles of neurology* (4th ed.) pp. 10–31. New York: McGraw-Hill. 1989c.

Arenas, A. M., Brenner, R. P., & Reynold, C. F. Temporal slowing in the elderly revisited. *American Journal of EEG Technology, 26*: 105–114. 1986.

Austin, E. J. Central nervous system trauma in the elderly. In S. Duckett (Ed.), *The Pathology of the Aging Human Nervous System*, (pp. 364–373). Philadelphia: Lea & Febiger. 1991.

Bradley, W. G., Daroff, R. B., Fenichel, G. M., & Marsden, C. D. The place of laboratory investigations in diagnosis and management. In W.G. Bradley, R.B. Daroff, G.M. Fenichel, & C.D. Marsden (Eds.), *Neurology in Clinical Practice*, (pp. 417–422). Boston: Butterworth-Heinemann. 1991.

Brinkman, S. D., Sarwar, M., Levin, H. S., & Morris, H. H. Quantitative indexes of computed tomography in dementia and normal aging. *Radiology, 138*: 89–92. 1981.

Brooke, M. H. Disorders of skeletal muscle. In W. G. Bradley, R. B. Daroff, G. M. Fenichel, & C. D. Marsden (Eds.), *Neurology in Clinical Practice* (pp. 1843–1886). Boston: Butterworth-Heinemann. 1991.

Chatrian, G. E. Coma, other states of altered responsiveness, and brain death. In D. D. Daly & T. A. Pedley (Eds.), *Current Practice of Clinical Electroencephalography*, (2nd ed pp. 425–487). New York: Raven Press. 1990.

Chi, T. L., & Bello J. A. White matter disease. In S. H. Lee, K.C.V.G. Rao & R. A. Zimmerman (Eds.), *Cranial MRI and CT*, (3rd ed., pp. 701–733). New York: McGraw-Hill. 1992.

Creasey, H., & Rapoport S. The aging human brain. *Annals of Neurology, 17*: 2–10. 1985.

Crook, T. H. Diagnosis and treatment of normal and pathologic memory impairment in later life. *Seminars in Neurology, 9*: 20–27. 1989.

Drachman, D. A., & Long, R. R. Neurological evaluation of the elderly patient. In M.L. Albert (Ed.), *Clinical Neurology of Aging* (pp 97–113). New York: Oxford University Press. 1984.

Duara, R. Structural and functional brain imaging in the elderly. In R. Katzman & J.W. Rowe (Eds.), *Principles of Geriatric Neurology* (pp. 89–143). Philadelphia: F.A. Davis. 1992.

Duckett, S. The normal aging human brain. In S. Duckett (Ed.), *The Pathology of the Aging Human Nervous System* (pp. 1–19). Philadelphia: Lea & Febiger. 1991.

Fine-Edelstein, J., & Babikian, V. The noninvasive evaluation of patients with cerebrovascular disease. In M. Fischer (Ed.), *Cerebral Vascular Diseases*. New York: Gower Publishing. In press.

Freedman, M., Knoefel, J., Naeser, M., & Levine, H. Computerized axial tomography in aging. In M.L. Albert (Ed.), *Clinical Neurology of Aging* (pp. 139–148). New York: Oxford University Press. 1984.

Gainotti, G. Neuropsychological features of normal aging and of degenerative dementia. In G. Pilleri & F. Tagliaviri (Eds.), *Brain Pathology, Vol I, Cerebral Ageing and Degenerative Dementias* (pp. 11–37). Bern, Switzerland: Brain Anatomy Institute. 1984.

Goldberg, H. I., & Lee, S. H. Stroke. In S. H. Lee, K.C.V.G. Rao, & R. A. Zimmerman (Eds.), *Cranial MRI and CT* (3rd ed. pp. 623–699). New York: Mc-Graw-Hill. 1992.

Greenspan, B. N., & Knoefel, J. E., Albert, M. L. Neurology and neurobiology of aging. *Current Opinion in Neurology and Neurosurgery, 3*: 123–127. 1990.

Hauser, W. A., & Hesdorffer, D. C. Incidence and prevalence. In *Epilepsy: Frequency, Causes and Consequences* (pp. 1–51). New York: Demos Publications. 1990.

Hayflick, L. Aging under glass. *Experimental Gerontology, 5*: 291–303. 1970.

Hill, T. C., Magistretti, P. L., Holman, B. L., Lee, R. G. L., O'Leary, D. H., Uren, R. F., Royal, H. D., Mayman, C. I., Kolodny, G. M., & Clouse, M. E. Assessment of regional cerebral blood flow (rCBF) in stroke using SPECT and N-isopropyl (I-123)-p-iodoamphetamine (IMP). *Stroke, 15*: 40–45. 1984.

Holman, B. L., & Devous, M. D. Functional brain SPECT: The emergence of a powerful clinical method. *The Journal of Nuclear Medicine, 33*: 1888–1904. 1992.

Hughes, J. R., & Cayaffa, J. J. The EEG in patients at different ages without organic cerebral disease. *Electroencelphalography and Clinical Neurophysiology, 42*: 776–784. 1977.

Jankowiak, J., Knoefel, J. E., & Albert, M. L. Vieillissement et maladie d'Alzheimer. In J.L. Signoret et J.J. Hauw (Eds.), *Demences et la maladie d'Alzheimer* (pp. 213–225). Paris: Medecine-Sciences Flammarion. 1991.

Jekyn, L. R. Examining the aging nervous system. *Seminars in Neurology, 9*: 82–87. 1989.

Katz, R. I., & Harner, R. N. Electroencephalography in aging. In M.L. Albert (Ed.), *Clinical Neurology of Aging* (pp. 114–138). New York: Oxford University Press. 1984.

Katzman, R., & Terry, R. Normal aging of the nervous system. In R. Katzman & J. Rowe (Eds.), *Principles of Geriatric Neurology* (pp. 18–58). Philadelphia: F.A. Davis. 1992.

Kaye, J. A., Grady, C. L., Haxby, J. V., Moore, A., & Friedland, R. P. Plasticity in the aging brain. *Archives of Neurology, 47*: 1336–1341. 1990.

Kemper, T. Neuroanatomical and neuropathological changes in normal aging and in dementia. In M.L. Albert (Ed.), *Clinical Neurology of Aging* (pp. 9–52). New York: Oxford University Press. 1984.

Kim, R.C., & Sung, J.H. Motor system degenerations. In S. Duckett (Ed.), *The Pathology of the Aging Human Nervous System* (pp. 159–171). Philadelphia: Lea & Febiger. 1991.

Kimura, J. Disease of the motor neuron. In *Electrodiagnosis in Disease of Nerve and Muscle: Principles and Practice,* (2nd ed. pp. 429–446). Philadelphia: F. A. Davis. 1989a.

Kimura, J. Diseases of the root and plexus. In *Electrodiagnosis in Disease of Nerve and Muscle: Principles and Practice,* (2nd ed. pp. 447–461). Philadelphia: F.A. Davis. 1989b.

Kimura, J. Myasthenia gravis and other disorders of neuromuscular transmission. In *Electrodiagnosis in Diseases of Nerve and Muscle: Principles and Practice,* (2nd ed. pp. 519–534). Philadelphia: F. A. Davis. 1989c.

Kimura, J. Myopathies. In *Electrodiagnosis in Diseases of Nerve and Muscle: Principles and Practice*, (2nd ed. pp. 535–557). Philadelphia: F. A. Davis. 1989d.

Kimura, J. Polyneuropathies. In *Electrodiagnosis in Disease of Nerve and Muscle: Principles and Practice*, (2nd ed. pp. 462–494). Philadelphia: F. A. Davis. 1989e.

Kirkwood, J. R. Atrophy, aging, and dementia. In *Essentials of Neuroimaging* (pp. 305–318). New York: Churchill Livingstone. 1990a.

Kirkwood, J. R. Spinal trauma. In *Essentials of Neuroimaging* (pp. 453–486). New York: Churchill Livingstone. 1990b.

Kirkwood, J. R. Spine. In *Essentials of Neuroimaging* (pp. 365–452). New York: Churchill Livingstone. 1990c.

Kirkwood, J. R. Techniques and anatomy. In *Essentials of Neuroimaging* (1–40). New York: Churchill Livingstone. 1990d.

Kirkwood, J. R. White matter disease. In *Essentials of Neuroimaging* (299–304). New York: Churchill Livingstone. 1990e.

Lange, D. J. Electrodiagnostic studies of neuromuscular disease: A primer for clinicians. In L.P. Rowland (Ed.), *Merritt's Textbook of Neurology*, (8th ed. pp. 3–18). Philadelphia: Lea & Febiger. 1991.

Manchester, D., Woollacott, M., Zederbauer-Hylton, N., & Marin, O. Visual, vestibular, and somatosensory contributions to balance control in the older adult. *Journal of Gerontology, 44*: 118–127. 1989.

Markand, O. N. Electroencephalogram in dementia. *American Journal of EEG Technology, 26*: 3–17. 1986.

Markand, O. N. Organic brain syndromes and dementias. In D. D. Daly & T. A. Pedley (Eds.), *Current Practice of Clinical Electroencephalography*, (2nd ed. pp. 401–423). New York: Raven Press. 1990.

Moran, M. G., Thompson, T. L., & Nies, A. S. Sleep disorders in the elderly. *American Journal of Psychiatry, 145*: 1369–1378. 1988.

North American Symptomatic Carotid Endarterectomy Trial Collaborators. Beneficial effect of carotid endarterectomy in symptomatic patients with high-grade carotid stenosis. *New England Journal of Medicine, 325*: 445–453. 1991.

Pedley, T. A., & Emerson, R. G. Clinical neurophysiology: Electroencephalography and evoked potentials. In W. G. Bradley, R. B. Daroff, G. M. Fenichel, & C. D. Marsden (Eds.), *Neurology in Clinical Practice* (pp. 429–451). Boston: Butterworth-Heinemann. 1991.

Plum, F., & Posner, J. B. The pathologic physiology of signs and symptoms of coma. In *The Diagnosis of Stupor and Coma*, (3rd ed. pp. 1–86). Philadelphia: F. A. Davis. 1980.

Poirier, J., Gray, F., & Escourolle, R. Traumatic lesions of the central nervous system. In *Manual of Basic Neuropathology*, (3rd ed. pp. 57–64). Philadelphia: W. B. Saunders. 1990.

Polich, J., & Starr, A. Evoked potentials in aging. In M.L. Albert (Ed.), *Clinical Neurology of Aging* (pp. 149–177). New York: Oxford University Press. 1984.

Prinz, P. N., Vitiello, M. V., Raskind, M. A., & Thorpy, M. J. Geriatrics: Sleep disorders and aging. *New England Journal of Medicine, 323*: 520–526. 1990.

Rao, K.C.V.G. The CSF spaces (hydrocephalus and atrophy). In S. H. Lee, K.C.V.G. Rao, & R. A. Zimmerman (Eds.), *Cranial MRI and CT*, (3rd ed. pp. 227–294). New York: McGraw-Hill. 1992.

Sabin, T. D. Biological aspects of falls and mobility limitations in the elderly. *Journal of the American Geriatric Society, 30*: 51–58. 1982.

Sanders, D. B., Howard, J. F. Disorders of neuromuscular transmission. In W. G. Bradley, R. B. Daroff, G. M. Fenichel, & C.D. Marsden (Eds.), *Neurology in Clinical Practice*, (pp. 1819–1842). Boston: Butterworth-Heinemann. 1991.

Sax, D. S., & Vonsattel, J. P. Case records of the Massachusetts General Hospital: Chorea and progressive dementia in an 88–year-old woman. *New England Journal of Medicine, 326*: 117–125. 1992.

Smirniotopoulos, J. G., & Lee, S. H. Primary tumors in adults. In S. H. Lee, K.C.V.G. Rao, & R. A. Zimmerman (Eds.), *Cranial MRI and CT*, (3rd ed. pp. 295–380). New York: McGraw-Hill. 1992.

Vital, C., & Vital, A. Peripheral neuropathy. In S. Duckett (Ed.), *The Pathology of the Aging Human Nervous System* (pp. 393–430). Philadelphia: Lea and Febiger. 1991.

Vitiello, M. V., & Prinz, P.N. Sleep and sleep disorders in normal aging. In M.J. Thorpy (Ed.), *Handbook of Sleep Disorders* (pp. 139–151). New York: Marcel Dekker. 1990.

Wald, S. L. Disorders of cerebrospinal fluid circulation and brain edema. In W. G. Bradley, R. B. Daroff, G.M. Fenichel, & C.D. Marsden (Eds.), *Neurology in Clinical Practice* (pp. 1211–1238). Boston: Butterworth-Heinemann. 1991.

Weintraub, S., & Mesulam M. Mental state assessment of young and elderly adults in behavioral neurology. In M. Mesulam (Ed.), *Principles of Behavioral Neurology* (pp. 71–123). Philadelphia: F.A. Davis. 1985.

Wolfson, L. Falls and gait. In R. Katzman & J.W. Rowe (Eds.), *Principles of Geriatric Neurology* (pp. 281–299). Philadelphia: F.A. Davis. 1992.

Wolfson, L., & Katzman, R. The neurologic consultation at age 80. II: Some specific disorders observed in the elderly. In R. Katzman & J. Rowe (Eds.), *Principles of Geriatric Neurology* (pp. 339–355). Philadelphia: F.A. Davis. 1992.

Wolpert, S. M. Neuroimaging. In W.G. Bradley, R. B. Daroff, G.M. Fenichel, & C. D. Marsden (Eds.), *Neurology in Clinical Practice* (pp. 493–541). Boston: Butterworth-Heinemann. 1991.

Zimmerman, R. A. Craniocerebral trauma. In S. H. Lee, K.C.V.G. Rao, & R. A. Zimmerman (Eds.), *Cranial MRI and CT*, (3rd ed. pp. 509–538). New York: McGraw-Hill. 1992.

Chapter Ten

Dialysis in the Geriatric Population

Theodore I. Steinman

What are the indications for dialysis in the elderly population? When examined closely, the answer is the same no matter what the age of the individual; age alone should not be an exclusion criterion. The purpose of renal replacement therapy is for the patient to derive overall benefit from treatment, and this is not age-dependent; the corollary being that therapy should be withdrawn when the patient ceases to derive benefit. With this proviso one needs to assess how patients will do with dialytic support because chronic hemodialysis can offer good quality of life to some of the elderly (Rothenberg, 1990; Steinmann, 1991). Uremia per se can produce mental status changes that make it appear the patient is nonfunctional and has no chance for reasonable recovery of cognitive functioning (Steinman, 1978).

Only by careful observation after a course of dialysis can one assess an individual's chance of recovery to the point of a positive interaction with his or her environment. Based on the patient's initial presentation, the judgment of health care providers about patients' chances to recover sufficiently to enjoy their environment and participate in their life is difficult at best. Therefore, health care providers must be cautioned about refusing dialytic support based on pretreatment judgment about a patient's nonviability (Steinman, 1991). Those responsible for health care budgeting will have to allow for the cost of treating our elderly population with renal replacement therapy if these individuals will derive benefit from therapy (Horina, Holzer, Reisinger, Krejs, & Neugebauer, 1991).

DEMOGRAPHICS OF THE END STAGE RENAL DISEASE POPULATION

The issue of providing dialysis for the elderly is with us now and will be an ever-increasing problem with the graying of our population. It is projected that by the year 2000 approximately 25% of all Americans will be older than age 65. When the ESRD program was started in 1973 (under the auspices of Public law 92–603), the median patient age was 46 years. Twenty years later the median age of new patients has increased to 61 years, and the total ESRD population now exceeds 200,000 (growing about 10%/year). The U.S. Renal Data System has collected the most precise information about the ESRD population, and all of the following data, figures and tables are from their 1991 Annual Report (U.S. Renal Data System, 1991).

INCIDENCE OF ESRD BY AGE

Forty percent of new dialysis patients are over age 65 years; 33% of this new population have diabetes mellitus (DM) (90% have Type II, and only 10% have Type I DM), and 27% have hypertension. There has been an increase in the incidence of treated ESRD patients over the past 12 years, with the highest incidence in the 65–74 year old age bracket (Figure 10.1). However, the most dramatic rate increase (fourfold) occurred in the age group over 74 years (Table 10.1). A total of 41,317 patients were registered as starting ESRD therapy during the year 1989, and this accounts for an overall rate of 166 new cases per million population (12 per million in the age range 0–19 years and 590 per million among patients aged 65–74 years).

Growth reached a high of 17.9% from 1988 to 1989 in patients aged more than 75 years in contrast to a 3% growth for young adults. The incidence per million population for patients ages 65–74 years increased by 5.3% from 1987 to 1988 but by 13.2% from 1988 to 1989 (the most recent year with full demographic data) (see Figure 10.2).

SURVIVAL PROBABILITIES IN ESRD PATIENTS

Survival is a measurable outcome for patients receiving renal replacement therapy. Mortality for the ESRD population is high rela-

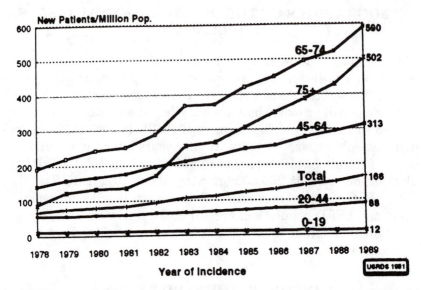

FIGURE 10.1 Incidence rates per million population of treated ESRD, by age, 1978–89, unadjusted (Medicare patients only.)

tive to the general population. As expected, the number of deaths increases more rapidly with each increasing age group. Renal replacement therapy can prolong life, but the expectations are limited (Figure 10.3). In the U.S. population life expectancy after age 59 is over 20 years. For the ESRD population after age 59, life expectancy is only 4.2 years, and this compares to 4.3-year survival for a patient of the same age with colon cancer. The patient over 85 years with ESRD has a 25% chance of dying within the first 90 days after initiation of dialysis. For the group aged 65–69 years,

TABLE 10.1 Treated ESRD Incidence Counts and Rates by Age Group, 1989

Age	Count	Percent of Total	Incidence per Million*
Total	41,317	100.0%	166
0-19	861	2.1%	12
20-44	8,740	21.2%	88
45-64	14,561	35.2%	313
65-74	10,727	26.0%	590
75 +	6,428	15.6%	502

*Incidence rates are unadjusted.

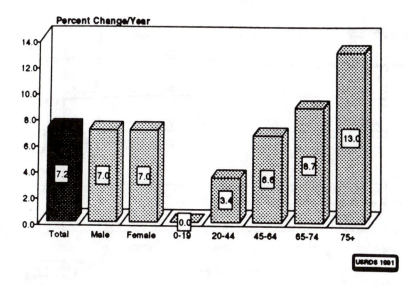

FIGURE 10.2 Change in ESRD incidence rates for the years 1984–86 versus 1987–89 by total, sex, and age. total rate adjusted for age, race, and sex. Rates by sex adjusted for age and race. Rates by age adjusted for sex and race. Percent annual compound rates of change are shown. (Medicare patients only.)

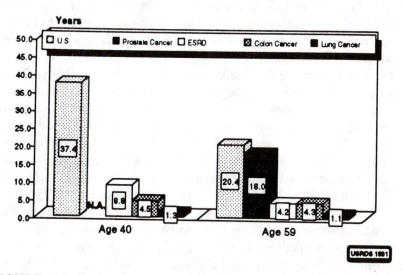

FIGURE 10.3 Expected remaining lifetime in years at age 40 and age 59 for ESRD population, 1989, and for prostate cancer population, colon cancer population, lung cancer population, and general U.S. population, 1988.

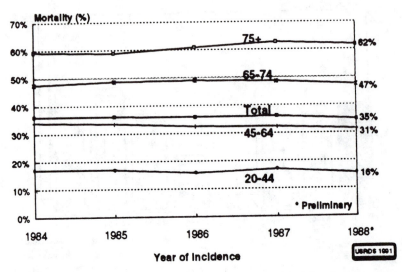

FIGURE 10.4 Two-year mortality rates (after 90 days) for four age groups, adjusted for race, sex, and primary diagnosis. Incident cohort is 1984–88. (Medicare patients only, preliminary.)

mortality drops to 11% in the first 90 days, with a survival rate of 70% at 1 year. This reflects the high incidence of comorbid conditions in the elderly, which leads to a higher death rate shortly after initiation of treatment.

For the 5 years 1984–1989, there was no change in the 2-year mortality for all age groups; patients 65–74 years old had a 47% mortality, and it rose to 62% mortality for patients 75 years and older (Figure 10.4). Myocardial infarction and other cardiac diseases are the most common causes of death, with septicemia and withdrawal from dialysis being the second and third most common reported causes for death in patients over 64 years. Patients with DM withdrew from dialysis three times more commonly than those with other diseases that cause ESRD. The treatment modality data for patients over age 65, in 1989, showed the following: 81.8% receive center hemodialysis, 9.1% receive continuous ambulatory/continuous cycling peritoneal dialysis (CAPD/CCPD), 2.7% have a functioning transplant, and 1.4% receive home hemodialysis.

EXPENDITURES FOR ESRD BENEFICIARIES

In addition to increased mortality risks, ESRD patients experience greater morbidity; hospitalization for dialysis patients strongly

TABLE 10.2 Annual Expenditures for ESRD Patients (1989) Data)

Total Expenditures—$6 billion
   4.4 billion Federal
   2.6 billion State, Private

Per capita—$30,900

1984–1989—annual increase of 13.4%

In-patient expenditures—$42,000/patient/year
   9x higher than all Medicare enrollees

Increasing costs due to increased number of beneficiaries—0.6%/patient/year
   increase (1984–1988)

correlates with the age of the patient and the presence of diabetes. Median number of days per year hospitalized after 1 year on dialysis for the patient over 65 years is 15 days. This represents a five-fold increase over the same age group without ESRD. This translates to an estimated Medicare payment per capita of $30,900 (federal only, 1989). Total medical payments in 1989 for care of the ESRD population, from all sources (federal, state, private), was approximately $6 billion. Inpatient expenditures per person receiving dialysis were almost $42,000 per year in 1989, nine times higher than for all Medicare enrollees (Table 10.2). The federal government pays 72% of this total ($4.4 billion) and the amount shows an 11% increase in payments over the previous year, with an annual increase of 13.4% over the previous 5 years. The Prospective Payment Assessment Commission's 1992 Annual Report to Congress shows that during 1984–1989 the total Medicare expenditures grew about 9% annually (less than the rate for ESRD services). A large part of the growth for ESRD beneficiaries was due to an increase in the number of enrollees, not an increase in expenditures per patient. While the number of people qualifying for ESRD benefits increased by an average of 9.5% annually from 1984 to 1989, the total Medicare population grew at only 2% a year over the same five year period. The proportion of ESRD beneficiaries over age 65 with diabetes or hypertension, the group with the highest expenditures, have increased at the fastest rate.

The payment rate for dialysis has remained essentially the same since 1983, increasing only 0.6% per patient per year over the 5-year period 1984 to 1989. The prospective Composite Rate Payment

System has controlled Medicare expenditures for dialysis services. However, total spending for dialysis patients continues to grow rapidly because of the increase in the number of beneficiaries who are sicker and use a greater volume of Medicare services.

MEDICAL COMPLICATIONS OF DIALYSIS IN THE ELDERLY

Consistently improving technology makes the dialytic process easier, but the patient population receiving dialysis has become older and more seriously ill because of more comorbid conditions. Patients are being kept alive for longer periods of time, and this allows for the underlying medical problems to become major clinical issues. This is reflected by more frequent and longer hospitalizations than occurred a decade ago. In addition to the medical problems that occur with normative aging, there are several specific issues that affect the elderly renal-failure patient on dialysis. The following discussion will be limited to medical problems specifically seen in the older dialysis population.

Cardiovascular

Hypertension is commonly present in elderly patients with ESRD. As a consequence of long-standing hypertension there is a high incidence of hypertensive heart disease. An increase in left ventricular (LV) muscle mass is seen in the older patients sustained by dialysis, which increases with the duration of dialysis. The enlarged heart, a consequence of concentric and eccentric hypertrophy, can improve by normalizing both volume and pressure overload (Leenen, Smith Khanna, & Oreopoulos, 1985). Restoration of blood pressure to normal can improve LV performance, and aggressive antihypertensive therapy may prevent deterioration in patients who have normal LV function at the start of dialysis. Cardiac dysfunction may present greater problems in the patient on hemodialysis than in one on peritoneal dialysis since the latter often permits better control of hypertension. However, the hemodynamic advantages of CAPD over intermittent hemodialysis are not translated into prolonged survival (Huting & Schutterle, 1992). Survival appears to be independent of the modality of therapy as long as cardiac function can be improved. Older patients with angina pectoris tend not to survive but mortality does not appear to be related to duration of CAPD, arterial blood pressure, hemoglobin, serum creatinine, blood urea nitrogen, or parathyroid hormone concentrations. Patients who have the poorest survival have a lower mean LV ejection fraction, higher LV end-systolic volume index, and a shorter mean LV ejection time (Huting & Alpert, 1992), as measured by echocardiography.

Uremia per se appears to produce a cardiomyopathy that improves with any form of dialysis but does not totally reverse until successful kidney transplantation. It is unclear whether this uremic cardiomyopathy represents the consequences of volume/pressure overload or is a distinct entity related to renal failure. Because older patients rarely receive a kidney transplant, their shortened life span might be due to the continued cardiovascular abnormalities that are directly related to uremia.

Consequences of accelerated atherosclerosis lead to premature death in the ESRD population. Hyperlipidemia, especially hypertriglyceridemia, often accompanies chronic renal failure, and these lipid abnormalities are thought to accelerate the atherosclerotic process. It is not known whether treatment of these lipid abnormalities with medication can improve life expectancy in the ESRD population, and a carefully controlled study is needed.

Because of progressive vascular disease with aging and the acceleration of atherosclerotic disease as a consequence of chronic renal failure, both maintenance of a patent vascular access and hemodynamic instability become major problems during dialysis. Autonomic insufficiency also occurs progressively with aging and is accelerated in the presence of DM (both Type I and Type II) (Zoccali, Mallamaci, Ciccarelli, Parlongo & Satnitro, 1992). Hypotension, frequently refractory to volume repletion, creates problems with long-term fluid management in the afflicted patient population. The physiological adaptative increase in peripheral vascular resistance to a decrease in vascular volume caused by ultrafiltration is blunted (Table 10.3). Thus, ultrafiltration during the dialysis procedure is not well tolerated because baroreceptor reflexes are attenuated. Volumetric ultrafiltration therefore becomes an important therapeutic modality in the dialysis prescription in elderly patients. Such volumetric control of fluid removal is a critical component because the weight loss must be achieved slowly and evenly throughout the dialytic process. There is no evidence that biocompatible membranes, compared to standard cellulosic membranes, ameliorate these hemodynamic problems. Repeated episodes of hy-

TABLE 10.3 Dialysis-Related Cardiovascular Complications

Left ventricular hypertrophy (LVH)
—both concentric and eccentric hypertrophy

Accelerated atherosclerotic disease
—role of ESRD-associated hyperlipidemia
—angina pectoris precipitated by dialysis

Uremic cardiomyopathy

Autonomic insufficiency
—especially in diabetics
—blunted physiologic adaptation to fluid removal

potension that prevent necessary ultrafiltration during the hemodialytic procedure are often the major factors necessitating a switch to CAPD, and this option should be explored in all patients who have problems with hemodynamic instability during hemodialysis.

Gastrointestinal

There is an increased incidence of gastrointestinal bleeding in the ESRD patient (Rosenblatt, Crake, Fadem, Welch, & Lifschitz, 1982). Peridialysis bleeding has been shown to be related to hypotension that occurs during the dialytic process because the drop in blood pressure alters the gastric mucosal barrier (Shapiro, Shillman, Steinman, & Silen, 1978). The modality of anticoagulation does not appear to play a role in this bleeding diathesis. Therefore, avoiding hypotension becomes a major therapeutic goal of dialysis in the patient at risk for bleeding. There appears to be less gastrointestinal bleeding with peritoneal dialysis than with hemodialysis because blood pressure changes are not as marked. Frequent causes for gastrointestinal bleeding in the renal failure patient are angiodysplasia/arteriovenous malformations (AVM) and erosive esophagitis (Zuckerman, Cornette, Clouse, Harter, 1985). While all of the other known causes for gastrointestinal bleeding occur in the uremic patient, the marked increased incidence of bleeding from the above makes it important to consider these diagnoses that appear to be more prevalent with advancing years (Table 10.4). Endoscopic photocoagulation is often necessary to stop the bleeding, but the recurrence rate is high. Angiodysplasia is the

TABLE 10.4   Causes for Gastrointestinal Bleeding in Dialysis Patients

Bleeding during dialysis related to hypotension-altered gastric mucosal
barrier

Angiodysplasia/Arteriovenous malformations

Erosive esophagitis

Peptic ulcer disease

Rectal ulcers

most frequent source of recurrent bleeding in patients with renal
failure. In addition, massive hemorrhage from rectal ulcers has
been noted in elderly chronic dialysis patients (Goldberg, Hoffman,
& Wombolt, 1984).

Nutrition

Malnutrition is a much greater problem for the older patient on dialysis than is overeating. A diet history can identify patients with
an inadequate protein intake. Poor dietary intake occurs because of
many factors: anorexia, nausea/vomiting (especially on dialysis
days), changes in smell and taste, socioeconomic status that inhibits food purchases, inadequate understanding of the dietary instructions, food fadism beginning beforehand and/or with the development of renal failure (Steinman, 1992; Steinman & Mitch, 1989).
It is important to question the dialysis patient about problems with
chewing (i.e., loose teeth, ill-fitting dentures), dysphagia, abdominal pain, early satiety, postprandial fullness, diarrhea, or constipation. By paying attention to detail one can frequently avert
problems.

Signs of malnutrition are seen in the first year of dialysis in two
thirds of patients, more commonly if the patient is maintained by
hemodialysis rather than peritoneal dialysis (Vujic, Petrovic, & Ra-
donvanovic, Popovic, 1991). The elderly patient on chronic hemodialysis commonly has evidence of malnutrition with low-calorie
intake, but there appears to be no overall correlation between nutritional status and socioeconomic status (Fierro & Barria, 1989).

Malnutrition can be avoided in patients if they adhere to their
prescribed diet with adequate protein and calorie intake (Car-

TABLE 10.5   Approach to Malnutrition in Dialysis

Take a detailed diet history

Provide specific diet prescription
  —Protein 1.0–1.4 g/kg/day
  —Calories 38–45 kcal/kg/day

Provide supplements
  —Multivitamins (with iron and folate)
  —Glucose polymer (polycose)
  —Fish protein
  —Intradialytic parenteral nutrition

Provide adequate dialysis

---

vounis, Carvounis, & Hung, 1986). Maintenance hemodialysis patients have normal energy expenditures and approximate normal requirements for maintenance of protein balance, body weight and body fat. It is recommended that the chronic dialysis patient, of any age, eat a minimum of 1 g protein per kilogram per day, and an intake of 1.4 g protein per kilogram per day should be the goal. Nitrogen balance, many plasma amino acids values, changes in body weight, midarm circumference, midarm muscle area, and body fat all correlate with energy intake. An average intake of about 38 kcal per kilogram of desirable weight per day is necessary to maintain nitrogen balance in the chronic dialysis patient (Marckmann, 1988), but it is more desirable for the chronic dialysis patient to consume between 40–45 kcal/kg/day. Dietary supplements may help to meet this goal.

Energy supplementation with a glucose polymer (Polycose) is said to have a beneficial effect on the nutritional status of hemodialysis patients (Allman et al., 1990), as well as body fat and lean body mass, without significant effect on plasma triglycerides, urea, or creatinine. A fish protein supplement was found to increase body weight in elderly patients maintained on dialysis and restore abnormal plasma amino acid profiles and amino acid ratios to normal (Tietze & Pedersen, 1991). Intradialytic parenteral nutrition (IDPN) has been suggested as a way to help correct the protein-calorie malnutrition in the elderly because this form of nutritional supplement may increase spontaneous eating (Cano et al., 1990). Despite a high fat content in the IDPN feedings there appears to be no adverse effect on plasma lipid levels (Table 10.5).

It is not known if conventional dialysis therapy with a relatively liberal diet can result in improved nutritional parameters, but adequate nutrition in the elderly remains a concern. Strong efforts should be made to increase protein intake to more than the levels earlier accepted as adequate. It is not yet known if the resulting improvement in nutritional parameters can be translated into decreased morbidity and mortality.

Adequate nutrition of dialysis patients can be achieved only if there is a sufficient amount of dialysis. A thorough study by Lindsey and Spanner (1989) suggests that, without adequate dialysis clearances nutritional intake remains less than prescribed, and this ultimately results in negative nitrogen balance. A greater degree of efficiency may be achieved with biocompatible membranes (those that do not activate complement) than with standard cellulosic membranes.

Dialysis itself is a catabolic event. Net protein degradation and negative nitrogen balance occur during hemodialysis. With the dialytic process there is a removal of amino acids, peptides, glucose metabolites (pyruvate, lactate), and glucose (if a glucose-free dialysate is used). It has been shown that fasting patients, on the average, lose about 7 g of free amino acids and about 2–3 g of peptides or bound amino acids during hemodialysis (Wolfson, Jones, & Kopple, 1982). An increase in energy expenditure occurs with dialysis, with resultant net protein degradation occurring with the procedure (Farrell & Hone, 1980). It is common practice for patients not to eat during the dialysis procedure, and nutrient losses must be replaced from endogenous stores. Lipolysis is stimulated under these circumstances and accentuated by the use of heparin to prevent clotting during the dialytic process. If the energy intake is low, protein wasting may occur and at the same time stimulate gluconeogenesis (Steinman & Mitch, 1989). Therefore, it is critical to have a dialysis prescription that allows effective urea clearance, no matter what dialyzer membrane is employed. The end result is that chronic dialysis patients with a poor nutritional status have a highly increased mortality (Marckmann, 1989).

When anthropometry, transferrin levels, and relative body weight mass are used as measures of nutrition, there appears to be no systematic difference between patients on hemodialysis and those treated with CAPD (Slomowitz, Monteon, Grosvenor, Laidlaw, & Kopple, 1989). Frequent assessment of the nutritional status is mandatory for optimal nourishment because it has been shown that the hemodialysis patient has a loss of muscle mass and an increase in total body fat when followed over a 3-year period (Biasioli, Petrosino, Cavallini, Zambello, & Porena, 1992). Muscle wasting is a common event in patients with chronic renal failure; this is due to both reduced net synthesis and increased oxidation rates of protein in a postabsorptive state (Berkelhammer et al., 1987).

Musculoskeletal

Renal osteodystrophy is a common event in the dialysis population, and the incidence of the problem increases with the duration of dialysis. In addition to secondary hyperparathyroidism, there are also problems with aluminum-induced bone disease, iron-induced bone disease, and beta-2–microglobulin–induced amyloidosis. Severe destructive bone disease with a fatal cervical spondyloarthropathy has been described in long-term dialysis patients, related both to amyloid deposition in the bone and to long-standing hyperparathyroidism (Allard et al., 1992). After 10 years of hemodialysis, dialysis-associated arthropathy is likely to occur no matter what type of dialysis membrane is used, and the prevalence of this disorder increases with the patient's age and duration of dialysis. Carpal tunnel syndrome is a common event that increases with duration of dialysis and is due to amyloid deposition induced by beta-2–microglobulin (Kessler et al., 1992). Crystal-induced inflammation has been known for many years to produce a painful pseudogout syndrome in the chronic renal failure patient treated by dialysis (Moskowitz, Vertes, Schwartz, Marshall, & Friedman, 1969).

Genitourinary

Acquired cystic disease of the kidney is noted in patients maintained on hemodialysis for many years. Renal cell carcinoma of the clear cell type has been shown to develop from these cystic areas. Atypical epithelial hyperplasia, a precursor of renal cell carcinoma, has been identified as arising from these cystic areas (Lin, Saklayen, Ehrenpresis, & Hillman, 1992). Although the incidence of renal cell carcinoma arising in acquired cystic disease of the kidney is on the rise, the issue of how to manage these patients is unsettled at this time.

QUALITY-OF-LIFE ISSUES

Some elderly patients on dialysis are easy to care for because they readily accept their current situation. They feel grateful for extension of their life, having fulfilled many of life's objectives. These patients accept their loss of vision, decreased hearing, short-term memory loss, and problems with ambulation with a certain degree of resignation and dignity. The extension of life is accepted in the form of compliance with the medical regimen and a great deal of independence. A survey showed patients over age 65 years (mean age 72) scored better on life satisfaction than did patients under 55 years and those aged 55–64. These elderly patients reported less stress with dialysis treatment than did younger patients (Winearls, Oliver, & Auer, 1992). Most older patients express satisfaction with life while philosophically accepting the limits of treatment. Any extension of quality of life is appreciated as patients begin to understand the death alternative to dialytic care. In contrast, the younger patient initiating dialysis may be resentful about the development of a debilitating disease in the prime of life, and this can be expressed as noncompliance with their medication and/or dialysis schedule. These younger patients tend to focus on loss and limitation caused by their ESRD.

An opposite response in other elderly patients may be described as "giving up," becoming completely dependent upon others for their care. They exhibit no desire and make no attempt to help themselves in any way, with both overt and covert signs of depression. This totally dependent group of patients frequently feels isolated because of loss of loved ones. Subsequently, they make the most demands on the dialysis staff and generate the most frustration among caregivers because their helplessness is not supported by objective criteria. A large study of the elderly on dialysis showed more functional disability, less frequent walking for exercise, decreased ability to do the things they would like to do, and lower levels of perceived mastery over their lives than occurred in the young patients (Kutner & Brogan, 1992). This elderly group on dialysis were more likely to report a need for health-related aides or services. The residual impairments of disabled elderly persons challenge rehabilitation professionals to address quality-of-life issues.

The goal of any dialysis team is to foster as much independence as is possible. However, natural prejudice against the aged is as evident in the dialysis unit as elsewhere. Caregivers naturally assume that older patients, as defined by physical appearance, apathy, depression, chronological age, or nearness to death, want to be totally cared for both on and off dialysis (Boag & Genevay, 1992). It is critical that the staff caring for the aged patient not assume this prejudicial stance but encourage independence. It is often easier and quicker to provide the care than to allow independence and encourage participation of the patient in his or her own care.

A positive attitude to initiation of dialysis is essential. It is acceptable to discontinue dialysis if the patient does not derive overall benefit from treatment. Repeated discussions with competent patients will generally lead to the patient's asking to stop dialysis if life is a miserable existence. Nephrologists agree about the management of requests to withdraw dialysis in competent patients or incompetent patients with clear prior wishes; they disagree about the management of incompetent patients with unclear prior wishes (Singer, 1992). Decisions to withhold dialysis are more frequent than decisions to withdraw it. Starting dialysis is not a commitment to continuing this treatment indefinitely if the patients are not enjoying their existence. The best approach is to empower patients to make decisions about their life. They usually will make decisions their caretakers can support. The same discussion can be held with the family of the incompetent patient. To keep a patient "existing" on dialysis is not quality care. Again, repeated conversations are necessary to determine the patient's advance directives. To improve advance directives it is recommended that the physician explicitly ask patients how strictly they want their advance directives followed and what factors they want considered in making decisions (Hammes, Dahlberg, & Colvin, 1991; Kjellstrand, 1992; Neumann, 1991; Riley & Pristave, 1992; Sehgal, 1992).

SHOULD DIALYSIS BE RATIONED ON THE BASIS OF AGE?

If rationing is employed, then it is important to make the process explicit, visible, specific, systematic, and acceptable. How to allocate resources thoroughly and responsibly is the major issue (Barnes, Johnson, Kent, & Thacker, 1992; Slepian, 1991). Should we adopt a nationwide Oregon Health Plan, which utilizes a published index to stratify competing claims to health care? The comparative benefits of each service to the population is the guiding principle in this process, with the emphasis on overall health rather than the treatment of disease (Porter, 1991). A model needs to be developed that balances individual rights versus societal and financial commitment in supplying the tax dollars for health care for all society, not just those currently on Medicaid. To ration resources on the basis of age would be a a draconian approach. Currently, we ration patient access to services through our insurance coverage rather than rationing services (Rubin, 1991). Practice guidelines are essential in the area of dialysis because of the need to have a uniform approach to everyone. Although age is not now a limiting factor for accepting patients for dialysis, financial support in days of cost containment is becoming an issue. Should we treat all patients who would benefit from dialysis? No individual can make that decision in isolation. If our society decides that renal replacement therapy for elder citizens is too costly, then let it be made explicit. Nephrologists should not proceed without guidelines and make decisions in a vacuum while dealing with government/societal financial pressures. An unwritten, unspoken policy is not acceptable.

References

Allard, J. C., Artze, M. E., Porter, G., Chandur-Mnaymneh, L. de Velasco R., & Perez G. O. Fatal destructive cervical spondyloarthropathy in two patients on long-term dialysis. *Am J Kidney Dis, 19*: 81–85. 1992.

Allman, M. A., Stewart, P. M., Tiller, D. J., Horvath, J. S., Duggin, G. G., & Truswell, A. G. Energy supplementation and the nutritional status of hemodialysis patients. *Am J Clin Nutr, 51*: 558–562. 1990.

Barnes, J. N., Johnson, P. T., Kent, R. E., & Thacker, J. Age and dialysis. *Lancet, 339*: 432. 1992.

Berkelhammer, C. H., Baker, J. P., Leiter, L. A., Uldall, P. R., Whittall, R., Slater, A., & Wolman, S. L. Whole-body protein turnover in adult hemodialysis patients as measured by 13C-leucine. *Am J Clin Nutr, 46*: 778–783. 1987.

Biasioli, S., Petrosino, L., Cavallini, L., Zambello, A., & Porena, P. Is it possible to improve the nutritional status of dialysis patients? *Clin Ter, 140*: 23–30. 1992.

Boag, J., & Genevay B. The impact of aging on dialysis: Human and technical considerations. *Dialysis and Transplantation, 21*: 124–127. 1992.

Cano, N., Labastie-Coeyrehourg, J. Lacombe, P., Stroumza, P., di Costanzo-Dufetel, J., Durbec, J. P., Coudray-Lucas, C., & Cynober, L.: Perdialytic parenteral nutrition with lipids and amino acids in malnourished demodialysis patients. *Am J Clin Nutr, 52*: 726–730. 1990.

Carvounis, C. P., Carvounis, G., & Hung, MH. Nutritional status of maintenance hemadialysis patients. *Am J Clin Nutr, 43*: 946–954. 1986.

Farrell, P. C., & Hone, P.W. Dialysis-induced catabolism. *Am J Clin Nutr, 33*: 1417–1422. 1980.

Fierro, J. A., & Barria, M. S. Nutritional assessment of patients on chronic hemodialysis: What is our reality? *Rev Med Chil, 117*: 766–772. 1989.

Glicklich, D. Acquired cystic kidney disease and renal cell carcinoma: A review. *Seminars in Dialysis, 4*: 273–283.1991.

Goldberg, M., Hoffman, G. C., & Wombolt, D. G. Massive hemorrhage from rectal ulcers in chronic renal failure. *Ann Intern Med, 100*: 397. 1984.

Hammes, B. J., Dahlberg, P., & Colvin, E. Advance directives by dialysis patients: A practical approach to tough ethical decisions. *Nephrol News Issues, 5*: 18–22. 1991.

Horina, J. H., Holzer, H., Reisinger, E. C., Krejs, G. J., & Neugebauer, J. S. Elderly patient and chronic hemodialysis. *Lancel, 339*–183. 1991.

Huting, J., & Alpert, M. A. Progression of left ventricular hypertrophy in end-stage renal disease treated by continuous ambulatory peritoneal dialysis depends on hypertension and hypercirculation. *Clin Cardiol, 15*: 190–196. 1992.

Huting, J., & Schutterle, G. Cardiovascular factors influencing survival in end-stage renal disease treated by continuous ambulatory peritoneal dialysis. *Am J Cardiol, 69*: 123–127. 1992.

Kessler, M., Netter, P., Azoulay, E., Mayeux, D., Pere, P., & Gaucher, A. Dialysis-associated arthropathy: a multicentre survey of 171 patients receiving hemodialysis for over 10 years. The Cooperative Group on Dialysis-associated Arthropathy. *Br J Rheumatol, 31*: 157–162. 1992.

Kjellstrand, C. M. Who should decide about your death? *JAMA, 267*: 103–104. 1992.

Kutner, N. G., & Brogan, D. J.: Assisted survival, aging, and rehabilitation needs: comparison of older dialysis patients and age-matched peers. *Arch Phys Med Rehabil, 73*: 309–315. 1992.

Leenen, F. H., Smith, D. L., Khanna, R., & Oreopoulos, D. G. Changes in left ventricular hypertrophy and function in hypertensive patients started on continuous ambulatory peritoneal dialysis. *Am Heart J, 110*: 102–106. 1985.

Lin, J. I., Saklayen, M., Ehrenpresis, M., & Hillman, N. M. Acquired cystic disease of kidney associated with renal cell carcinoma in chronic dialysis patients. *Urology, 39*: 190–193. 1992.

Lindsey, R. M., & Spanner, E. A hypothesis: the protein catabolic rate is dependent upon the type and amount of treatment in dialyzed uremic patients. *Am J Kidney Dis, 13*: 382–389. 1989.

Marckmann, P. Nutritional status and mortality of patients in regular dialysis therapy. *J Intern Med, 226*: 429–432. 1989.

Marckmann, P. Nutritional status of patients on hemodialysis and peritoneal dialysis. *Clin Nephrol, 29*: 75–78. 1988.

Marckmann, P., Skott, H. C., & Jorgensen, K. A. A longitudinal study of the nutritional status of chronic dialysis patients. *Ugeskr Laeger, 152*: 812–814. 1990.

Moskowitz, R. W., Vertes, V., Schwartz, A., Marshall, G., & Friedman, B. Crystal-induced inflammation associated with chronic renal failure treated with periodic hemodialysis. *Am J Med, 47*: 450–460. 1969.

Neumann, M. E. Advance directives: a sign of the times. *Nephrol News Issues, 5*: 42–43. 1991.

Porter, G. A. The Oregon Health Plan. *American Kidney Fund Newsletter, 3*: 4–6. 1991.

Prospective Payment Assessment Commission 1992 Annual Report to Congress, Washington, DC.

Riley, J., & Pristave, R. Patient Self-Determination Act hope to make decisions on continuation of care easier. *Nephrol News Issues, 6*: 32–34. 1992.

Rosenblatt, S. G., Crake, S., Fadem, S., Welch, R., & Lifschitz, M. D. Gastrointestinal blood loss in patients with chronic renal failure. *Am J Kidney Dis, 4*: 232–236. 1982.

Rothenberg, L. S. Ethical concerns for the elderly with ESRD. *Advances in Peritoneal Dialysis, 6*: 6–10. 1990.

Rubin, R. J. Health care rationing. *The nephrologist response. American Kidney Fund Newsletter, 3*: 1–3. 1991.

Sehgal, A., Galbraith, A., Chesney, M., Schoenfeld, P., Charles G., & Lo, B. How strictly do dialysis patients want their advance directives followed? *JAMA, 267*: 59–63. 1992.

Shapiro, N., Shillman, J. J., Steinman, T. I., & Silen, W. Gastric mucosal permeability and gastric acid secretion before and after hemodialysis in patients with chronic renal failure. *Surgery, 83*: 528–535. 1978.

Singer, P. A. Nephrologists' experience with and attitudes towards decidions to forego dialysis. The End-Stage Renal Disease Network of New England. *J Am Soc Nephrol, 2*: 1235–1240. 1992.

Slepian, F. Health care rationing. The case for rationing. *American Kidney Fund Newsletter, 3*: 1–3. 1991.

Slomowitz, L. A., Monteon, F. J., Grosvenor, M., Laidlaw, S. A., & Kopple, J. D. Effect of energy intake on nutritional status in maintenance hemodialysis patients. *Kidney Int, 35*: 704–711. 1989.

Steinman, T. I. Patients selection means back to the Dark Ages. *Nephrology News and Issues, 6*: 37. 1991.

Steinman, T. I. Right to life versus quality of life: Who decides? *Nephrology News and Issues, 5*: 12–14. 1991.

Steinman, T. I. Nutritional management of the chronic hemodialysis patient. *Seminars in Dialysis, 5*: 155–158. 1992.

Steinman, T. I., & Mitch W. E.: Nutrition in dialysis patients. In: Maher JF, ed. Replacment of Renal Function by Dialysis. Dordrecht, Holland: Kluwer Academic Publishers. 1088–1106. 1989.

Steinman, T.I., & Yager, H. M. Catatonia as a manifestation of uremia. *Am Intern Med, 89*: 74–75. 1978.

Tietze, I. N., & Pedersen, E. B.: Effect of fish protein supplementation on amino acid profile and nutritional status in hemodialysis patients. *Nephrol Dial Transplant, 6*: 948–954. 1991.

U.S. Renal Data System: USRDS 1991 Annual Data Report. Bethesda, MD. National Institutes of Health, NIDDK, 1991.

Vujic, D., Petrovic, M., Radovanovic, L. J., & Popovic, J. Comparative overview of the nutritional status of patients on hemodialysis and peritoneal dialysis. *Srp Arh Celok Lok, 119*: 194–197. 1991.

Winearls, C. G., Oliver, D. C., & Auer, J. Age and dialysis. *Lancet, 339*: 432. 1992.

Wolfson, M., Jones, M. R., & Kopple, J. D. Amino acid losses during hemodialysis with infusion of amino acids and glucose. *Kidney Int, 21*: 500–506. 1982.

Zoccali, C., Mallamaci, E., Ciccarelli, M., Parlongo, S., & Salnitro, F.: The influence of autonomic failure on plasms ANF concentration in uremic patients on chronic hemodialysis. *Clin Nephrol, 37*: 198–203. 1992.

Zuckerman, G. R., Cornette, G. L., Clouse, R. E., & Harter, H. R. Upper gastrointestinal bleeding in patients with chronic renal failure. *Ann Intern Med, 102*: 588–592. 1985.

Chapter Eleven

Joint Replacement in the Aged

Isadore G. Yablon and David J. Covall

One of the commonest causes of disability in the elderly population is degenerative arthritis. Joints permit locomotion and function because of the presence of a unique tissue called hyaline cartilage. It is this viscoelastic tissue that provides the joints with a smooth glistening surface, which has a coefficient of friction approximately 1/5 of that of ice on ice (Salter, 1983). Hyaline cartilage also acts as a shock absorber, resisting compressive forces and thereby enabling us to enjoy an active life.

Articular cartilage, however, is subject to the mechanical effects of wear and tear, especially if it has been damaged or subject to increased contact loads. Further, with aging, certain biochemical changes occur that make it less resilient and more viscous (Mankin, 1982). This results in a thinning and gradual wearing away of the articular surface. Unfortunately, cartilage does not contain any pain endings, so this degenerative process is painless (Bullough, 1992). Sometimes, if the degenerative process is more acute, an inflammatory response may occur within the lining of the joint, the synovium. This will evoke pain because the synovium is richly innervated by sensory nerves, but more often than not the degenerative process is slow and painless. As the subchondral bone loses its articular cartilage covering, it is subject to greater stresses and therefore becomes harder or eburnated. This can result in pain because the subchondral bone is richly innervated by pain fibers.

In the early phases of arthritis conservative measures may offer some relief (Table 11.1). If the patient is obese, weight reduction

TABLE 11.1   Treatment of Osteoarthritis

Encourage weight reduction
Exercise as tolerated
Activity modification
Ambulatory assistive devices
Braces
NSAID
Physiotherapy
Surgery

may be beneficial. Exercise as tolerated helps to maintain muscle tone and may improve the health of the remaining articular cartilage. Modifying activities, ambulatory assistive devices and braces may often offer relief of pain. Nonsteroidal antiinflammatory medication has proved to be of some value, but it must be remembered that all of these measures are temporary and will serve only to slow the degenerative process (Brandt & Slowman-Kovacs, 1986). In the final analysis we still do not know what triggers the wear-and-tear phenomenon and why some patients will develop degenerative arthritis and others will not. Recent evidence suggests that a genetic factor may be involved (Harris, 1986; Peyron, 1986).

There are, of course, other predisposing factors for joint degeneration (Bullough, 1992; Harris, 1986) (Table 11.2). Trauma, infection, rheumatoid arthritis, and diabetes all may have a direct deleterious affect upon articular cartilage. Diabetic patients often suffer from a neuropathy in which protective sensation to the joint is markedly diminished. Because of this, the particular joint or joints are subject to greater than normal stresses without the benefit of protective muscle splinting. Such repeated trauma results in what is called a neuropathic joint, known as a Charcot joint.

Some joints undergo degenerative changes when their blood sup-

TABLE 11.2   Predisposing Factors for Osteoarthritis

Congenital abnormalities (Congenital Dislocation of Hip, Clubfeet)
Recurrent hemarthrosis (hemophilia)
metabolic (gout, Calcium Pyro Phosphate Disorder (CPPD)
Incongruity (2' to A Vascular Necrosis (AVN), slipped capital femoral
    epiphysis, legs-calves-perthes)
Malalignment (genu carum)
Instability Anterior Cruciate Ligament (ACL) deficiency)
Inflammatory disorders (Rheumatoid Arthritis, Ankylosing Spondylitis (AS)

ply is interfered with causing avascular necrosis. A prime example is the hip. This could be idiopathic (Hungerford & Zizik, 1983) or could follow a fracture through the femoral neck. In this case, the blood supply to the bone underneath the articular cartilage may be directly interfered with, resulting in death of the bone. This contributed to a collapse of the subchondral tissue. Because the cartilage loses its underlying support, it develops cracks and fissures that cause the destruction of the joint.

Although there are many forms of surgical treatment to help restore function to a degenerated joint, this chapter will concern itself with joint replacement.

HISTORY

The principle behind joint replacement is to remove the diseased bone and articular cartilage and to insert a prosthesis. The major problem facing the early investigators was that of obtaining a biologically compatible material. One of the earliest attempts was made by the Judet brothers of France, orthopedic surgeons, who developed a nylon prosthesis to replace the femoral head (Judet & Judet, 1950). The nylon, however, showed a high degree of wear and caused a foreign body inflammatory response in the hips in which it was used. In the 1950s, the Moore and the Thompson prostheses were developed by their respective inventors (Moore, 1952; Thompson, 1954). Both of these were made of a stainless steel alloy and were used to replace the femoral head.

Because only one part of the joint—namely the femoral head—was replaced, such an operation was called a hemiarthroplasty. However, the acetabulum forms the other part of the hip joint, and very often it is involved as well. It was not long, therefore before attention was directed to this portion of the joint. Subsequently, in the mid-1960s two early models became available to restore the whole hip joint. One was called a McKee-Farrar (McKee, 1970) prosthesis after the two British orthopedic surgeons who developed it, and the other was called the Charnley prosthesis, designed by another famous British orthopedic surgeon (Charnley, 1979).

The early investigators faced many problems, and the first concerned itself with the anchoring of the prosthetic components. The results with the Moore and Thompson prostheses were not entirely satisfactory because loosening of the stem occurred. The Moore prosthesis tried to overcome this problem by having two fenestrations within the femoral stem in the hope that, once inserted into the femoral canal, bone would grow through these fenestrations and thereby create a so-called biological anchor (Moore, 1952). This, however, did not occur because although bone did grow through the fenestrations, it was generally not sufficient to create a solid support to prevent micromotion of the prosthesis. To address this problem John Charnley (1979) introduced the use of methyl methacrylate, which is a cold-curing cement. This enables the components to be securely anchored and revolutionized the development of better and more diverse prostheses.

The next problem was to determine what was the best articulating surface. The McKee-Farrar prosthesis had a metal femoral head articulating with a metal acetabular cup. The Charnley prosthesis used a metal femoral head which articulated with a teflon acetabular cup. Charnley reasoned that the coefficient of friction would be less for metal on plastic as opposed to metal on metal. He was right: the McKee-Farrar prosthesis and subsequent similar models did not become very popular. Charnley had problems in the beginning because there was excessive wear of the Teflon component, so he began to use high-density polyethylene, which proved to be quite satisfactory (Charnley, 1979; Muller, 1992). Today almost all of the prosthetic components have a metal femoral head articulating with a plastic acetabular cup.

Once the initial problems with the total hip replacement components were addressed and overcome it was only natural that progress would be made with regard to replacing other diseased joints. The knee was next, and in the early 1960s a Toronto orthopedic surgeon, David MacIntosh (1966) introduced a metal replacement for the medial tibial condyle. This was not cemented and inserted in a free fashion. Obviously, the success rate was not high, but it did lead to the modern era of total knee arthroplasty. Using Charnley's concepts, Gunston (1971) designed a prosthesis based on the polycentric motion of the human knee. Leonard Marmor (1976), an American orthopedic surgeon, developed a modular knee system. This system stem had two components for the femoral condyles and two components for the tibial plateaus, which were cemented in place. However, because diseases of the knee frequently involved the cruciate and collateral ligaments, the modular components failed to address knee instability. The subsequent models took this into account and consisted of a single unit to replace both femoral condyles and a single unit to replace both tibial plateaus.

This enables some stability to be built into the prosthesis with remarkable success. Today almost any joint can be replaced with variable results as will be seen.

CURRENT CONCEPTS

General Considerations

Joint replacement is indicated in a functional patient whose joint has been destroyed by any of the arthritides, trauma, or infection. It is important to be extremely careful when doing a total joint replacement in the latter situation because the introduction of a foreign body such as a prosthesis may activate an infection even if it has been quiescent for years. It can be done, but one must be certain that the infection has been eradicated and that the patient be given antibiotics for a number of months after the surgery.

Hip

As mentioned previously, one can do a hemoarthroplasty or a total joint replacement, depending on the pathology. Obviously, if only the head is involved, as is often the case with a fracture or avascular necrosis, then only that portion of the joint need be replaced. Although the older Thompson and Moore prosthetic designs are still available and indicated in a specific population, many orthopedic surgeons would select a bipolar implant instead (Marcus, 1992). This is a device that theoretically allows motion between the prosthetic head, femoral prosthesis, and acetabulum; older devices allowed motion only between the femoral head and acetabulum (Giliberty, 1983). The bipolar prostheses, whether cemented or press-fit, have more satisfying results than the Moore prosthesis because of the aforementioned feature; that is, they tend to produce less acetabular pain (Figure 11.1a and 11.1b).

When both the femoral head and acetabulum are destroyed, then a hip replacement is indicated. Most of the implants consist of a metal femoral component that articulates with a metal-backed acetabular plastic cup (Figure 11.2).

At this writing, more and more orthopedic surgeons are getting away from using cement, especially with regard to the acetabular cup. There have been a number of problems with polymethylmethacrylate cement even though it has greatly enhanced the use of

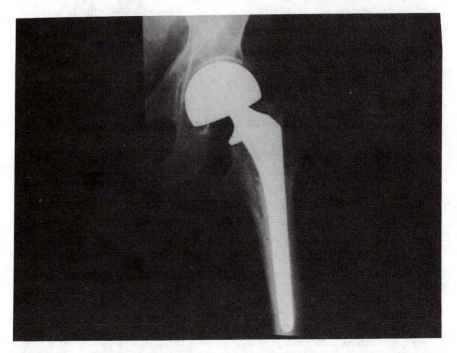

FIGURE 11.1A Bipolar endoprosthesis. Anteroposterior radiograph of the left hip of an 82-year-old male who underwent a hemo-arthroplasty for a displaced femoral neck fracture.

implanting articular components. Cement basically does two things; it distributes the weight-bearing load more evenly across the bone, and it helps to secure the fixation of the components. It must be understood that cement is not a glue; in fact, the cement is not at all sticky. It acts by anchoring itself to the bone by infiltrating the cancellous interstices. Even though cement works, it has been found that aseptic loosening does occur and increases over time (Callaghan, 1992). Further, should infection supervene, the presence of cement can make an otherwise difficult complication even more formidable. Alternative means of anchoring the prosthetic components have been developed, especially for the younger population with their heavier and greater demands. The most common ways of doing this consist of porous-coating the proximal portion of the femoral components and the metal backing of the acetabular components with titanium or a suitable cobalt-chromium alloy (Figure 11.3a and 11.3b). The microscopic pores allow for the in-

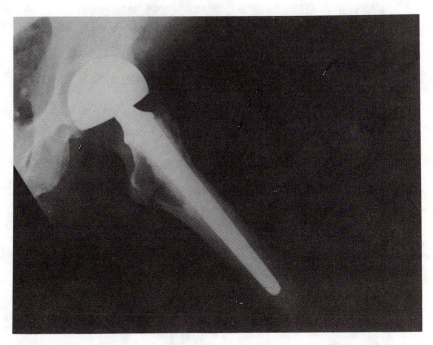

FIGURE 11.1B Lateral radiograph of the hip shown in Figure 11.1A.

growth of cancellous bone once the components have been inserted and allow for a biological anchor to occur (Engh, Bobyn, & Glassman, 1987). More recently the components have been coated with hydroxyapatite, which appears to stimulate the ingrowth of bone to stabilize the prosthesis (Cook, Thomas, Kay, & Jarcho, 1988). The results to date have been satisfactory, but it is still too early to determine whether porous coating or hydroxyapatite is superior to cement (Figures 11.4a, 11.4b and 11.4c).

Knee

There are a number of different models available to address specific problems regarding the knee. If only the medial or lateral compartment is involved, then a unicompartmental can be done. In almost all instances it is the medial compartment rather than the lateral one that is involved. This is because even with a normal valgus angle more weight is borne on the medial side, so it is only

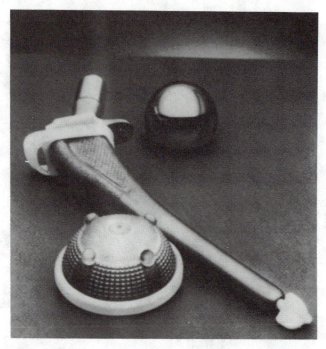

FIGURE 11.2 Example of femoral and acetabular prosthetic components. Courtesy of Howmedica, Rutherford, New Jersey.

natural that this joint space will wear out more quickly. The type of component that is available consists of a metal moon-shaped prosthesis that fits over the femoral condyle and a corresponding tibial component which consists of high-density polyethylene attached to a metal base. These components may be inserted and anchored with or without cement.

In most instances, however, the medial, lateral, and patellar areas are involved, and all of these require replacement. The implants available consist of a single metal prosthesis that fits over the distal end of the femur and a plastic-on-metal tibial component. The femur is cut and reshaped using special jigs and a power-driven saw to conform accurately to the shape of the femoral prosthesis. Similarly, the tibial component is shaped to accept the tibial prosthesis (Laskin & Rieger, 1989). As in the hip, the components are made to be inserted with or without the use of cement. When the patella is involved, which is almost always the case, the diseased articular cartilage is removed down to the sub-

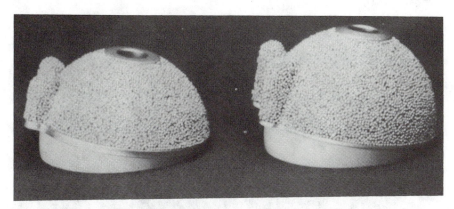

FIGURE 11.3A   Porous coated PCA acetabular cup.
Courtesy of Howmedica, Rutherford, New Jersey.

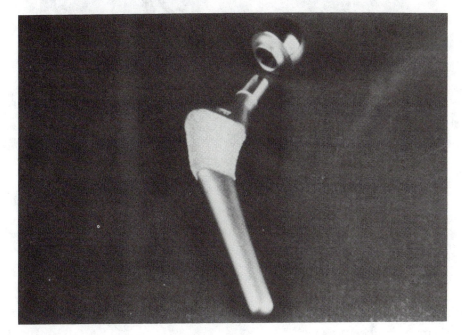

FIGURE 11.3B   Porous coated PCA femoral stem.
Courtesy of Howmedica, Rutherford, New Jersey.

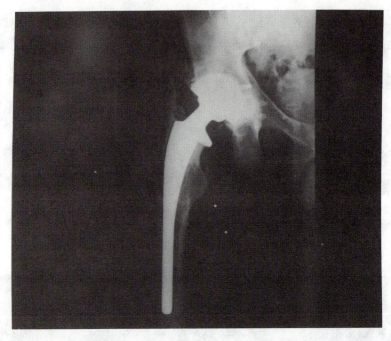

FIGURE 11.4A AP radiograph of right hip of a 38-year-old white male who is 7 years status post right total hip arthroplasty with loosening of the femoral component.

chondral bone, and the articular surface is replaced with a plastic button which articulates with the femoral prosthesis (Figure 11.5a, 11.5b & 11.5c).

The anterior cruciate ligament must generally be sacrificed to permit the tibial component to be properly seated. To compensate for any instability as a result of the loss of this ligament the components are designed to be somewhat constrained. This is made possible by contouring the tibial component in such a way as to prevent excessive rotation and forward gliding. This design can be further modified in instances where the posterior cruciate ligament is absent as well.

Occasionally, gross instability of the knee is present in which both cruciates and the medial and lateral collateral ligaments are either torn or attenuated. This may occur after severe trauma or more commonly in advanced cases of rheumatoid arthritis. In such instances a hinge prosthesis is available. This is a totally constrained device which allows for only flexion and rotation. Because

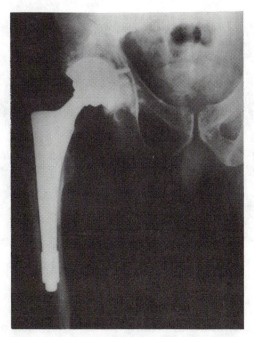

FIGURE 11.4B AP radiograph after revision of the loose hip in Figure 11.4A with a hydroxyapatite Osteolok (Howmedica, Rutherford, New Jersey) femoral cementless stem.

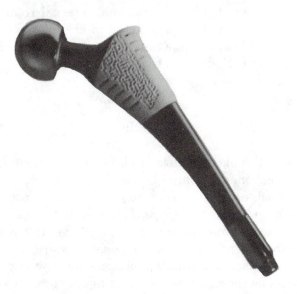

FIGURE 11.4C C) An example of the hydroxyapatite osteolok.
Courtesy of Howmedica, Rutherford, New Jersey.

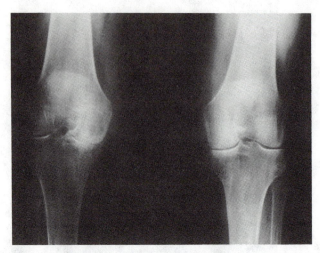

FIGURE 11.5A AP radiograph of bilateral knees of a 68-year-old woman with rheumatoid arthritis.

the femur must rotate internally as full extension occurs and because the hinge prostheses have lacked this compensatory mechanism they have not been very successful and have shown as relatively high incidence of loosening and breakage. Some of the more recent models have taken this terminal internal rotation mechanism into account and have attempted to incorporate this in their design. Nevertheless, a hinge prosthesis should be used with caution and only in patients who will not be making a heavy demand on their knees.

Ankle

Total ankle arthroplasties have not been very successful. Although there are components available, the long-term results have not been that good, especially when compared to the results of ankle fusions (Jensen & Kroner, 1992). A typical total ankle prosthesis consists of a dome-shaped metal component that fits over the talus and a rectangular polyethylene component that replaces the tibial plafond. The reason total ankle replacements have not enjoyed the same success as those in the knee and hip is not fully understood. It is likely that there is a biomechanical reason or problem has not as yet been solved.

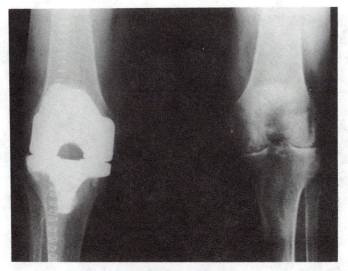

FIGURE 11.5B

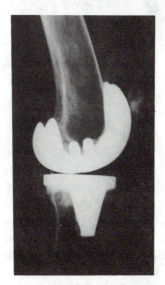

FIGURE 11.5C

AP lateral radiographs of same patient in Figure 11.5A after right total knee arthroplasty.

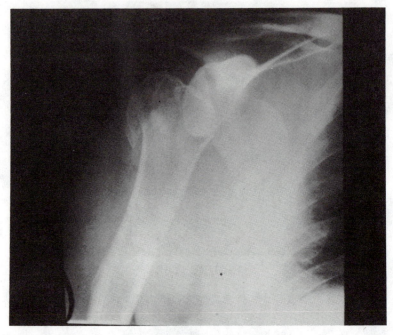

FIGURE 11.6A AP radiograph of the right shoulder of a 62-year-old man who suffered a four-part fracture/dislocation of his proximal humerus.

Shoulder

Prosthetic replacement of the shoulder has been relatively successful. Because the shoulder is a non-weight-bearing joint, it is not always necessary to replace the glenoid. Indeed most operations really consist of a hemiarthroplasty in which only the humeral part is replaced (Neer, 1988). However, when the glenoid is damaged as well, it can be resurfaced. As with the hip and knee, cemented and noncemented components are available, depending on the surgeon's choice. The most common indication for a total shoulder replacement in the elderly is trauma that damages the humeral head and glenoid to such a degree that good reduction is not possible (Figure 11.6a & 11.6b). Other indications are degenerative and rheumatoid arthritis (Craig, 1988).

Elbow

Total elbow replacement is not very common (Goldberg, Figgie, Inglis, & Figgie, 1988). The reason for this is that the upper extrem-

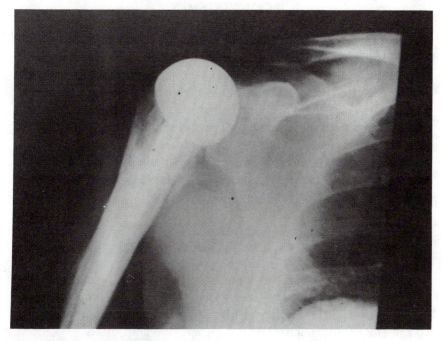

FIGURE 11.6B AP radiograph of the same patient in Figure 6A after a right shoulder hemo-arthroplasty.

ity can still be quite functional even if the elbow is ankylosed in some degree of flexion due to the fact that compensatory motion can be achieved in the shoulder and wrist. However, when the patient is suffering from severe pain secondary to either degenerative or rheumatoid arthritis, a total elbow replacement can be considered. These prostheses fall into three categories: unconstrained, semiconstrained, and constrained. In the unconstrained models the distal humerus is replaced by a metal component that articulates against either a metal or plastic ulnar component and occasionally a radial head replacement. This could be used in an otherwise structurally sound joint. The more commonly used semiconstrained prosthesis is essentially a "sloppy" hinged prosthesis with relatively good results when utilized in a moderately damaged joint. Finally, the constrained type consists of a replacement for the distal humerus and proximal ulna and is hinged. It is rarely used today except in severely damaged unstable joints (Leber & Malone, 1988).

CONCLUSION

Total joint replacement in the elderly has vastly improved the quality of life in this age group as well as being cost-effective (Boettcher, 1992). In prior years patients who were crippled by the various forms of arthritis were either bed-ridden or wheelchair bound. Obviously, with their activity being restricted they succumbed to the complications of inactivity. The development of total joint replacement has enabled these patients to lead more productive and enjoyable lives. Great strides have been made but further work is necessary and in fact is being done to improve the results obtained to date.

• *Editor's Comment* •

This chapter describes in some detail the various methods and prostheses available to replace joints. The authors emphasize the improvement of the quality of life that joint replacement can bring to the elderly incapacitated by degenerative joint disease.

To provide additional information on the risks and benefits of arthroplasty, the editors conducted a MEDLINE search on articles published during the past 3 years on joint replacements in the aged. There were 202 references found, dealing with this broad subject. An analysis of 40 articles on hip replacement and of 39 papers on knee replacement yielded the following information.

Hip replacement: The end results of total hip replacement employing different types of prostheses and different techniques ranged from a high incidence of good and excellent results in 97% of hips followed for 10 years (Papenfus et al., 1992) to a low in 6–12 years of 50% (Boetcher, 1992). The largest series of patients involved 3,777 hips in persons over 80 years old, receiving three different types of prostheses. Good results were obtained in 95% of the survivors alive after the operation for 3–9 years (Lindestrand et al. 1992). However, caution is advised in proceeding with hip replacement in the elderly. Pettine et al. (1992), in studying infectious complications, found good outcomes in 15 patients aged 52 years or younger and failures in 19 patients older than 65 years. Greenfield et al. (1993) caution that coexisting diseases in the aged explain the different rate of recovery from hip replacement, which is more prolonged in the aged.

Knee replacement: The end results of knee replacement range from a high of 98% favorable results in over 3 years (Eskola et al. 1991; Groh et al. 1991) to a low of 71% (Hohl et al. 1992). The 61 patients in this latter group were over 80 years old. The largest multicenter study involved 12,118 patients and showed a high success rate. However, it also included serious infectious complications, and there were 22 amputations necessitated by failed joint replacements (Bengtson & Knudson, 1991). The many reports on joint revisions after complications (Dendrinos et al., 1991; Rand, 1992; Scott, 1991) suggest that a careful weighing of risk versus benefit is essential before making the decision to replace a knee joint. In the very old, even the nondemented, there is the added problem of frequent postoperative delirium (Williams-Russo et al., 1992).

References for Editor's Comment

Bengtson, S., & Knutson, M. *Acta Orthop. Scan*, *62*(4): 301–11. 1991.
Boetcher, W. G. *Clin. Orthop, and Related Research*, (*274*): 30–4. 1992.
Collins, D. M., & McKenzie, J. M. *Clin. Orthop. and Related Research*, (*269*): 9–15. 1991.
Dendrinos, G. K., et al. *Acta Orthop, Belgica*, 57(3): 1274–84. 1991.
Eskola, A., et al. *J. of Orthoplasty*, 7(3): 223–28. 1992.
Greenfield, S., et al. *Medical Care*, *31*(2): 141–54. 1993.
Groh, G. I., et al. *Clin. Orthop. and Related Research*, (*269*): 58–67. 1991.
Hohl, W. M. et al. *Clin. Orthop. and Related Research*, (*273*): 91–97. 1991.
Lindestrand, A., et al. *Acta Orthop, Scandinavica*, *63*(3): 256–9. 1992.
Papenfus, K., et al. *Clin. Orthop. and Related Research*, (*281*): 133–9. 1992.
Pettine, K. A., et al. *Clin. Orthop. and Related Research*, (*266*): 127–32. 1992.
Rand, J. A. *Clin. Orthop. and Related Research*, (*271*): 63–71. 1991.
Scott, R. D. *Clin. Orthoped, and Related Research*, (*271*): 96–100. 1991.

References

Boettcher, W. G. Total hip arthroplasties in the elderly. *Clinical Orthopedics*, *274*: 30. 1992.
Brandt, K. D., & Slowman-Kovacs, S. Nonsteroidal anti-inflammatory drugs in the treatment of osteoarthritis. *Clinical Orthopedics*, *213*: 84. 1986.
Bullough, P. G. *Atlas of orthopedic pathology*. New York: Glower Medical Publishing. 1992.
Callaghan, J. J. Total hip arthroplasty: Clinical perspective. *Clinical Orthopedics*, *276*: 33. 1992.
Charnley, J. Low friction arthroplasty of the hip: Theory and Practice. New York: Springer, Berlin-Heidelberg. 1979.
Cook, S. D., Thomas, K. A., Kay, J. F., & Jarcho, M. Hydroxyapatite-coated ti-

tanium for orthopedic implant applications. *Clinical Orthopedics, 232*: 225. 1988.

Craig, E. V. Total shoulder replacement. *Orthopedics, 11*: 1: 125. 1988.

Engh, C. A., Bobyn, J. D., & Glassman, A. H. Porous coated hip replacement: The factors governing bone ingrowth, stress, shielding and clinical results. *JBJS, 69B*: 45. 1987.

Giliberty, R. P. Hemi-arthroplasty of the hip using a low friction bipolar endoprosthesis. *Clinical Orthopedics, 175*: 86. 1983.

Goldberg, V. M., Figgie, H. E., Inglis, A. E., & Figgie, M. P. Total elbow arthroplasty: Current Concepts Review. *JBJS, 70A*: 778. 1988.

Gunston, F. H. Polycentric knee arthroplasty: Prosthetic simulation of normal knee movement. *JBJS, 53B*: 272. 1971.

Harris, W. H. Etiology of osteoarthritis of the hip. *Clinical Orthopedics, 213*: 20. 1986.

Hungerford, D. S., & Zizik, T. M. Pathogenesis of ischemic necrosis of the femoral head. In The Hip: *Proceeding of the Eleventh Open Scientific Session of the Hip Society*. The C. V. St. Louis: Mosby Co. 1983.

Jensen, N. C., & Kroner, K. Total ankle joint replacement: A clinical follow-up. *Orthopedics, 15*: 2: 236. 1992.

Judet, G., & Judet, R. The use of an artificial femoral head for arthroplasty of the hip. *JBJS, 32B*: 106. 1950.

Laskin, R. S., & Rieger, M. A. The surgical technique for performing a total knee replacement arthroplasty. *Orthopedic Clinic of North America, 20*: 31. 1989.

Leber, C., & Malone, C. P., Jr. Total elbow replacement. *Orthopedic Review, 27*: 9: 857. 1988.

MacIntosh, D. L. Arthroplasty of the knee. *JBJS, 48B*: 179. 1966.

Mankin, H. J. The response of articular cartilage to mechanical injury. *JBJS, 64A*: 640. 1982.

Marcus, R. E., Heintz, J. J., & Pattee, G. A. Don't throw away the Austin Moore. *Journal of Arthroplasty*, 7: 1: 31. 1992

Marmor, L. The modular knee. *Clinical Orthopedics, 120*: 86. 1976.

McKee, G. K. Development of total prosthetic replacement of the hip. *Clinical Orthopedics, 72*: 85. 1970.

Moore, A. J. Metal hip joint: A new self-locking vitallium prosthesis. *South Med J, 45*: 1015. 1952.

Muller, M. E. Lessons of 30 years of total hip arthroplasty. *Clinical Orthopedics, 274*: 22. 1992.

Neer, C. Articular replacement of the humeral head. *JBJS, 37A*: 215. 1988.

Peyron, J. G. Osteoarthritis: The epidemiologic viewpoint. *Clinical Orthopedics, 213*: 13. 1986.

Salter, R. B. *Textbook of disorders and injuries of the musculoskeletal system*. Baltimore: MD. Williams and Williams. 1983.

Thompson, F. R. Two and a half years' experience with a vitallium intramedullary hip prosthesis. *JBJS, 36A*: 489. 1954.

Chapter Twelve

Laparoscopic Surgery in the Aged

Desmond Birkett

Elderly patients have been known for some time to have a higher morbidity and mortality rate than younger patients, particularly when undergoing emergency procedures (Gardener & Palasti, 1990). However, the morbidity and mortality rate for both elective and emergency abdominal operations has improved over the past two decades due to improved anesthetic techniques, better understanding of critical care management of the elderly, and greater use of intensive care units. Nevertheless, elderly patients continue to have a higher morbidity and mortality than do younger patients because of a higher incidence of associated comorbidity factors such as pulmonary, renal, and vascular diseases (Herron, Jesseph, & Harkin, 1960). Even in those elderly patients in whom there are no overt comorbidity factors, the morbidity and mortality rates are higher because of nonevident compromise of the pulmonary, renal, and cardiac systems (Kaplan et al., 1972; Tandon & Tsapogas, 1975).

It is well recognized that any elderly patient will not handle trauma or recover from trauma as well as younger patients. A surgical operation is nothing more than controlled trauma, and the physiological responses to it are the same as those to trauma. Any operation that reduces the amount of trauma to a patient, young or old, is in the best interest of the patient.

Laparoscopy has played an important part in gynecological practice for many years, but by and large this is in a young healthy population. It is only since the first laparoscopic cholecystectomy in 1987 by Mouret of Lyon, France, and its development and popularization by Perissat in Bordeaux (Perissat, Collet, & Belliard, 1990) and Dubois in Paris that a significant number of elderly patients have undergone laparoscopic procedures. It has become extremely clear that patients who undergo laparoscopic cholecystectomy recover faster, have shorter hospital stays, and return to work sooner than do those patients who undergo open cholecystectomy (Glinatsis, Griffith, & McMahon, 1992). The two major differences between the two procedures are the lack of a large incision and the lack of retraction and handling of the intestines. It is this reduction of trauma combined with a lesser injury response that is responsible for a faster recovery. Elderly patients, with their known problem of comorbidity should benefit even more than younger ones from this lesser trauma.

GALLSTONE TREATMENT OPTIONS

The first cholecystectomy was performed in Berlin by Carl Langenbuch in 1886; a number of years later Courvoisier added common duct exploration for the management of common duct stones. Since then open cholecystectomy has been the "gold standard" for the management of gallstone disease, although this now seems to be changing. Over the years there have been many attempts to find a nonoperative method of treating gallstones. In the early 1970s gallstone dissolution with chenodeoxycholic acid was attempted (Sanzinger, Hoffman, Schoenfield, & Thistle, 1972). This did more for the understanding of the formation of gallstones than for the treatment of the disease. Only the small number of patients with small cholesterol stones in a functioning gallbladder benefited from this form of treatment (Schoenfield, Lachin, 1981). Other disadvantages were the length of time it took to dissolve the stones, the presence of symptoms in some patients until the stones were completely dissolved, and the high incidence of recurrence after the completion of treatment.

Stone dissolution using methyl-tert-butyl ether, perfused through a fine catheter placed in the gallbladder via a transhepatic route, was described by Thistle et al. (1989). This was highly effective at dissolving cholesterol stones but was labor-intensive, taking up to 24 hours to complete stone dissolution and suffering from the problem of stone recurrence since the gallbladder was left in place.

Extracorporeal shockwave lithotripsy combined with ursodeoxycholic acid dissolution of the stone fragments was introduced by Sackmann et al. (1988) in the mid-1980s. This was received with great enthusiasm because of the appeal of a totally noninvasive ambulatory technique. However, the technique required a functioning gallbladder and noncalcified stones, no greater than three in number and no larger than 2 cm in diameter. It was shown, in a study of patients undergoing cholecystectomy for symptomatic gallstone disease, that only 19% of patients fitted these criteria. Also, of those that were eligible for this form of treatment only 80% were stone-free after 1 year of daily ursodeoxycholic acid therapy.

These attempts were followed by the start of the age of minimal access surgery, in which gallstone lithotripsy and stone extraction was performed via percutaneous access routes to the gallbladder, either transabdominal or transhepatic. The techniques were effective but left the gallbadder in place for the formation of recurrent stones. The development of this technology was soon eclipsed by the introduction of laparoscopic cholecystectomy in 1987, which soon became universally accepted as the preferable way of treating gallbladder stone disease.

LAPAROSCOPIC CHOLECYSTECTOMY

In 1987 Mouret performed the first laparoscopic cholecystectomy in Lyon; later that year Perissat in Bordeaux (Perissat et al., 1990) and Dubois in Paris championed the operation. The following year McKernan introduced the operation to the United States, after which it spread rapidly throughout the world and has now become the standard of care for symptomatic gallstone disease.

Indications for laparoscopic cholecystectomy are no different from what has now come to be called open cholecystectomy, they are the presence of symptomatic gallstones. There are basically few absolute contraindications to laparoscopic cholecystectomy, and these are severe pulmonary disease, such as chronic obstructive pulmonary disease, and severe heart disease. However, there are a series of relative indications depending on the experience and expertise of the operating surgeon. These are acute cholecystitis, previous upper abdominal operations, and pregnancy. Acute cholecystitis is being treated by laparoscopic cholecystectomy more often as the experience of surgeons increases. A history of previous upper abdominal operations gives rise to the chance of intraperitoneal adhesions, which make the operation more difficult but, with increasing experience and the improvement in equipment and techniques, more patients with a history of previous upper abdominal operations are undergoing safe and satisfactory laparoscopic cholecystectomy.

The operation of laparoscopic cholecystectomy is performed under a general anesthetic and sterile conditions. A 1-cm incision is made at the umbilicus, and a Veress needle, 2 mm in diameter and with a safety tip, is introduced into the peritoneal cavity and a pneumoperitoneum to 15 mm of mercury is created by insufflation with carbon dioxide. A 10-mm trocar and sheath, with a safety tip to prevent bowel and vascular injury, is introduced through the umbilical incision into the peritoneal cavity. The laparoscope with camera attached is passed through this sheath into the peritoneal cavity and, under direct vision, three other trocars and sheaths (two 5-mm and one 10-mm) are introduced into the peritoneal cavity for the placement of dissecting and cautery instruments, scissors, and retractors. The gallbladder is retracted and placed on the stretch to enable dissection of the cystic duct and artery. The cystic artery is clipped and divided, and the cystic duct, after cleaning, is opened and the catheter secured in place for a cholangiogram to define the anatomy and find stones in the common bile duct. Should stones be found, the common bile duct is explored through the cystic duct or by a direct choledochotomy of the common bile duct. After the cholangiogram and/or common duct exploration, the cystic duct is clipped off and divided, and the gallbadder is dissected out of the gallbladder bed and removed through one of the large trocar sites.

The patient is mobilized shortly after recovery from anesthesia, starts eating and drinking the evening of the operation, and is usually ready for discharge the next morning after a 1-night hospital stay. Patients return to work soon after the operation, with all patients back to their normal way of life 1 week from the time of the operation.

MANAGEMENT OF COMMON DUCT STONES

If stones are found in the biliary tree at the time of open cholecysytectomy, then the common bile duct is opened and the stones removed by baskets and balloon extraction and the help of choledochoscopy. Stones found on intraoperative cholangiography at the time of laparoscopic cholecystectomy are currently handled in one of three ways: postoperative endoscopic retrograde cholangiopan-creatography (ERCP) and papillotomy, conversion to an open opera-tion for common duct exploration, or laparoscopic common duct ex-ploration at the time of laparoscopic cholecystectomy via the cystic duct or via a choledochotomy with placement of a T-tube (Petelin, 1991; Stoker, Leveillee, McCann, & Maini, 1991). ERCP and papil-lotomy and, to a lesser extent, conversion to an open exploration is the more commonly accepted method of handling stones, but the former does require the patient to undergo two procedures, and the latter requires an open operation. Laparoscopic common duct ex-ploration at the time of cholecystectomy, the preferable method, is becoming more commonly performed as surgeons become comfort-able undertaking laparoscopic procedures.

RESULTS

Patients recover faster from laparoscopic cholecystectomy than from open cholecystectomy. Their hospital stay is shorter, they take fluids and solids faster, and they need less postoperative analgesia. We have found that in our population, with ages ranging from 19 to 82 years, the average length of stay is 1.6 days. In a study comparing open and closed cholecystectomy, the length of operation, time in hospital, and analgesia used in the postoperative period were compared. The la-paroscopic operation averaged 90 minutes, compared with the open operation that took 45 minutes; however, the length of hospital stay was significantly shorter in the laparoscopic group (2 days vs. 5 days) and the complication rate was 7.5% for the laparoscopic group, com-pared to 10% for open cholecystectomy group (Glinatsis et al., 1992). The most significant complication seems to be injury to the common duct, which is reported to be twice the open cholecystectomy rate (Moossa, Easter, Van Sonnenberg, Casola, & D'Agostino, 1992). There is evidence that injury is experience-related; in one study the injuries occurred early in the surgeon's learning curve. With a few precautions and the use of cholangiography at the time of cholecystectomy to de-fine the anatomy, the duct injury rate should be no higher than with open cholecystectomy.

OTHER LAPARSCOPIC OPERATIONS

Laparoscopic cholecystectomy is the best understood general surgi-cal laparoscopic procedure. With the current rapid expansion of la-

paroscopy, many other laparoscopic procedures are being introduced to replace open operations.

Laparoscopic appendectomy has been performed for some time.
However, except in females, where it may be useful in diagnosing
gynecological problems, it is hard to improve on the standard appendectomy through a small incision in the right lower quadrant of
the abdomen, from which the patient recovers quickly. Inguinal
hernia repair is being performed laparoscopically, but again it will
be hard to improve on the standard hernia repair that has been
performed under local anesthesia and as a day case with its good
results, but this procedure needs careful studying. Other procedures, such as laparoscopic Nissen fundoplication, that require a
significant open operation, are spreading, as well as colectomy and
abdominoperineal resection of the rectum.

Laparoscopic rectopexy with a sacral sling for rectal prolapse, an
operation performed almost exclusively in the elderly, is gaining
acceptance, as it also is a less stressful operation for the patient
than an open operation. Other procedures have been reported, such
as splenectomy, adrenalectomy, oversewing perforated ulcers, proximal gastric vagotomy and antrectomy and vagotomy for peptic ulcer disease, gastrojejunostomy and biliary enteric bypass for unre-
sectable carcinoma of the pancreas.

These procedures and others will be developed and refined over
the next few years and will play an important part in the management of elderly patients requiring abdominal operations.

DISCUSSION

A lesser degree of trauma and less physiological stress from a minimal access procedure are almost certainly the reasons for the rapid
recovery of patients undergoing laparoscopic cholecystectomy, an
operation that requires 1 day of hospitalization rather than the 3–5
day hospitalization of an open cholecystectomy. This more rapid recovery is also seen in the elderly patient population. The laparoscopic approach to the peritoneal cavity causes less operative stress
than an open operation. Recently, Griffith et al. (Griffith, Everitt,
Curley, & McMahon, in press) reported inhibition of T-cell prolifer-
ation and increase in C-reactive protein in patients undergoing an
open cholecystectomy compared to patients undergoing a laparoscopic cholecystectomy, suggesting the lesser reduction in the im-

munological competency and less operative stress. There are reports that there is no difference in the immunological changes after minilaparotomy cholecystectomy and laparoscopic cholecystectomy. This is almost certainly because a minilaparotomy through a small incision also causes minimal stress.

It must be remembered that it is not only laparoscopy that is the cause of minimal trauma but any operation performed through small wounds with minimal intraperitoneal trauma; however, the laparoscopic approach is the ultimate for small incisions and minimal trauma. The trauma response is almost certainly related to the amount of tissue injury resulting from the size of the incision and the amount of handling and retraction of the intestines. The smaller incisions of laparoscopy result in less impairment of pulmonary function, less atelectasis and hypoxia than occurs with the splinting associated with the larger subcostal incision of an open cholecystectomy. Putensen-Himmer et al. (Putensen-Himmer, Putensen, Lammer, & Lingnau, 1992) found that lung volumes, including postoperative forced vital capacity, residual capacity, and forced expiratory volume, were reduced less and returned to normal values sooner after laparoscopic cholecystectomy than after open cholecystectomy .

Although laparoscopic operations have great appeal because of the minimal physiological stress, there are groups of patients who may not be candidates for this approach. To define this more clearly, a better understanding of the physiological disturbances of laparoscopy are needed. The pneumoperitoneum to 15 mm of mercury has physiological effects that are now starting to be defined. The increased intraabdominal pressure on the diaphragm, altering pulmonary physiology by limiting excursion of the diaphragm, and the increased absorption of carbon dioxide from the peritoneal cavity may pose problems for patients with severe compromise of pulmonary function due to chronic obstructive pulmonary disease (Blobner, Felber, Gogleer, Weigl, & Jelen, 1992; McKinstry, Perverseff, & Yip, 1992). Currently, all general surgical laparoscopic procedures are performed under general anesthesia; however, with development and better understanding of the laparoscopic approach to the peritoneal cavity other methods of anesthesia may be used in the future.

The increase in intraabdominal pressure from the carbon dioxide is thought to reduce venous return to the heart and may compromise cardiac function. The effect of a pneumoperitoneum on cardiac function has been measured by monitoring patients undergoing laparoscopic cholecystectomy, using Swan-Ganz catheters. Mean arterial pressure and cardiac index fall 24% and 28%, respectively, and systemic peripheral resistance rises; these represent impairment in cardiac function. However, to date, no adverse effects have been reported as a result of this fall in cardiac performance (McLaughlin, Bonnell, Scheeres, & Dean, 1992; Noirot, Joris, Legrand, & Lamy, 1992). These changes may not be significant in patients being subjected to the minimal trauma and lowered physiological stress of a laparoscopic procedure compared to an open operation. New methods of retracting the abdominal wall to create a space in the peritoneal cavity large enough to perform the laparoscopic procedure are being developed, and these will do away with the need for a pneumoperitoneum. These new methods of abdominal wall retraction may not depress cardiac function to the same degree, but the abdominal wall retraction may cause more postoperative pain as a result of the pulling on the abdominal wall. The results of procedures performed with these instruments must be studied carefully before they become widely accepted.

All patients, including elderly patients seem to tolerate laparoscopic surgical procedures well; their hospital stay is short, and the recovery to a normal way of life is shorter than with open operations. Despite the theoretical pulmonary and cardiac disadvantages of laparoscopic operations, they seem to tolerate them better than open procedures. Theoretical disadvantages of a pneumoperitoneum will be overcome as a result of development and a better understanding of the laparoscopic approach to the peritoneal cavity. The introduction of this technique into general surgery is a major advance in the management of the surgical patient and is of a particular advantage to the elderly patient.

References

Blobner, M., Felber, A. R., Gogleer, S., Weigl, E. M., & Jelen S. Carbon dioxide uptake from pneumoperitoneum during laparoscopic cholecystectomy. *Anesthesiology*, 77: A37. 1992.

Danzinger, R. G., Hoffmann, A. F., Schoenfield, L. J., & Thistle, J. L. Dissolution of cholesterol gallstones by chenodeoxycholic acid. *N Engl J Med*, 286: 1–8. 1972.

Gardener, B., & Palasti, S. A comparison of hospital costs and morbidity between octogenarians and other patients undergoing surgical operations. *Surg Gynecol Obstet*, 171: 299–304. 1990.

Glinatsis, M. T., Griffith, J. P., & McMahon, M. J. Open versus Laparoscopic cholecystectomy: A retrospective study. *J Laparoend Surg, 2:* 81–86. 1992.

Griffith, J., Everitt, N., Curley, P., & McMahon, M. Laparoscopic versus "open" cholecystectomy-reduced influence upon immune function and the acute phase response. *Surg Endosc.,* In press.

Herron, P. W., Jesseph, J. E., & Harkin, H. N. Analysis of 600 major operations in patients over 70 years of age. *Ann Surg, 152:* 686–98. 1960.

Kaplan, M. S., West, J. W., & Stemmer, E. A., et al. Surgical management of upper gastrointestinal bleeding in the aged patient. *Am J Gastroenterol, 58:* 109–23. 1972.

McKinstry, L. J., Perverseff, R. A., & Yip, R. W. Arterial and end-tidal carbon dioxide in patients undergoing laparoscopic cholecystectomy. *Anesthesiology, 77:* A107. 1992.

McLaughlin, J. G., Bonnell, B. W., Scheeres, D. E., & Dean, R. J. The adverse hemodynamic effects related to laparoscopic cholecystectomy. *Anesthesiology, 77:* A70. 1992.

Moossa, A. R., Easter, D. W., Van Sonnenberg, E., Casola, G., & D'Agostino, H. Laparoscopic injuries to the bile duct. A cause for concern. *Ann Surg, 215:* 203–208. 1992.

Noirot, D., Joris, J., Legrand, M., & Lamy, M. Hemodynamic changes during pneumoperitoneum for laparoscopic cholecystectomy. *Anesthesiology, 77:* A69. 1992.

Perissat, J., Collet, D., & Belliard, R. Gallstones, laparoscopy, cholecystectomy, cholecystostomy, lithotripsy. *Surg Endosc, 4:* 1–5. 1990.

Petelin, J. B. Laparoscopic approach to common duct pathology. *Surg Lap & Endo, 1:* 33–41. 1991.

Putensen-Himmer, G., Putensen, C. H., Lammer, H., & Lingnau, W. Functional residual capacity, post-operative lung function, and gas exchange following open laparotomy or laparoscopy for cholecystectomy. *Anesthesiology, 77:* A1253. 1992.

Rossi, R. L., Schirmer, W. J., Braasch, J. W., Sanders, L. B., & Munson, J. L. Laparoscopic bile duct injuries. Risk factors, recognition, and repair. *Arch Surg, 127:* 5: 596–601. 1992.

Sackmann, M., Delius, M., Sauerbruch, T., Holl, J., Weber, W., Ippisch, E., Hagelauer, U., Wee, O., Brendel, W., Paumgartner, G. Shock-wave lithotripsy of gallstones: The first 175 patients. *N Engl J Med, 318:* 394–397. 1988.

Schoenfield, L. J., & Lachin, J. M., The Steering Committee, and The National Cooperative Gallstone Study Group: Chenodiol (chenodeoxycholic acid) for dissolution of gallstones: the National Cooperative Gallstone Study. *Ann Intern Med, 95:* 257–282. 1981.

Stoker, M. E., Leveillee, R. J., McCann, J. C. Jr., & Maini, B. S. Laparoscopic common bile duct exploration. *J Laparoend Surg, 1:* 287–293. 1991.

Tandon, R. K., & Tsapogas, M. J. Bleeding peptic ulcer. *NY J Med, 75:* 35–8. 1975.

Thistle, J. L., May, G. R., Bender, C. E., Williams, H. J., LeRoy, A. J., Nelson, P. E., Peine, C. J., Petersen, B. T., & McCullough, J. E. Dissolution of cholesterol gallbladder stones by methyl-*tert*-butyl ether administration by percutaneous transhepatic catheter. *N Engl J Med, 320:* 633–639. 1989.

Chapter Thirteen

Problems and Opportunities for the Diagnosis and Treatment of Prostatic Cancer

Mireille Grégoire, Michael A. O'Donnell and William C. DeWolf

Prostatic adenocarcinoma is the most common tumor diagnosed in men in the United States, with 132,000 new cases in 1992, and is the second most common cause of cancer deaths (Boring, Squires, & Tong, 1992). Although uncommon before age 40, the incidence of prostatic cancer rises markedly after age 60. Upon meticulous step-sectioning of prostate glands at autopsy, the prevalence of cancer ranges from 29% for males between ages 50 and 60 to 57% for males between ages 80 and 90 (Franks, 1954; Scott et al., 1969). Nevertheless, while the lifetime probability of being diagnosed with prostatic cancer is 9.5%, the lifetime risk of dying of prostatic cancer is only 2.9% (Seidman et al., 1985). Thus, not all prostatic adenocarcinomas become clinically significant. However, with current diagnostic modalities, indolent prostatic cancers cannot be distinguished from those that will progress. Prostate adenocarcinoma appears to have a slow doubling time estimated at 2 years, which could explain the appearance of clinically significant disease only in later life (Stamey & Kabalin, 1989).

In order to understand the diagnostic and therapeutic approaches to this cancer, first the anatomy of the normal prostate and then pathological staging and grading classifications will be reviewed briefly. Traditionally, the prostate had been divided into

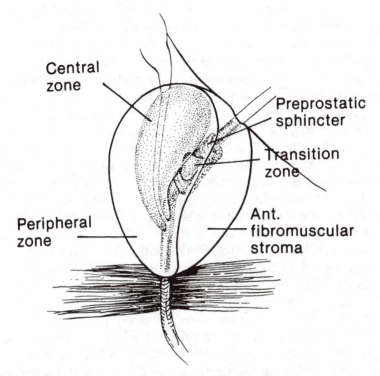

Central zone

Preprostatic sphincter

Transition zone

Peripheral zone

Ant. fibromuscular stroma

FIGURE 13.1 Prostate gland anatomy of the young adult male, adapted from McNeal's description (1968). The transitional zone often increases in size in older individuals (reproduced with permission).

five lobes. Although this classification has been abandoned, it is customary to refer the right and left lobes of the prostate to designate the corresponding areas of the gland on each side of the median sulcus on digital rectal examination. According to current nomenclature, the gland is divided into five zones based on anatomic and histologic characteristics (Figure 13.1) (McNeal, 1968): (1) the peripheral zone, comprising 70% of the gland, is the most frequent origin of prostatic cancer; (2) the central zone, comprising 25% of the gland, is located along the ejaculatory ducts; (3) the transition zone, accounting for about 4% of the normal young adult prostate, is the origin of benign hyperplasia; (4) the periurethral and (5) the anterior fibromuscular zones comprise the remaining 1% of glandular tissue.

Classically, the American Joint Committee on Cancer (AJCC) classification has been used for prostatic cancer staging. As it remains in broad use, it will be briefly reviewed. Localized disease includes stages A and B; Stage A_1 represents *well-differentiated*, clinically unsuspected, organ-confined carcinoma discovered during surgery for benign prostatic disease and comprising less than three foci of adenocarcinoma. Stage A_2 disease is also organ-confined but diffusely present in the gland. A small amount of *poorly-differentiated* adenocarcinoma is also classified as Stage A_2. Stage B_1 carcinoma is palpable, less than 1.5 cm, and confined to one lobe of the gland. On the other hand, Stage B_2 represents neoplasia in excess of 1.5 cm or involving both lobes of the prostate. Nonlocalized disease is classified within stages C and D. C_1 represents prostatic capsular invasion, whereas C_2 represents contiguous organ invasion. Pelvic lymph node metastases are classified as D_1, whereas D_2 represents distant metastases. However, more recently, the Organ Systems Coordinating Center (OSCC) of the National Cancer Institute has devised a new staging system, which incorporates features of both the TNM and AJCC systems (Table 13.1, Figure 13.2).

Carcinomas of the prostate are usually graded according to the Gleason system, which is based on low-power microscopic glandular characteristics of the tumor rather than on cellular anaplasia. The tumor characteristics are ranked from 1 to 5; 1 is the least and 5 the most disruption of normal glandular configuration (Figure 13.3) (Gleason, 1977). The sum of the Gleason grade of the largest and second largest areas of tumor is called the Gleason score, which reflects the overall tumor aggressiveness (Gardner et al., 1988).

SCREENING AND DIAGNOSIS

Digital rectal examination (DRE), combined with digitally guided biopsies when appropriate, has been the primary modality of diagnosis of prostatic cancer for many decades. By DRE alone, clinical studies have demonstrated cancer detection rates between 0.8% and 1.4% in the general population (Seidman et al., 1985). However, in a recent study of 2,425 men screened for prostatic cancer, 88 (3.6%) were diagnosed with the disease, using a combination of DRE, prostatic specific antigen (PSA) and/or transrectal ultrasound (TRUS) (Babaian et al., 1992). Of the 88 patients with cancer, half were diagnosed by DRE, underlining the limits of DRE as a sole diagnostic tool (Figure 13.4). Despite this limitation, DRE remains a useful clinical tool because of its low cost and risk.

TABLE 13.1 **Organ systems coordinating center for clinical staging of prostate cancer (reproduced with permission).**

Primary Tumor(T)	
TX	Anatomic relationships indefinable (e.g., prior total prostatectomy)
TA	Digitally unrecognizable cancer (confirmed histologically and substaged if traditional TUR cancer)
TA1	≤ 5% of total surgical specimen and of low to medium grade
TA2	> 5% of specimen, any grade, or ≤ 5% of specimen with any high grade
TAX	TA, but not A1 or A2
TAX-TRUS	*Detected by ultrasound, confirmed by biopsy*
TAX-PSA	*Detected by PSA, testing confirmed by biopsy*
TAX-Asym	*Detected by DRE as a normal feeling but asymmetric prostate*
TB	Digitally palpated cancer, organ-confined
TB	≤ ½ of one lobe, regardless of location
TB2	> ½ of one lobe but not > 1 lobe
TB3	> 1 lobe or bilaterally palpable cancer
TBX	Palpable, organ-confined cancer, not otherwise characterized
TBX-asym	*Abnormally firm (non-nodular)*
TBX-sym	*Abnormally firm (non-nodular)*
TBC*	Palpable cancer extending beyond prostate capsule
TC1	Extension beyond margin unilaterally (may include seminal vesicle)
TC2	Extension bilaterally (may include seminal vesicle)
TC3	Extension into bladder, rectum, levator muscles, or pelvic side walls
Lymph Node Status (N)	
N0 (C and/or H)	No regional lymph node metastases, clinically (C) and/or histologically (H)
N1 (H)	Microscopic regional lymph node metastasis, proved histologically
N2 (C and/or H)	Gross regional lymph node metastases
N3 (C and/or H)	Extraregional lymph node metastases
NX	Minimal requirements have not been met
Distant Metastases (M)†	
M0	No evidence of metastases
M1	Elevated acid phosphatase only (three consecutive elevations)
M2 (V and/or B)	Visceral (V) and/or bone (B) metastases
MX	Minimal requirements not met

*TBC, in addition to the TC categories, requires TB specification of the extent of the intracapsular cancer.

†Excludes lymph nodes.

Abbreviations: TUR, transurethral resection: TRUS, transrectal ultrasound; PSA, prostate-specific antigen; DRE, digital rectal examination.

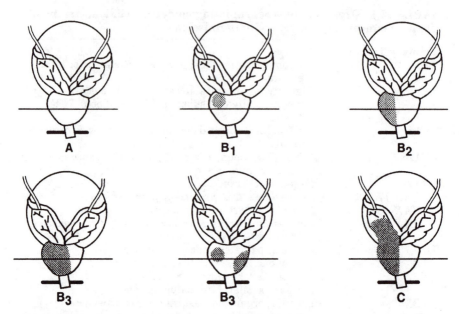

FIGURE 13.2 Palpable findings on digital examination for clinical stages TA, TB, and TC. (reproduced with permission).

Fortunately, new technologies can now complement DRE and improve our diagnostic abilities.

Prostatic specific antigen (PSA), a tumor marker, has dramatically altered our approach to prostatic cancer diagnosis; its high sensitivity (68%), especially with respect to localized disease, makes measurement of prostatic acid phosphatase, the former prostatic cancer serum marker, rarely necessary (Oesterling, 1991). PSA is a serine protease exclusively produced by the epithelial cells of the prostatic acini and is involved in the liquefaction of seminal coagulum. PSA is prostate specific but *not* prostatic cancer–specific; that is to say, benign prostatic hyperplasia (BPH) and acute bacterial prostatitis can also elevate PSA levels. Serum levels less than 4.0 ng/ml (4.0 mg/l) represent the normal range using the Hybritech assay. Care should be taken with respect to timing of blood sampling for PSA because increases in serum PSA levels can occur after DRE (twofold), cystoscopy (fourfold), and prostate needle biopsy (55-fold), even in the presence of a benign prostate. As the clinical half-life of serum PSA varies between 2 and 3 days (Oesterling et al., 1988; Stamey et al., 1987), it is recommended to wait

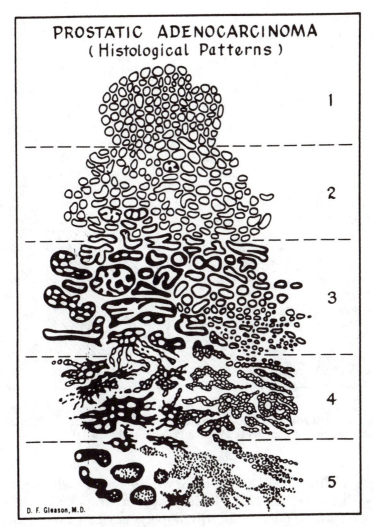

FIGURE 13.3 Gleason histological grading of prostatic carcinoma. (reproduced with permission).

1 week after DRE and 4 weeks after biopsy or TURP, before drawing PSA serum levels (Stamey & McNeal, 1992). In fact, serum PSA should ideally be drawn prior to any prostatic manipulation.

In a recent study, an increased PSA serum level was noted in 15% of 1,249 men. Irrespective of the DRE, when the PSA serum level ranged between 4.0 and 10.0 ng/ml (4.0–10.0 mg/l), a quarter of them had prostatic cancer. When the PSA serum level was above

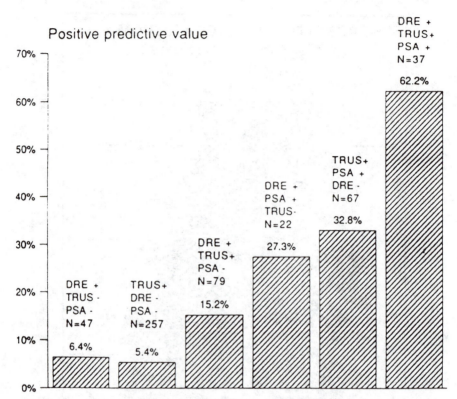

FIGURE 13.4 Positive predictive values according to combination of transrectal ultrasound (TRUS), digital rectal examination (DRE), and prostate-specific antigen (PSA). Positive PSA defined as >4.0 ng/ml.

10.0 ng/ml (10.0 mg/l), half of them were diagnosed with prostatic cancer (Brawer et al., 1992). Patients with a serum PSA level less than 4.0 ng/ml (4.0 mg/l) can still harbor a prostatic cancer, dictating a thorough workup in any patient with a suspicious rectal examination (Table 13.2) (Labrie et al., 1992). PSA serum levels tend to increase with advanced stages of prostatic cancer although there is much overlap with BPH, making accurate staging by serum PSA alone difficult (Figure 13.5) (Oesterling, 1991). It is still not clear if PSA alone is sufficient to diagnose or stage prostatic cancer adequately.

Transrectal ultrasonography (TRUS) is another modality used to help diagnose prostatic cancer. The prostate can be visualized in either transversal or longitudinal fashion (Figure 13.6) (Spinack & Resnick, 1991). For the physician experienced in the use of TRUS,

TABLE 13.2 Serum PSA levels and the distribution of presence and absence of prostate cancer in a randomized population of 1002 men 45 to 80 years old. (reproduced with permission).

No. Pts.	Serum PSA Levels (μg./l.)	Cancer Present No.	(%)	Cancer Absent No.	(%)
11	Greater than 30	10	(90.9)	1	(9.1)
6	20.1–30	5	(83.3)	1	(6.7)
18	10.1–20	3	(16.7)	15	(83.7)
60	5.1–10	17	(28.3)	43	(71.7)
29	4.1–5	6	(20.7)	23	(79.3)
67	3.1–4	5	(7.5)	62	(92.5)
52	2.6–3	3	(5.8)	49	(94.2)
68	2.1–2.5	2	(2.9)	66	(97.1)
125	1.6–2.0	0	(0)	125	(100)
187	1.0–1.5	2	(1.1)	185	(98.9)
379	Less than 1.0	4	(1.1)	375	(98.9)
Totals 1,002		57		945	

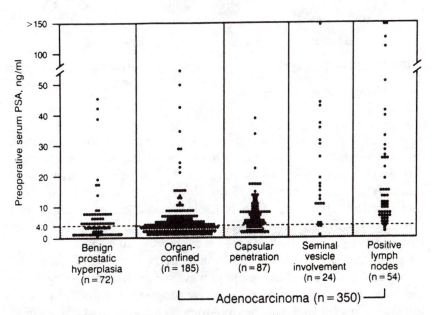

FIGURE 13.5 Preoperative serum PSA level as function of prostate histology. Adenocarcinoma patients underwent radical prostatectomy for clinically organ-confined cancer. (reproduced with permission).

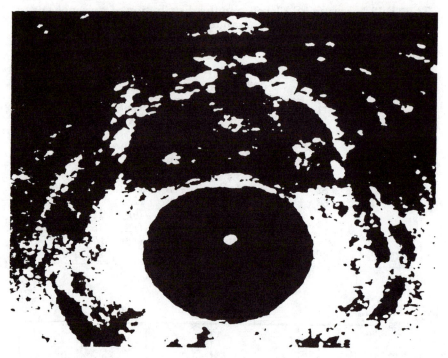

FIGURE 13.6 Transverse ultrasound image of normal prostate. Central black area represents rectum with probe in it. Arrows indicate prostate capsule. (reproduced with permission).

it provides clear visualization of the gland's anatomy. Approximately one third of early prostatic cancer will appear isoechoic, two thirds as hypoechoic, and only 1% as a hyperechoic lesion (Shinohara, Wheener, & Scardino, 1989). However, prostatic ultrasound is not specific; it is not suitable as a sole method for screening of prostatic cancer (Pontes et al., 1985). It is nevertheless useful to survey the prostate for suspicious areas (and biopsy them) in the absence of anomalies on DRE when serum PSA is elevated (Figure 13.7) (Cooner, 1992). Ultrasonography, whether transrectal or transabdominal, can also be used to measure prostatic volume. This information is useful because it can help determine if prostatic enlargement (BPH), as indicated by volume, is responsible for an increase in serum PSA value. This is measured by the PSA index, also known as PSA density, which is calculated by dividing the serum PSA value by the estimated volume of the prostate gland. Preliminary data suggest that a PSA index greater than 0.15 is as sensi-

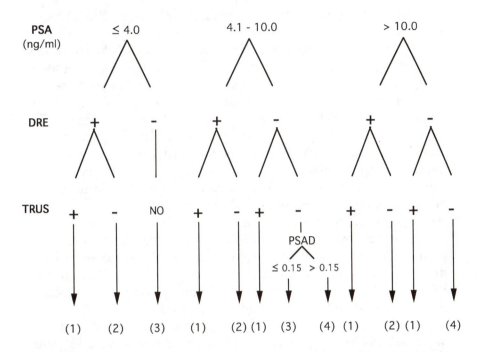

FIGURE 13.7 Algorithm for prostate cancer detection. PSA: prostate specific antigen (Hybritech immunoradiometric assay); DRE: digital rectal examination; TRUS: transrectal ultrasound; PSAD: Prostate specific antigen density. (1) Biopsy of lesion visualized by TRUS. (2) Biopsy of palpable lesion. (3) Annual DRE and serum PSA. (4) Systematic ultrasound-guided biopsies of the prostate gland. (reproduced with permission).

tive as a serum PSA level greater than 4.0 ng/ml (4.0 mg/l) and even more specific for cancer detection (Catalona, 1992). PSA index may prove to be a helpful adjunct to our diagnostic modalities in the near future, especially in patients with minimally increased serum PSA levels and an enlarged prostate.

Prostatic biopsy is the *sine qua non* for establishing the diagnosis of prostatic cancer. It can be performed as an outpatient procedure, without anesthesia, in about 10 minutes. Although pointing the biopsy needle to the suspicious area by digital guidance is commonly used, ultrasound probes can be loaded with a needle whose path of biopsy will be precisely established by the ultrasound apparatus. This allows precise biopsies of a small suspicious area. The technique, although simple, requires a prebiopsy self-administered enema as well as oral Gram-negative antibiotic coverage. Although unusual, complications such as urinary retention, hemorrhage, and sepsis can occur after prostate biopsy.

With the advent of these new diagnostic modalities, the question of large-population screening arises. The ideal low-cost, low-morbidity, highly sensitive and specific screening test has yet to be designed; serum PSA has too low a diagnostic accuracy (64%) to meet these requirements (Oesterling, 1991). To make matters more difficult, there is some question about whether screening should be done at all. Autopsy prevalence of prostatic cancer is relatively high, yet only a minority of cancers progress to clinical significance. In other words, many cancers do not need treatment and hence no diagnostic screening. Moreover, as with any screening strategy, the question always arises to what extent screening really increases survival rather than just prolonging the time one is aware that the cancer is present. The definitive answer is not known. In a recent study of 2,425 men screened with DRE, serum PSA, and TRUS, the cancer detection rate was only 2.4% (Mettlin et al., 1991). At this time, therefore, it appears that mass screening is not warranted (Thompson, 1990). However, it is the current recommendation of the American Urological Association that male patients under the care of a practitioner and between 50 and 80 years should undergo a yearly DRE and serum PSA. Under these circumstances, the algorithm proposed by Cooner (1992) seems logical and practical (Figure 13.7). It is based on the prostatic cancer detection rate as it relates to serum levels of PSA and DRE, on one hand, and the number of biopsies and ultrasound examinations required to detect a cancer using these modalities (Cooner, 1991).

STAGING

Serum PSA, DRE, and TRUS are helpful in assessing the clinical stage of the disease. Only patients with prostate-confined cancer can be expected to be cured of their disease. Unfortunately, these modalities, either alone or in combination, have a limited ability to predict the local extent of the cancer. Organ confinement was pathologically confirmed in only 40% of radical prostatectomy specimens at Stanford University (Stamey & McNeal, 1992). On the other hand, serum PSA has been a very useful adjunct in the diagnosis of metastatic prostatic cancer. Until recently, all patient candidates believed to harbor localized cancer underwent a radionuclide bone scan to rule out distant metastasis. However, in a recent study, only 2.7% of patients with serum PSA levels below 20.0 ng/ml (20.0 mg/l) demonstrated metastasis on bone scan; none of the patients had any bony metastasis with PSA levels less than 10.0 ng/ml (10.0 mg/l) (Chybowski et al., 1991). The authors of this study have concluded that bone scans for patients with serum PSA levels less than 10.0 ng/ml (10.0 mg/l) are no longer justified. A consensus has not been reached on abandoning bone scans in patients with a serum PSA level between 10.0 and 20.0 ng/ml (10.0–20.0mg/l). Currently, there is no need for routine computed tomography or magnetic resonance imaging in staging patients with prostatic cancer. Definitive pelvic lymph node status is best achieved at the time of surgery. Recently, laparoscopic techniques have been used successfully to retrieve pelvic lymph nodes and have been shown to be as reliable as conventional surgery (Parra, Andrus, & Boullier, 1992). As more urologists become proficient with this new approach, laparoscopy should become more widely used for this purpose, especially in those cases selected for radiation therapy, as will be discussed below.

TREATMENT OF PROSTATIC CANCER

Organ-confined disease

Before assigning a patient with clinically localized prostatic cancer to a definitive treatment, one has to consider the long doubling time of most of these cancers and the fact that most patients diagnosed with adenocarcinoma of the prostate are elderly and are often afflicted with other diseases. In other words, the morbidity and mortality caused by the prostatic cancer itself, its treatment, other concomitant diseases must be considered in order to estimate the patient's life expectancy. Although this represents a difficult task, general guidelines do exist. Historical series have documented a median time to progression of 17.5 years in Stage TA_1, 4.75 years in Stage TA_2 (Lowe & Listrom, 1988), whereas the median time to local and metastatic progression is estimated at 48 and over 138 months respectively, for untreated Stage TB_1 (Whitmore, Warner, & Thompson, 1991). In view of these facts, it is wise to consider definitive treatment of prostatic cancer in those with a life expectancy of at least 10 years. Should such a patient, who is not treated at the time of presentation, develop progressive disease, local symptoms can be adequately controlled by hormonal therapy and/or transurethral resection of the prostate (TURP). Metastases are treated by hormonal therapy (see following section). The earlier concerns that TURP may hasten cancer dissemination have not been substantiated (Paulson & Cox, 1987).

For patients deemed good candidates for definitive therapy, two types of treatment exist: radiation and radical prostatectomy. Radiation can be given in two forms: by locally implanted radioactive seeds (brachytherapy) and by external beam (teletherapy). Only a few specialized centers offer brachytherapy, using mainly I-125 and Au-198. In general, external beam therapy and radical prostatectomy have achieved better local control than brachytherapy alone (Smalley & Noble, 1992). For stages TB, radiation offers overall 5– and 10–year survival rates of about 80% and 60%, respectively (Bagshaw, Cox, & Ramback, 1990; Hanks, 1991). The relapse-free 5– and 10–year survival rates are 64% and 42%, respectively (Hanks, 1991). These data are difficult to compare with those obtained in surgically treated patients, as radiation patients rarely undergo a staging pelvic lymphadenectomy. Radiation patients may therefore harbor more widespread disease than is clinically evident.

Another concern with radiation is the significance of a positive prostate biopsy following treatment. In a series of 27 consecutive patients followed for a mean of 5.2 years, 93% had a positive biopsy (Kabalin et al., 1989). Whether a positive biopsy following definitive irradiation of Stage TB portends a local recurrence remains to be clearly demonstrated. At this time, Stage TC disease is best treated by irradiation. It is also an adequate treatment for Stage TB prostate cancer in elderly patients not otherwise surgical candidates. Morbidity caused by radiation therapy may include gastrointestinal symptoms, impotence, and urinary frequency. Currently, new protocols are examining the role of hormonal therapy in association with radiation as a means to improve upon local control of the disease. Moreover, with the advent of laparoscopic lymph node dissection, improved staging may delineate groups of patients likely to benefit from radiation therapy.

Surgery has been more commonly performed since the advent of the nerve-sparing radical prostatectomy. This technique allows for better visualization of the pelvic anatomy, hence reducing blood loss by improving control of the blood vessels and reducing incontinence by allowing a more accurate anastomosis between the blad-

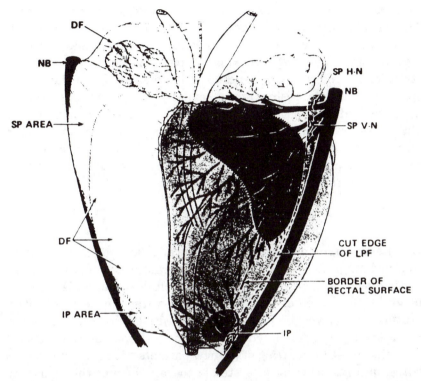

FIGURE 13.8 Distribution of nerve branches to prostate - right posterolateral view. NB: neurovascular bundle; SP: superior pedicle; IP: inferior pedicle; DF: Denonvilliers fascia; LPF: lateral pelvic fascia. (reproduced with permission).

der neck and the remaining urethra. Moreover, the technique preserves the posterolateral neurovascular pedicle which contains the nerve fibers controlling erections (Figure 13.8) (Walsh, 1988). Although nerve-sparing radical prostatectomy, by virtue of its reduced morbidity, has been broadly used, long-term data are available only for patients prior to the nerve-sparing era. The overall 10–year survival of surgically treated stages TB_1 and TB_2 is 75%, while 10–year disease-free survival rate is 69% (Frohmüller, Theiss, & Wirth, 1991). When the cancer invades the prostatic capsule or the seminal vesicles, the 10–year disease-free survival rate drops to 41%. Since only 40% of patients undergoing nerve-sparing radical prostatectomy have pathological organ-confined disease (Stamey & McNeal, 1992), the technique, which limits surgical dissection, may therefore not always be an adequate cancer operation. Definitive answers are expected with long-term follow-up series. The role of radical prostatectomy for stages TC with or without pelvic lymph node involvement also remains controversial. Specific complications following radical prostatectomy can lead to urethral strictures, urinary incontinence, and impotence. Using the nerve-sparing technique, postoperative sexual potency was preserved in about two thirds of patients potent prior to surgery (Quinlan et al., 1991). Preservation of sexual function is better attained in younger patients; those older than 70 tend to fare more poorly. In summary, radical prostatectomy appears to give better results in patients with pathologically prostate-confined cancer.

Advanced Disease

Despite attempts to detect prostate cancer at an ever earlier organ-confined stage, 25%–30% of patients currently have distant metastatic disease (Stage D_2) at the time of clinical diagnosis (McCullough, 1988). Another 30% of patients with clinically localized prostate cancer will be found to have positive lymph nodes (Stage D_1) at the time of pelvic lymphadenectomy (Donahue et al., 1990). Overall, an estimated 75% of all new patients with prostate cancer will require some form of systemic therapy during the course of their disease (Stamey & McNeal, 1992), and more than 34,000 patients each year in the United States will suffer and die as a direct consequence of their disease (Boring, et al., 1992).

Once prostate cancer metastasizes, there is little evidence to suggest that any form of conventional therapy will significantly affect patient survival (Eisenberg, Bezerdjian, & Kalash, 1987). Treatment, therefore, is usually directed at palliation. However, because many patients remain largely asymptomatic until late in the course of their disease, therapy has traditionally been delayed until the onset of symptoms. Roughly, one quarter of patients will suffer from local spread of the tumor, resulting in bladder outlet or ureteral obstruction. The overwhelming majority progress systemically with skeletal (usually vertebral) metastases (Steinberg, Epstein, Piantodosi, & Walsh, 1990). Spinal involvement may extend into the epidural space, threatening extrinsic compression and paraplegia in 5% (Flynn & Shipley, 1991). Only very late in the course is there involvement of the liver or lungs. When patients with metastatic disease are treated in this expectant fashion, approximately 10% will die within 6 months and 50% within 3 years. Ten percent, however, will survive over 10 years (Schroeder, Klihn, & deJong, 1986). Adverse prognostic factors include high tumor volume, high Gleason grade, nondiploid DNA histogram, and advanced age (Byer & Corle, 1987; Winkler et al., 1988).

The mainstay of palliative therapy is androgen withdrawal. Overall, 60%–80% of men with Stage D_2 disease will respond favorably to this approach. Unfortunately, due to the emergence of androgen resistance, 35%–40% will fail during the first year, and 50% will fail by 15 months (Sogani & Fair, 1987). Long-term responses are possible, however, and may be predicted in many cases by a significant and sustained fall in serum PSA (Siddall et al., 1986).

Methods to achieve androgen ablation include surgical castration and medical blockade. Since the testes provide 95% of the circulating androgen, bilateral orchiectomy remains a direct and rapid means of achieving androgen ablation. This surgery can be performed with minimal morbidity and mortality and obviates the concern over patient compliance. Concern over potency loss, hot flashes, and the psychological and physical disfigurement associated with the procedure, however, have led to the development of nonsurgical alternatives to orchiectomy.

Five distinct classes of androgen ablative drugs form the mainstay of medical therapy. The synthetic estrogen diethylstilbestrol (DES), at oral doses of greater than 3 mg/day, produces castrate testosterone levels largely through feedback inhibition of the pituitary and hypothalamus. Despite its low cost and ease of use, DES has been associated with significant cardiovascular toxicity (Glashan & Robinson, 1981). Painful breast enlargement and impotence have also limited its use. A lower dose, 1 mg/day, does reduce cardiovascular risk while maintaining efficacy but fails to achieve castrate testosterone levels. A group of related compounds, progestins, work in a similar manner on the pituitary and hypothalamus but lose efficacy over time and are not recommended for clinical use.

The second class of drugs comprises gonadotropin releasing hormone (GnRH) agonists, peptide analogs that function by desensitizing the pituitary to release gonadotropins. These agents must be administered in a monthly intramuscular or subcutaneous depot form. Although as effective as castration in reducing circulating androgens, they also cause impotence and hot flashes. An important consequence of their use is an initial flare of testosterone release during the first week of therapy, increasing bone pain and the potential for spinal cord injury. Often an antiandrogen (see below) is started simultaneously and continued for the first 2 weeks of therapy to abrogate this phenomenon. The GnRH agents are also quite costly, averaging over $400 for each monthly injection.

Antiandrogens act as competitive inhibitors of the intracellular steroid receptor in androgen-sensitive cells and come in two forms. Flutamide, a nonsteroidal competitor, has the advantage of preserving erectile function. Breast tenderness, diarrhea, three-times-a-day dosing, and high cost are some of its disadvantages. Cyproterone acetate is a steroidal antiandrogen lacking the erection-preserving effects of flutamide. Neither agent is recommended as monotherapy, however, because of failure to achieve long-term androgen blockade (Labrie et al., 1987; Robinson, 1987).

The fourth class of agents reduces serum testosterone by nonselectively inhibiting steroidogenesis in both the testes and the adrenal glands. Ketoconazole is the prototype member in this group. It causes a significant drop in serum androgen within 4–8 hours of a 400-mg oral dose. This rapid androgen decline is particularly useful when an impending spinal cord compression is suspected. Dosing must continue three times a day, and liver failure is reported to occur in 1/16,000 cases (Trachtenberg & Pont, 1983). Monitoring the patients for signs of adrenal insufficiency during therapy must also be performed.

The final and newest class of agents is represented by finasteride, an inhibitor of the enzyme 5–a-reductase. This enzyme is responsible for the conversion of testosterone into dihydrotestosterone, the active intracellular androgen in the prostate. Like flutamide, finasteride preserves erectile potency; however, it also is not recommended as monotherapy. Its very low incidence of side effects and once-a-day dosing make it an appealing alternative to antiandrogens as an adjunctive agent, but its clinical efficacy in this regard has not yet been definitively established.

With the availability of agents that act on both gonadal and adrenal androgens and the recognition of differing degrees of androgen dependence by prostate cancer cells, two new approaches in the treatment of prostate cancer are under investigation. The first involves total androgen blockade achieved by combining an antiandrogen with either orchiectomy or a GnRH agent. The second involves institution of androgen therapy at the time of initial diagnosis. Studies with both approaches suggest a modest benefit

(4–6 months) in terms of a progression-free interval and survival for a selected group of patients (Crawford et al., 1990; Kramolowsky, 1988). Such therapy must be carefully weighted against the untoward side effects, added cost, and expected benefit for the individual patient.

Once androgen resistance occurs, most patients enter a terminal downward spiral measured in months. Although hormonal therapy appears ineffective during this time, it is important that it not be discontinued because of the risk of precipitating an androgen-driven rebound flare. Therapy at this point is directed at palliating specific symptoms. Local outlet obstruction can be managed by a limited prostatic resection. Localized bone pain is amenable to focal radiation treatment. More diffuse bone pain often responds to either hemibody irradiation or to strontium-89 radiotherapy (Kuban et al., 1989; Lewington et al., 1991). A new compound of drugs, termed biphosphonates, may also be effective in palliating bone pain by inhibiting bone turnover (Clarke, Holbrook, McClure, & George, 1991). Terminal pain relief with epidural and long-acting narcotics is also appropriate. Above all, it is important to maintain the patient's dignity during this difficult time and work with him and the family in delivering compassionate and effective palliative terminal care.

CONCLUSION

Prostatic cancer is prevalent in this country. The lifetime risk of being diagnosed with this disease is 9.5%, and the risk of dying from it is 2.9% (Seidman et al., 1985). For most patients, the disease seems to progress slowly, although it is by no means benign. In general, organ-confined prostatic cancer is best suited to curative treatment. Therefore, in general, early diagnosis of patients at risk of dying from prostatic cancer offers the best chance of cure, as long as the life expectancy of the patient exceeds 10 years. Currently, diagnosis is best achieved by digital rectal examination and serum prostatic-specific antigen complemented by prostate biopsy. In general, drawing serum prostatic-specific antigen or biopsying the prostate for screening purposes is not recommended in asymptomatic patients older than 80 years, for they would rarely benefit from aggressive treatment of their prostatic cancer.

Accepted treatments for localized prostatic cancer include radiotherapy and radical prostatectomy. However, it appears from recent studies that radiotherapy may not be curative. On the other hand, radical prostatectomy can be considered curative only if the cancer is confined within the prostate gland at surgery. Of all patients believed to have localized disease by clinical assessment, only 40% will have truly organ-confined prostatic cancer (Stamey & McNeal, 1992). Moreover, the ideal therapy for locally advanced disease remains elusive. On the other hand, palliative therapy for metastatic prostatic cancer has been available for 50 years. Metastatic prostatic cancer remains best treated by hormonal manipulation, which can be achieved by either surgical or medical castration. The ideal treatment of prostatic cancer metastatic only to the pelvic lymph nodes is still unclear and awaits the results of further clinical studies. Both basic and clinical research are still needed to understand the biology of this tumor, optimize therapy, and create new ones. Therefore, the practicing clinician must keep in mind that diagnostic and therapeutic modalities are still evolving, and best care requires that he or she remain vigilant for these changes.

Further Readings

Walsh, P. C., Retik, A. B., Stamey, T. A., Vaughan, E. D. Campbell's Urology. Philadelphia: W. B. Saunders. Chapter 29. 1992.

References

Babaian, R. J., Mettlin, C., & Kane, R., et al. The relationship of prostate-specific antigen to digital rectal examination and transrectal ultrasonography; Findings of the American Cancer Society National Prostate Cancer Detection Project. *Cancer, 69*: 1195. 1992.

Bagshaw, M. A., Cox, R. S., & Rambak, J. E. Radiation therapy for localized prostate cancer: Justification by long-term follow-up. *Urol Clin North Am, 18*: 787. 1990.

Boring, C. C.; Squires, T. S., & Tong, T. Cancer Statistics 1992. *CA, 42*: 19. 1992.

Brawer, M. K., Chetner, M. P., & Beatie, J., et al. Screening for prostatic carcinoma with prostate specific antigen. *J Urol, 147*: 841. 1992.

Byer, D. P., & Corle, D. K Hormone therapy for prostate cancer: Results of the Veterans Administration Cooperative Urological Research Group studies. *NCI Monogr, 7*: 165. 1987.

Catalona, W. J. *PSA Staging and Monitoring. Paper presented* at the Urologic Cancer Course organized by Harvard Medical School, Boston, Sept. 1992.

Chybowski, F. M., Larson Keller, J. J., & Bergstrahl, E. J. et al. Predicting radionuclide bone scan findings in patients with newly diagnosed, untreated prostate cancer: Prostate specific antigen is superior to all other clinical parameters. *J Urol, 145*: 313. 1991.

Clarke, N. W., Holbrook, I. B., McClure, J., & George, N. J. Osteoclast inhibition by pamidronate in metastatic cancer: A preliminary study. *Br J Cancer, 63*: 3;420. 1991.

Cooner, W. H. Prostate-specific antigen, digital rectal examination, and transrectal ultrasonic examination of the prostate in prostate cancer detection. *Mongr Urol, 12*: 3. 1991.

Cooner, W. H. *Early detection of prostate cancer using DRE, PSA, and ultrasound.* Paper presented at the Urologic Cancer Course organized by Harvard Medical School, Boston, Sept. 1992.

Crawford, E. D., Blumenstein, B. A., & Goodman, P. J., et al. Leuprolide with and without flutamide in advanced prostate cancer. *Cancer, 66*: 15;1039. 1990.

Donohue, R. E., Mani, J. H., & Whitesel, J. A., et al. Intraoperative and early complications of staging pelvic lymph node dissection in prostatic adenocarcinoma. *Urology, 35*: 223. 1990.

Eisenberger, M. A., Bezerdjian, L., & Kalash, S. A critical assessment of the role of chemotherapy for endocrine-resistant prostatic cancer. *Urol Clin North Am, 14*: 40;695. 1987.

Flynn, D., & Shipley, W. U. Management of spinal cord compression secondary to metastatic prostate cancer. *Urol Clin North Am, 18*: 145. 1991.

Franks, L. M. Latent carcinoma of the prostate. *J Path Bact, 68*: 603. 1954.

Frohmüller, H., Theiss, M., & Wirth, M. P. Radical prostatectomy for carcinoma of the prostate: Long-term follow-up of 115 patients. *Eur Urol, 19*: 279. 1991.

Gardner, W. A. Jr, Coffey, D., & Kam, J. P., et al. A uniform grading system for prostate cancer. *Hum Pathol, 19*: 119. 1988.

Glashan, R. W., & Robison, M. R. G. Cardiovascular complications in the treatment of prostate cancer. *Br J Urol, 53*: 624. 1981.

Gleason, D. F. Histologic grading and clinical staging of prostatic carcinoma, In M. Tannenbaum *Urologic Pathology: The Prostate* (pp. 171–198). Philadelphia: Lea and Febiger. 1977.

Hanks, G. E. Radiotherapy or surgery for prostate cancer? Ten and fifteen-year results of external beam therapy. *Acta Oncol, 30*: 231. 1991.

Kabalin, J. N., Hodge, K. K., & McNeal, J. E., et al. Identification of residual cancer in the prostate following radiation therapy: Role of transrectal ultrasound guided biopsy and prostate specific antigen. *J Urol, 142*: 326. 1989.

Kramolowsky, E. V. The value of testosterone deprivation in stage D1 carcinoma of the prostate. *J Urol, 139*: 1242. 1988.

Kuban, D. A., Delbridge, T., & el-Mahdi, A. M., et al. Half-body irradiation for treatment of widely metastatic adenocarcinoma of the prostate. *J Urol, 141*: 3; 572. 1989.

Labrie, F., Luthy, I., & Velleux, R., et al. New concepts on the androgen sensitivity of prostate cancer In G. P. Murphy, S. K. Khoury; R. K: ⅓uss; C. Chatelain; & L. Denis (Eds.); *Proceedings of Second International Symposium on Prostate Cancer: Prostate Cancer, Part A. Research, Endocrine Treatment and Histopathology.* New York, Alan R. Liss, Inc., Pp. 145–172. 1987.

Labrie, F., Dupont, A., & Suburu, R., et al. Serum prostatic specific antigen as pre-screening test for prostate cancer. *J Urol, 147*: 846. 1992.

Lewington, V. J., McEwan, A. J., & Ackery, D. M., et al. A prospective, randomized double-blind crossover study to examine the efficacy of strontium-89 in pain palliation in patients with advanced prostate cancer metastatic to bone. *Eur J Cancer, 27*: 8; 954. 1991.

Lowe, B. A., & Listrom, M. B. Incidental carcinoma of the prostate: An analysis of predictors of progression. *J Urol, 140*: 1340. 1988.

McCullough, D. L. Diagnosis and staging of prostate cancer. In D. G. Skinner & G. Lieskovsky (Eds.); *Diagnosis and Management of Genitourinary Cancer* (pp. 405–416). Philadelphia: W. B. Saunders. 1988.

McNeal, J. E. Regional morphology and pathology of the prostate. *Am J Clin Pathol, 49*: 347. 1968.

Mettlin, C., Lee, F., & Drago, J., et al The American Cancer Society National Prostate Cancer Detection Project: Findings on the detection of early prostate cancer. *Cancer, 67*: 2949. 1991.

Oesterling, J. E. Prostate specific antigen: A critical assessment of the most useful tumor marker for adenocarcinoma of the prostate. *J Urol, 145*: 907. 1991.

Oesterling, J. E., Cahn, D. W., & Epstein, J. I., et al. Prostate specific antigen in the preoperative and postoperative evaluation of localized prostatic cancer treated with radical prostatectomy. *J Urol, 139*: 766. 1988.

Parra, R. O., Andrus, C., & Boullier J. Staging laparoscopic pelvic lymph node dissection: Comparison of results with open pelvic lymphadenectomy. *J Urol, 147*: 875. 1992.

Paulson, D. F., & Cox, E. B Does transurethral resection of the prostate promote metastatic disease? *J Urol, 138*: 90. 1987.

Pontes, J. E., Eisenkraft, S., & Watanabe, H., et al. Preoperative evaluation of localized prostatic carcinoma by transrectal ultrasonography. *J Urol, 134*: 289. 1985.

Quinlan, D. M., Epstein, J. I., & Carter, B. S., et al. Sexual function following radical prostatectomy: Influence of preservation of neurovascular bundles. *J Urol, 145*: 998. 1991.

Robinson, M. R. G Complete androgen blockade: The EORTC experience comparing orchiectomy versus orchiectomy plus cyproterone acetate versus low-dose stilbestrol in the treatment of metastatic carcinoma of the prostate. In G. P. Murphy, S. Khoury, R. K: ⅓uss, C. Chatelain, & L. Denis (Eds.), *Proceeding of Second International Symposium on Prostate Cancer. Prostate Cancer, Part A. Research, Endocrine Treatment and Histopathology.* (pp. 383–390). New York: Alan R. Liss. 1987.

Schroder, F. H., Klihn, J. G, & deJong, F. H. *Metastatic cancer of the prostate managed by Buserelin acetate versus Buserelin acetate plus cyproterone acetate.* Paper presented at annual meeting of The American Urological Assocation, New York. 1986.

Scott, R., Mutchnik, D. L., & Laskowski, T. Z., et al. Carcinoma of the prostate in elderly men: Incidence, growth characteristics, and clinical significance. *J Urol, 101*: 602. 1969.

Seidman, H., Mushinski, M. H., & Gelb, S., et al. Probabilities of eventually developing or dying of cancer: United States 1985. *CA, 35*: 36. 1985.

Shinohara, K., Wheener, T. M., & Scardino, P. T. The appearance of prostate cancer on transurethral ultrasonography: Correlation of imaging and pathological examinations. *J Urol, 142*: 76. 1989.

Siddall, J. K., Hetherington, J. W., & Cooper, E. H., et al. Biochemical monitoring of carcinoma of prostate treated with an LH-RH analogue (Zoladex). Br J Urol, *58*: 672. 1986.

Smalley, S. R., & Noble, M. J. Prostate brachytherapy: Part 2. Clinical results, complications, and salvage therapy. *AUA update series, XI*: 34. 1992.

Sogani, P. C., & Fair, W. R. Treatment of advanced prostate cancer. *Urol Clin North Am, 14*: 353. 1987.

Spinack, J. P., & Resnick, M. I. Ultrasound (imaging). In J. Y. Gillenwater, J. T. Grayhack, S. S. Howards, & J. W. Duckett (Eds.), *Adult and Pediatric Urology* (pp. 161–188). St. Louis. Mosby Year Book. 1991.

Stamey, T. A., & Kabalin, J. N. Prostate specific antigen in the diagnosis and treatment of adenocarcinoma of the prostate: I. Untreated patients. *J Urol, 141*: 1070. 1989.

Stamey, T. A., & McNeal, J. E. Adenocarcinoma of the prostate, In P. C. Walsh, A. B. Retik, T. A. Stamey, & E. D. Vaughan (Eds.), *Campbell's Urology.* (pp. 1159–1221). Philadelphia: Saunders. 1992.

Stamey, T. A., Yang, N., & Hay, A. R., et al. Prostate-specific antigen as serum marker for adenocarcinoma of the prostate. *N Engl J Med, 317*: 909. 1987.

Steinberg, G. D., Epstein, J. I., Piantodosi, S., & Walsh, P. C.: Management of stage D1 adenocarcinoma of the prostate: The Johns Hopkins Experience, 1974 to 1987. *J Urol, 144*: 1425. 1990.

Thompson, I. M. Screening for carcinoma of the prostate. *AUA update series,* 9: 29. 1990.

Trachtenberg, J., & Pont, A. Ketoconazole: A novel and rapid treatment for advanced prostate cancer. *J Urol, 150*: 152. 1983.

Walsh, P. C. Radical retropubic prostatectomy with reduced morbidity: An anatomic approach. *NCI monogr, 7*: 133. 1988

Whitmore, W. J. Jr., Warner, J. A., & Thompson, I. M., Jr. Expectant management of localized prostatic cancer. *Cancer, 67*: 1091. 1991.

Winkler, H. Z., Rainwater, L. M., & Myers, R. P., et al. Stage D1 prostate adenocarcinoma. Significance of nuclear DNA ploidy patterns studied by flow cytometry. *Mayo Clinic Proc, 63*: 103. 1988.

Chapter Fourteen

Advanced Cancer Treatment of the Elderly

Wallace L. Akerley, III and Paul Calabresi

Although cancer strikes all ages and causes more premature deaths than any other illness in the United States (Mettlin, 1989), it remains overwhelmingly an affliction of middle and later years (Seer Program, 1984). Cancer incidence plotted against age (Figure 14.1) demonstrates a low risk of developing cancer during the first years of life, which increases exponentially with age after the first decade. Despite the appearance of a declining slope after the eighth decade, there is no plateau, and the rate continues to rise. The exponential doubling time of this slope between the second and eighth decades of life is relatively constant at 8 years. This implies that an individual will experience a doubling of cancer risk every 8 years, and a population will double its overall annual cancer incidence if the median age of the population increases by 8 years.

This relationship between cancer and aging has special meaning for the United States and other industrialized countries, where a rising median population age places proportionally more people into age categories with greater risk of developing cancer. In the United States the proportion of those of greater age is rapidly expanding due to a combination of a declining birthrate and extended survival. In the past two decades, the population older than 65 years grew by 56%, and in the next two decades, those older than 80 years are expected to double in number (Kennedy, 1988). These trends have resulted in a rising, non-age-adjusted cancer in-

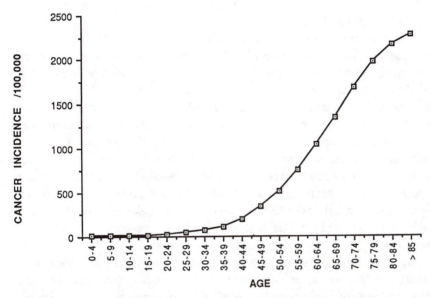

FIGURE 14.1 The incidence of cancer in the United States plotted as a function of age. The data are from the Surveillance, Epidemiology and End Results (SEER) Program during 1978–1981.

cidence that promises continued pressure on a health care system already financially strained (Brown, 1990).

ADVANCED CANCER TREATMENT

All forms of cancer treatment are, by their very nature, advanced therapeutic technologies because the selective eradication of a cancer from the composite cancer–host interface cannot yet be achieved without risking disruption of normal tissues. Despite improvements in therapy, an element of treatment-induced destruction of normal host tissue or transient organ dysfunction can be anticipated, even with well-tolerated and successful treatment. Therapies directed toward the local eradication of a cancer are frequently complicated by local adverse effects, whereas those designed to control widespread systemic cancer are often associated with global, systemic imbalances that risk lethal potential. In this respect, all forms of cancer therapy represent a delicate balance between therapeutic efficacy and therapeutic toxicity (physical and emotional) that must be thoughtfully weighed whenever any treatment is contemplated.

A major reason that cancer treatment represents such a formidable task is the absence of a clearly defined separation or border between the cancer and normal host tissues. Malignant cells have the ability to infiltrate directly into surrounding normal tissue or metastasize to distant, noncontiguous sites via blood vessel or lymphatic pathways. When the tumor grows directly into adjacent normal tissues, a clear demarcation between the tumor and host may appear obvious; however, the invasive process is frequently more insidious, as slender fingers of innocent-appearing tumor cells can often be found interdigitating themselves within the presumed normal tissue. In this case, the boundaries are ill-defined and functionally nonexistent, as if spread through systemic, metastatic pathways.

Surgery and radiation are local and regional cancer treatments designed to control or cure cancer at a specific location. To cure, these therapies must eradicate all existing tumor. Due to the absence of a well-demarcated tumor border, these therapies attempt physically to remove or destroy all gross tumor plus a rim of surrounding normal tissue, which may be inhabited by unrecognized cancer cells. The resulting morbidity of these procedures is largely dependent upon the size of the tumor, the preexisting damage caused by the tumor, and the amount of normal tissue that must be removed to improve the chances of complete tumor eradication. The degree of morbidity may be minimal, with little functional impairment, or it may be far greater, necessitating complete removal of organs or limbs. These therapies can also be associated with systemic complications such as infection, myelosuppression after radiation, or anesthetic risks during surgery.

Systemic treatments with chemotherapy, hormones, or biologics may be associated with a temporary or permanent multiorgan dysfunction that may affect any or all of the body's systemic vital functions. Immune suppression, inhibition of hematopoiesis, infection, bleeding, gastrointestinal upset, and mucositis are the most frequent concerns, but dysfunction of the renal, pulmonary, hepatic, cardiovascular, or nervous systems may also occur. The toxicity profile of hormonal cancer therapy, although generally less intimidating than other systemic treatments, can also be associated with dire systemic complications as tightly controlled endocrine feedback loops have been disrupted. Even control of pain with narcotics or other analgesics can be associated with respiratory, neurologic, gastrointestinal, or renal adverse effects. These potential complications highlight the expertise required to maintain the delicate homeostatic balance of the host during all forms of cancer treatment, which, though routinely practiced, cannot be taken for granted.

GLOBAL ORGAN FUNCTION

The human body has a substantial built-in redundancy or functional reserve capacity that allows one not only to maintain normal homeostasis but also to withstand the unexpected physiologic or emotional stresses encountered in everyday life. The challenges of a cold or pneumonia seldom overcome a fully competent physiologic reserve, but the demands of cancer treatments or the cancer itself can generate a wide range of stresses that may overwhelm even the most capable of reserve capacities. The art of successful cancer treatment is to estimate global organ function, and the science is to assure that it is not exceeded by therapy. The difficult parameter complicating this equation is organ function because it is neither fixed for all individuals nor constant over time, even within a particular individual.

The diagnosis of overt organ dysfunction is easily discerned through patient symptomatology and routine testing. The greater challenge is diagnosing and estimating the more subtle changes affecting the reserve capacity only. These changes are clinically silent in an unstressed state and must be specifically measured by a directed laboratory evaluation when clinical circumstances dictate a need for a specific, critical organ reserve. Comorbid disease and age are the major factors influencing organ dysfunction.

A disease is generally organ-based and characterized by varying degrees of dysfunction of a dominantly involved organ, whereas the deleterious effects of age are usually more heterogeneous. Gross dysfunction of a single organ system is usually due to a coexisting disease such as stroke, atherosclerotic heart disease, or emphysema. Although the prevalence of such illnesses may increase with increasing age, they are not necessarily an obligatory feature of aging. Their symptom complexes may frequently overlap with symptoms associated with aging, but their pathogeneses, natural histories, and treatments are discrete. An accurate diagnosis is essential for rational patient care because it determines prognosis, guides treatment, and defines the upper limits of specific organ function. Additionally, disease-specific therapy may correct, improve, or at least prevent an illness from following a progressive course.

Age is also associated with diminished organ function, but the relationship is variable, and a causal mechanism for all of its touted effects is not yet clearly defined. Consequently, before a diagnosis of age-related organ dysfunction is made, one must first exclude all alternative specific disease etiologies. The process of aging is commonly thought of as "chronic wear and tear," with changes that are usually quite insidious, slowly progressive, and irreversible. They likely represent the cumulative effects of multiple processes triggered by both genetic and environmental agents.

Chronologic age is the most frequently used method to quantify age, but chronologic age and physiologic age, as measures of global organ function, often differ. Many chronologically elderly individuals are physiologically able to live independently and manage the responsibilities of full-time employment long after their peers have retired or considered alternative living arrangements to support their personal care. Although both groups of individuals may be healthy, in the sense that they do not have any identifiable specific illnesses, the latter group, who may require ancillary assistance for self-care, exemplify the cumulative effects of subtle multiorgan dysfunction that is associated with aging. This contrast emphasizes the important distinction of variability between physiologic and chronologic age. Unfortunately, there is no ideal biomarker of physiologic age (Mooradian, 1992), and surrogates must be used to define it as a measure of global organ function in the elderly.

Performance status evaluation using the scales of Karnofsky or Zubrod are used by oncologists to rate a patient's overall functional status. Though designed specifically to gauge cancer-related morbidity, they serve reasonably as surrogate markers or indirect measures of global organ function. These scales rate patients' overall ability or inability to function independently in their usual daily activities by evaluating their capacities to work, to care for themselves, and to ambulate at a particular instance of time. Those who live independently and by definition have a good performance status demonstrate a relatively high level of overall global organ function, whereas those with a poor performance status, who require social or medical assistance, all share some element or elements of organ system failure. Though performance status may overlook moderate variations in functional reserve and adaptive compensations, such as adjustments in life-style or medications unrelated to the cancer, it provides a reproducible, quantitative surrogate marker of global organ function that is reflective of coordinated organ competence (Schag, Heinrich, & Ganz, 1984).

AGING AND CANCER TREATMENT

Numerous functional alterations are associated with aging, but most do not interfere with one's capacity to tolerate the stresses of cancer treatment. Stereotypic changes of aging, such as loss of skin elasticity and depigmentation of hair, are cosmetic only and have no bearing on vital organ function or treatment. Those important changes that do affect vital organ function, however, do not necessarily all hinder one's ability to undergo treatment if the deficiency is insignificant relative to the unused silent functional reserve or if the organ or particular function is unlikely to be stressed by the specific treatment. For example, pulmonary flow parameters decline predictably with age, whereas the functions of oxygenation and acid–base homeostasis are rigidly maintained. An isolated deficiency of forced expiratory vital capacity would not change the risk–benefit ratio for most types of chemotherapy but would be of critical importance when considering surgical lung resection or radiation therapy because a further decline of this parameter can be anticipated as a direct consequence of these latter treatments. Finally, the most common change of vital organ function due solely to age is "no change at all" (Rowe, 1985), which includes peripheral blood counts, acid–base balance, fasting glucose levels, and many endocrine functions. The functional reserves of the organ systems most germane to cancer medicine are those likely to be affected as a direct consequence of the treatment and the organs involved in drug metabolism and clearance (liver and kidney).

The renal system is of particular importance when considering the effects of age and certain antineoplastic chemotherapy because the kidney is a dominant organ of drug elimination, its function is known to decline with advancing age, and substantial degrees of renal dysfunction can be tolerated without symptoms. Glomerular filtration decreases with age at the rate of approximately 10 ml per minute per decade of age after the third decade of life. This renal dysfunction is classically identified by noting a consequent rise in serum creatinine. In the elderly, it is important to realize that this expected increase in serum creatinine may frequently be masked by age-related decreases in muscle mass, resulting in decreased creatinine production. This opposing force tends to make the serum creatinine a less than adequate marker of renal function in the elderly, and significant dysfunction may go unrecognized despite history and screening tests. Consequently, older patients may be at increased risk for developing unanticipated chemotherapeutic toxicity due to delayed drug clearance if more sensitive testing is not performed.

The liver shares an equally important role in the metabolism and clearance of chemotherapeutic agents; however, age-related changes of liver function are of limited scope and seldom become an issue during cancer treatment. Decreased hepatic blood flow has been associated with age (Bressler, 1985), but clinical drug toxicity is unusual because drug metabolism, the rate-limiting step of hepatic elimination, is adequately maintained at the cellular level. Enhanced toxicity as a result of hepatic dysfunction occurs only when there is substantial destruction of the liver by tumor or a coexisting primary disease of the liver. Liver function can be adequately screened by routine testing of liver enzymes and markers of synthetic function.

The bone marrow is the organ system most commonly affected as a direct consequence of cytotoxic chemotherapy. The density of hematopoietic elements in the bone marrow decreases with age, suggesting that the myelopoietic reserve may be limited (Baldwin, 1988), but this has been clinically difficult to substantiate. The basal blood counts monitored by a CBC do not change with age, and if drug dosing is corrected for variations in renal drug clearance and performance status, little difference is seen in myelotoxicity (Gelman & Taylor, 1984).

The kidney, although involved in drug clearance, is also frequently an innocent target of dose-related chemotoxicity. Cisplatin, a drug common to many of the chemotherapeutic regimens used in nonhematopoietic cancers, causes renal dysfunction in a variable but generally predictable fashion. In aged patients, there is an 2 ml/min loss of glomerular filtration per dose of therapy, compared to an 8 ml/min loss of glomerular filtration per dose that occurred in a younger peer group. Although the elderly patients were known to have a decrease in their renal function due to age, the younger patients showed a greater loss of renal function per dose of cisplatin, which resulted in proportionally equivalent toxicity for both young and old (Hrushesky, Shimp, & Kennedy, 1984).

Most toxicities of treatment are modality-specific and proportional to dose. If any part of an organ is removed surgically, then the remaining organs must have an adequate physiologic reserve to sustain the function of the predicted void. The same is true for systemic therapies, although the anticipated toxicity is often more diffuse and frequently affects multiple organ systems. In this respect, the elderly, who may have latent compromise of organ function as a result of aging, may be at higher risk for dose-related toxicity if attention is not paid to pretreatment organ reserves.

OUTCOME

In most instances, older patients with a wide variety of nonhematopoietic cancers demonstrate comparable treatment outcomes compared to their less senior peers, but elderly patients with acute leukemia (Champlin, Gajewski, & Golde, 1989; Ellison et al., 1991), non-Hodgkin's lymphoma (Vose et al., 1988), and Hodgkin's lymphoma (Guinee, 1991) demonstrate decreased survival with advancing age. The reason for the dichotomy between nonhematopoietic and hematopoietic cancers remains elusive. It is possible that the greater intensity of treatment for leukemia and lymphoma (chemotherapy at the highest tolerable dose) results in a narrower margin of safety for the elderly who may have unrecognized deficiencies of vital organ function. Alternatively, the tumors in the elderly may display a more aggressive biology because they are genetically different from those found in younger patients.

In a retrospective analysis of 19 separate chemotherapy trials by the Eastern Cooperative Oncology Group—which treated cancers of the lung, colon, rectum, stomach, head/neck, kidney, and ovary, as well as melanoma—the clinical outcomes of patients of more than or less than 70 years of age were compared and found to be similar in terms of toxicities, benefits of therapy, and survival (Begg & Carbone, 1983). A similar retrospective analysis of patients with metastatic breast cancer from five clinical trials performed by the Piedmont Oncology Group showed that response rates, disease progression, survival, and toxicity were not affected by age (Christman, Muss, & Stanley, 1992). All patients evaluated were ambulatory, and capable of self-care, and demonstrated adequate hematologic, renal, and hepatic function.

At the same time, it must be understood that the outcomes of these trials may not necessarily always correlate with those of the general medical community because clinical trials often study a population of patients different from those seen in the community, and these trials are frequently asked retrospectively to answer questions for which they were not originally designed. To answer a specific question accurately in a controlled experiment, one must strive to limit the number of variables to the one of primary interest. In a clinical trial, like those described, where therapy is the primary variable of interest, the effects of all other potentially confounding variables, such as coexisting illness or organ dysfunction, are minimized or eliminated, if possible, during the design of the trial. This is done by rigidly adhering to predefined eligibility criteria that specify a minimum standard for organ function, clinical performance, and non-life-threatening concurrent diseases. The eligible patients are, by definition, similar in their pretreatment characteristics, but older patients do not fit these criteria as frequently as younger patients do, so the population studied may be proportionally different from the community population. As an example, only 13% of the more than 6000 patients evaluated in the ECOG analyses were older than 69 years. Therefore, a trial conclusion may be less generalizable to an older population than to a younger population. On the other hand, one should not automatically discard a study's applicability to an older patient population because many older patients do indeed fit the criteria used to define a trial's eligibility.

APPROACH TO CANCER TREATMENT OF THE AGED

The approach to cancer treatment of the elderly can and should be unbiased by age if care is taken to address each aspect of patient care that is routinely considered in all patients. There are differences between older and younger patient populations, but the variations are not restricted to either age group. In every patient with a suspected cancer, an accurate histologic diagnosis and careful staging to determine the extent of disease must first be obtained. Together, these give an indication of the natural history of the disease and the likelihood of response to specific treatments. Then, an evaluation of organ function is performed to determine which of the diagnostic and treatment options can be tolerated by the patient. With this information, a deliberate and careful discussion should take place with the patient, regarding life's goals, prognosis, treatment options, potential toxicities and expected outcomes, before reaching a treatment decision that best suits the patient's particular needs.

First and foremost, an accurate histologic diagnosis by an experienced pathologist must be confirmed in all patients with suspected cancer. A clinical diagnosis without biopsy confirmation is frequently incorrect and is always too general to identify a potentially favorable histologic subclass. Lymphoma, germ cell tumors, and hematologic neoplasms may be curable regardless of extent of disease, many low-grade tumors have a favorable prognosis without therapy, and many cancers demonstrate extended survival with relatively nontoxic therapy, so it is critical that a diagnosis of cancer be subclass-specific. Failure to obtain a histologic diagnosis because of age, concurrent disease, difficult tumor location, or other bias leaves patients uninformed and unable to participate meaningfully in their own care. It may deny the patient an opportunity for a disease-specific cure, extended survival, or effective palliation. Worse yet, it may allow the patient to be subjected to an ineffective therapy with inherent toxicity that may possibly shorten survival or decrease quality of life.

Clearly, no aspect of cancer treatment can reasonably be considered without an accurate histologic diagnosis, but a surgical biopsy in certain instances can be associated with significant risks. Fortunately, several alternative methods of histologic diagnosis, including cytologic examination of exfoliated cells in secretions or scrapings, fiberoptic-assisted biopsy, and stereotactic fine-needle aspiration, can be considered in these situations. A conclusive diagnosis of a specific neoplasm by one of these minimally invasive procedures can obviate the risks of general anesthesia and the morbidity of major surgery. When the procedure confirms the suspected malignancy, the advantage is formidable. The addition of immunohistochemistry and cell surface phenotyping has added considerably to the diagnostic yield. Unfortunately, a benign or nonspecific diagnosis is difficult to interpret because it is impossible to determine if the cancer cells were not sampled or if the lesion was truly benign. In these situations, the procedure must be repeated or be followed by the gold standard, large-sample incisional biopsy. The great advantages and potential disadvantages of minimal invasiveness are similar for both young and old.

Staging is the next important step in patient evaluation because it provides a mechanism for accurate comparison of an individual's disease with the published clinical experience to give an indication of prognosis, the effectiveness of various treatments, and their potential toxicities. Staging is performed by defining the locations and spread of the tumor in terms of direct tumor invasion, lymphatic extension, and metastatic blood-borne spread. All cancers are broadly staged in a similar manner, but tumor-specific modifications are added to reflect the discrete natural history of specific cancers. Accordingly, the process of staging is initiated in a general way during the evaluation of the patient's history and physical findings but is later refined when the histologic diagnosis has been confirmed. Staging is the same for young and old. With this information in hand, a list of appropriate therapies can be determined and their historical outcomes and toxicities listed.

Next, a baseline evaluation of organ function is performed. Initially, organ function is evaluated in a general way during the history, physical, and laboratory evaluation. After the stage and site-specific diagnosis have been confirmed, the evaluation is refined to determine more precisely the functional reserve of the organs likely to be affected by the potential therapies under consideration. If the disease is limited in spread and a locally destructive therapy is planned, then attention is directed to the task of predicting residual function of the organ after therapy. Alternatively, if the disease is widespread and drug therapy is contemplated, then attention is directed to the organ systems responsible for drug clearance and those that may be at risk from systemic drug toxicity. In the elderly, the same procedure is followed, but efforts are made to quantitate the degree of dysfunction because a cursory exam will frequently miss silent deficiencies of the functional reserve. For example, if renal function is being evaluated, a creatinine clearance should be performed rather than just a serum creatinine, and for cardiac function a radionucleotide angiogram should be considered in place of an electrocardiogram.

The measurement of performance status completes the data collection. As the quantitative equivalent of the clinician's estimate of "how the patient looks," it complements the information gained through staging and baseline organ function. First, as a measure of cancer-related morbidity, it provides prognostic information related to survival and response to treatment that acts as a further refinement of staging. Second, as a cumulative measure of global organ function due to cancer-related morbidity and comorbidity from other concurrent diseases, it gives an indication of the global physi-

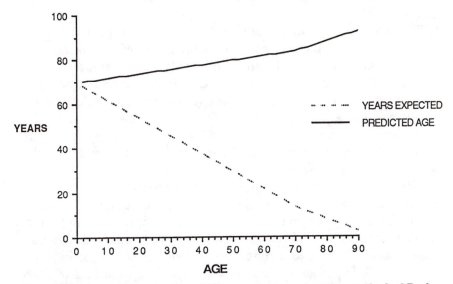

FIGURE 14.2 Approximation of life expectancy using the method of Beck, 1982. The dotted line represents years of life expectancy and the solid line represents the predicted age of death. For example, a 70-year-old person is expected to live an additional 13½ years and expire at 83 years of age. Note, life expectancy decreases with increasing age, but the predicted age of survival increases.

ologic, functional reserve, which helps to define the limits of therapy that the patient may safely endure.

Life expectancy is also to be considered, even though it is frequently given undue emphasis and, on occasion, leads to inappropriate conclusions. Life expectancy does decrease with absolute age, but the relationship is nonlinear (Figure 14.2; Beck, Kassirer, & Pauker, 1982). It is clear that an incurable cancer will shorten a young patient's predicted long survival based on age alone, but this statement is often true for the elderly, too. It is sometimes incorrectly assumed that when a person has achieved the anticipated median life expectancy, there is no more. In fact, this older person has a greater probability of achieving a greater absolute age than any younger person of the same sex, culture, and social economic status. For example, a 70–year-old person is expected to live an additional 13½ years. If these additional years are achieved, then this 84–year-old can expect an additional median 6 years of life, and so on. In this case, a poor outcome from cancer would certainly shorten this patient's life expectancy and decrease the quality of life.

With this information, a candid discussion takes place with the patient and/or family to discuss the implications of the disease, the prognosis, the relative risks and benefits of different therapies, and the patient's life goals. The types of treatments tolerated, the efficacy of treatment, the goals of therapy, and the patient's expectation (Cassileth et al., 1980) may differ between the young and old, so the patient should be encouraged to take an active role in the treatment decision. Most patients, regardless of age, want to take an active role in their therapy.

Clinical cancer trials designed specifically to examine the issue of treatment of the expanding population of senior Americans should be considered. In the absence of a clinical trial, a deliberate, positive approach should be taken with each patient to individualize therapy, taking into account the patient's stage, physiologic reserve, coexisting diseases, quality of life, and expectations of therapy. In that way the patient can choose a therapeutic option that will match personal goals and satisfy the risk–benefit quotient. In most situations, the decision will be a compromise that has been thoughtfully considered by both the patient and physician. Cancer treatment of the aging is an issue that has been clearly recognized by the National Cancer Institute and the President's National Cancer Advisory Board as an area of high priority.

References

Baldwin, J. Hematopoietic function in the elderly. *Arch Intern Med, 148*: 2544–6. 1988.

Beck, J., Kassirer, J., & Pauker S. A convenient approximation of life expectancy. *Am J Med, 73*: 883–888. 1982.

Begg, C., & Carbone, P. Clinical trials and drug toxicity in the elderly: The experience of the Eastern Cooperative Oncology Group. *Cancer, 52*: 1986–1992. 1983.

Bressler, R. Drug use in elderly patients, P223–5. In D. Lipschitz, (moderator) *Cancer in the Elderly: Basic science and clinical aspects. Ann Intern Med, 102*: 218–28. 1985.

Brown, M. Special Report: The national economic burden of cancer, an update. *JNCI, 82*: 1811–14. 1990.

Calabresi, P. & Scheim, P. Medical oncology (2nd ed.), New York: McGraw Hill. 1993.

Cassileth, B., Zupkis, R., & Sutton-Smith, K. et al. Information and participation preferences among cancer patients. *AIM, 92*: 832–6. 1980.

Champlin, R., Gajewski, J., & Golde D. Treatment of acute myeloid leukemia in the elderly, pp. 51–56. In W. Ershler, (Ed.), *Cancer in the elderly, 16*: 1. 1989.

Christman, K., Muss, H., Case, L., Stanley, V. Chemotherapy of metastatic breast cancer in the elderly: The Piedmont Oncology Experience. *JAMA, 268*(1): 57–62. 1992.

Ellison, R., Mick, R., & Cuttner, J., et al. The effects of postinduction intensification treatment with cytarabine and daunorubicin in adult acute leukemia: A prospective randomized clinical trial by the CALGB. *J Clin Oncol, 9*: 2002–15. 1991

Gelman, R., & Taylor S. Cyclophosphamide, methotrexate and 5–fluorouracil chemotherapy in women more than 65 years old with advanced breast cancer: The elimination of age trends in toxicity by using doses based on creatinine clearance. *J Clin Oncol, 2*: 1404–13. 1984.

Guinee, V. The prognosis of Hodgkin's disease in older adults. *J Clin Oncol, 9*: 947–53. 1991.

Hrushesky, W., Shimp, W., & Kennedy, B. Lack of age dependent cisplatin nephrotoxicity. *Am J Med, 16*: 579–84. 1984

Kennedy, B. Aging and cancer. *J Clin Oncol, 16*: 1903–11. 1988.

Mettlin, C. Trends in years of life lost to cancer: 1970–85. *Ca, 39*(1): 33–39. 1989.

Mooradian, A. Biological and functional definitions of the older patient, (pp. 39–44). In N. Tchekmedyian, D. Cella, A. Mooradian, (Eds.), *Care of the Older Cancer Patient. Oncology, 6*: 2 Supplement. 1992.

Rowe, J. Health care of the elderly. *N Engl J Med, 302*: 827–35. 1985.

Schag, C., Heinrich, R., & Ganz, P. Karnofsky performance status revisited: Reliability, validity and guidelines. *J Clin Oncol, 2*: 187–93. 1984.

Seer Program. *Cancer incidence and mortality in the United States.* NIH Publication No. 85–1837. 1984.

Vose, J., Armitage, J., & Weisenburger, D., et al. The importance of age in survival of patients treated with chemotherapy for aggressive non-Hodgkin's lymphoma. *J Clin Oncol, 6*: 1838–44. 1988.

Chapter Fifteen

The Progress and Promise of Effectiveness Research in Aged Patients

Claire W. Maklan

This chapter focuses on a new kind of research—variously called patient outcomes research or medical effectiveness research—that seeks to inject "rationality" into a wide range of health care decisions by expanding the scientific information and range of perspectives that are brought to bear. Effectiveness research has implications not only for the rational use of advanced diagnostic and therapeutic technologies and not exclusively for elderly persons (i.e., the chief concerns of this volume) but also for the rational use of ordinary clinical procedures and services that are or are not implemented, every day, in patients of all ages.

Readers should know at the outset that effectiveness research starts with a heavy dose of skepticism about current medical practice. It has emerged from several decades of health services research that documents dramatic variations in clinical practice from one geographic region to another (Chassin et al., 1986; Wennberg, Freeman, & Culp, 1987). These variations—for instance, in rates of hospital admission for low back pain—are usually attributed to the lack of clinical consensus about what treatment is correct. Effectiveness research focuses on "reasonably held but inadequately tested theories of treatment" (Wennberg et al., 1987) and assesses the outcomes of alternative clinical strategies. It seeks to differentiate those clinical interventions with demonstrable and beneficial effects from those with adverse, equivocal, improbable, or unimportant effects. Simply put, effectiveness research focuses on determining which of the available clinical options is best.

Effectiveness research has attracted considerable interest within both government and private research and health professional organizations. Hopes are high that it will lead to improved health outcomes for individuals and a more effective and cost-effective health care system (Relman, 1988; Roper, Winkenwerder, Hackbarth, & Krakauer, 1988). This chapter reviews the purpose, methods, and issues addressed by federally funded effectiveness research and some of the early findings. The selected examples focus on clinical topics that are pertinent to the rational use of health services for elderly persons.

WHAT IS "RATIONALITY" IN HEALTH CARE?

Before attempting to illustrate the potential of particular effectiveness studies to contribute to rational health care, it is necessary to present some ideas about what constitutes a rational health care decision. (The concept of effectiveness will be explored in the next section.)

Rational decisions, regarding health care or other concerns, "proceed from" and are "consistent with reason and intellect" (*Roget's Thesaurus*, 1988). Thus, rationality in health care is dependent on the quantity and quality of clinical and other information that is available and the validity of the process by which physicians and others transform that information into a decision they can implement. In a sense, rationality is relative. If we can increase the amount and accuracy of available information and improve the processing of that information, we should be able to make decisions that are both more rational and more consistently rational.

The following types of information are fundamental to rational health care decisions:

- Scientific information about the effectiveness of the proposed treatment.
- Scientific information about the relative effectiveness of alternative treatments.
- Scientific information that is relevant to the population of interest (here, elderly patients).

A pragmatic approach requires us to acknowledge the fact that economic disparities, limited resources, and sometimes legal and regulatory requirements present serious challenges to the implementation of health care decisions that are based on science alone. While working toward a more equitable health care system, we must recognize the dilemma of reaching decisions that are rational but not feasible. Thus, rational health care decisions must, temporarily at least, also explicitly incorporate information about

- availability of needed providers and facilities
- access to treatment
- cost

With so many kinds of informational requirements (and with constant change in what is "known"), it is unrealistic to expect either that all pertinent information will be available for all issues or that health care decision makers could possess and process it. Indeed, we have long been aware of the limits of medical science and/ or any individual's personal grasp of it. We must admit the fact that some diseases have no known cause, some have no known cure. Further, we accept the fact that some procedures are experimental.

A recent focus of concern is the frequent unavailability or poor quality of scientific information about the effectiveness and relative effectiveness of treatments that are in everyday use, treatments whose value has generally been assumed (Eddy & Billings, 1988; Roper et al., 1988). We have tuned into the reality that, without first undergoing adequate evaluation, many treatments and procedures have been adopted into practice; they have become the community standard and what patients expect.

Among physicians, geriatricians especially can list far too many examples of treatments and practices that are in wide use despite the lack of evidence regarding effectiveness for their patients. On the one hand, there are common treatments whose effectiveness in general, or in elderly people in particular, remains unevaluated or unsettled. Examples include

- treatment of mild hypertension
- radical surgery for early prostate cancer
- estrogen replacement therapy

On the other hand, unasked and unanswered questions about the relative effects of alternative clinical strategies account for significant differences in observed practice patterns, associated differences in resource use, and frequently, differences in outcomes. The effectiveness of radical surgery for localized prostate cancer must be considered in the light of the outcomes of other, less risky procedures. The effectiveness of long-term estrogen replacement therapy to prevent osteoporosis must be considered in the light of expected cardiovascular benefits and the possible increased risk of endometrial cancer.

FEDERALLY SPONSORED MEDICAL EFFECTIVENESS RESEARCH

Under an initiative known as the Medical Treatment Effectiveness Program (MEDTEP), the federal government has started to address many of the information gaps that impede rational clinical decision making. MEDTEP is a DHHS-wide program led by the newest component of the U.S. Public Health Service, the Agency for Health Care Policy and Research (AHCPR). The program supports research and other activities aimed at improving the effectiveness and appropriateness of health care by developing new scientific information and by facilitating its dissemination to all potential users.

To appreciate the relevance and timeliness of AHCPR's effectiveness research, it is essential to understand how AHCPR interprets the traditional concept of efficacy and the newer concepts of effectiveness, cost-effectiveness, and appropriateness.

Efficacy

A clinical therapy or procedure is usually said to be efficacious (i.e., to meet the test of efficacy) if it has the potential to produce observable clinical benefits, at least under ideal conditions. Studies to determine efficacy are usually controlled experiments in which selected health care providers follow specified protocols to care for selected patients. Efficacy is typically measured in terms of reductions in mortality and morbidity or physiological indicators of improved clinical status. A complicated surgical procedure may be deemed efficacious, regardless of whether it would have the observed effect in community practice, regardless of whether patients value its effect, and regardless of its effect relative to other modes of treatment. Similarly, a regimen for controlling blood glucose in diabetics may be deemed efficacious regardless of the feasibility of its implementation outside of a clinical trial.

Effectiveness

A therapy or procedure that is effective has exceeded tests of safety and efficacy and has proved its value in the "real world." Effectiveness studies explicitly acknowledge that health care is provided to patients who may have comorbidities and who certainly have diverse histories, resources, and expectations; this is provided by clinicians with different training, technical expertise, and interpersonal skills. This complexity is controlled statistically so that research findings can be generalized to health care as it is received and practiced in the community—not just in the best academic centers, in the hands of the most skilled physicians, and with compliant patients.

Effectiveness is measured in terms of outcomes that are experienced and understood by patients. Thus, in addition to morbidity, mortality, and objective clinical measures, effectiveness research focuses on patients' perceptions of symptom relief, functional status, quality of life, satisfaction with care, and cost.

Cost Effectiveness

Another concept that is key to understanding the potential of effectiveness research is cost effectiveness. To improve the quality of health care, it is necessary to reduce the utilization of care that is not beneficial and to increase access to care that is. Thus, effectiveness research is interested not just in absolute costs (direct and indirect, reimbursed and not) but in how the costs of care relate to outcomes in the short and long term. A cost-effective treatment is not necessarily inexpensive, not even necessarily the least expensive of the available alternatives. For patients with end-stage renal disease, for example, kidney transplant may be more cost effective than dialysis whether or not the total lifetime cost is lower.

Appropriateness

Closely related to effectiveness, and in some ways an extension of it, is the concept of appropriateness. Appropriateness incorporates considerations of values and preferences, and recognizes that these are subjective and idiosyncratic. AHCPR-sponsored effectiveness research is concerned with understanding and improving decisions about health care and the decision-making process, from the perspectives of patients, providers, and policymakers. In the same way that efficacious treatments are not necessarily effective, a highly effective treatment is not necessarily appropriate. Cataract extraction, while generally safe, efficacious, and effective, is not appropriate unless or until a patient values its potential benefits over the potential risks.

AHCPR's effectiveness studies are carried out primarily through peer-reviewed grants, plus a smaller number of competitive contracts. During MEDTEP's first 4 years, approximately 130 research projects have been undertaken. The rigorous methodological expectations for MEDTEP research help to ensure that the findings that ultimately emerge will accurately fill information gaps and help to resolve existing clinical controversies (AHCPR, 1990).

MEDTEP's broad research portfolio is depicted in Table 15.1. Clinical conditions under study include both acute and chronic diseases and disorders that may threaten life itself or the quality of life. The research agenda encompasses conditions pertinent to all age groups, with current studies ranging from childbirth and pediatric gastroenteritis to hysterectomy, osteoarthritis, ischemic heart disease, depression, and hip fracture. Though distinguished by differences in epidemiology, etiology, treatment, and prognosis, conditions in the MEDTEP portfolio are united by similarities along the following themes:

- Large numbers of people, especially elderly people, are affected.
- The human and economic costs are high.
- Clinical practice is known to vary, especially across geographic areas.
- Data for research are available or can be obtained.
- Medicare or Medicaid program is affected.

The existing clinical repertoire for these conditions includes both low- and high-technology procedures and strategies for prevention, diagnosis, treatment, and/or management. It encompasses medical, surgical, and pharmaceutical interventions, as well as the clinical services of nurses and allied health professionals. Also, signifi-

TABLE 15.1 Agency for Health Care Policy and Research
Effectiveness Research Portfolio, Projects Receiving Support During
Fiscal Year 1992

Condition or Procedure- Oriented Study Topics	Total No. Projects FY89-FY92	Active Projects in FY 1992
Chronic Cardiovascular Disease	7	4†
Obstetrical Practice	8	3†
Acute Myocardial Infarction	5	3†
Low Back Pain	2	2†
Community-Acquired Pneumonia	1	1†
Cataract	2	2†
Type II Diabetes and Retinopathy	4	3†
Emergency/Trauma, and Critical Care	6	5
Stroke Prevention	2	2†
Cancer (other than prostate)	5	5
Pediatric Conditions	5	4
Prostate Cancer	3	3
Birth Outcomes	2	2†
Biliary Tract Disease	2	1†
Benign Prostate Disease	3	3†
Total Knee Replacement	1	1†
Hip Fracture and Hip Replacement	1	1†
Schizophrenia	1	1†
Hysterectomy	3	2
Other Surgery	2	1
Other Clinical Condition**	9	4
Depression	1	1
Dental Conditions	3	2
Methodological Study Topics		
Methods for Effective Dissemination	9	8
Quality of Care Measurement	5	4
Practice Variations	9	5
Other Research Methods	8	5
Outcomes Measurement	4	3

*Topics are listed in order of total AHCPR investment during Fiscal Year 1992.

†One of these projects is a Patient Outcomes Research Team (PORT).

**"Other" includes one or more studies on each of the following: cerebral palsy, drug prescribing, drug-related illness, genital chlamydia, epilepsy, HIV infection, home care, and pain (other than back pain).

cantly, many MEDTEP projects are evaluating the effects of decisions to employ watchful waiting. Evaluation of outcomes for patients who choose monitoring, rather than immediate treatment, will provide needed information about the natural history of many diseases.

As carried out by AHCPR, effectiveness research employs several approaches that further distinguish it from other kinds of clinical research. First, while the research requires the clinical knowledge of primary care physicians and subspecialists, it also depends on a multidisciplinary perspective and commitment to incorporating the different concerns and skills of diverse research participants. The most complex MEDTEP projects are designed and carried out by highly skilled investigative teams that are expected to include academic and community physicians, health services researchers, epidemiologists, health economists, sociologists, biostatisticians, and others. Clinical knowledge and sensitivities must be joined by social science perspectives and expertise in a variety of special research methods, which typically include meta-analysis, survey research, decision analysis, assessment of functional status, and economic analysis. Some of the important advances expected from effectiveness research will be methodological ones.

Second, MEDTEP is distinguished by the serious emphasis placed on intensive, targeted dissemination of findings and clinical recommendations. Researchers are expected to develop and employ active and innovative methods for delivering information about outcomes to patients, physicians, and policymakers. In addition to all forms of print media, presentations, and continuing medical education, the results of effectiveness research are finding their way in new formats, including interactive video productions designed to inform patients about treatment options. MEDTEP also supports some research that is focused directly on developing improved dissemination strategies and on evaluating the effects of dissemination, in terms of changes in clinical practice and subsequent patient outcomes.

PROGRESS OF AHCPR EFFECTIVENESS RESEARCH

Patient Outcomes Research Teams (PORTS) are the largest and most complex of the MEDTEP projects to date. These are multidisciplinary studies that employ a combination of data sources and research methods to compare the outcomes of alternative clinical strategies for a selected disease or condition (Clinton, 1991; Raskin & Maklan, 1991). PORT assessments will lead to the development of clinical recommendations regarding rational use of particular treatments, incorporating better understanding of their relative benefits and risks for different groups of patients.

The following sections present some early published findings from the four PORTs that have been underway longest. Each of these 5–year projects is scheduled for completion in 1994.

Acute Myocardial Infarction (AMI) PORT

AHCPR's AMI PORT, at Harvard University, is studying the utilization of diagnostic and therapeutic interventions during and after hospitalization for AMI and the effects of these interventions on patient survival, health status, functional capacity, and quality of life (Pashos & McNeil, 1990). Specific interventions under investigation include cardiac procedures such as coronary angiography, coronary artery bypass graft (CABG) surgery, and percutaneous transluminal coronary angioplasty (PTCA), as well as drug therapies such as administration of thrombolytic agents, beta-blockers, heparin, calcium-channel blockers, and nitroglycerin.

Like all PORTs, this study involves a combination of powerful methodologies. To analyze variations in rates of coronary angiography and revascularization and subsequent patient outcomes and costs, the PORT is conducting retrospective analysis of national Medicare claims data and other billing data. Collection and analysis of primary data from medical records and surveys of patients with AMI from two states with different practice patterns will enable the PORT to examine more closely differences in outcomes and to describe case mix, process of care, and patient preferences. Decision modeling techniques will result in models for performance of elective coronary angiography and for administration of thrombolysis in the elderly during the period immediately following an AMI. Another contribution of this PORT is the development of "cumulative meta-analysis" to synthesize the results of published studies on the use of angiography, revascularization, fibrinolytic drugs, and other drug therapies.

Early descriptive findings of the AMI PORT, based on analysis of Medicare claims data, reveal significant sociodemographic and geographic differences in the utilization of various procedures. For example, the following patterns are observed: (1) for patients hospitalized with coronary heart disease, women are less likely than men to receive major diagnostic and therapeutic procedures, including coronary angiography, bypass surgery, and angioplasty (Ayanian & Epstein, 1991); (2) patients aged 65 to 74 have procedure rates more than five times higher than patients over age 80 (Udvarhelyi et al., 1991).

Using meta-analysis, the AMI PORT has demonstrated the lag between availability of certain treatments and recognition of their lifesaving effects by clinical experts writing review articles and medical textbooks. Specifically,

- By 1973, there was sufficient cumulative evidence to show that thrombolytic therapy reduces mortality in AMI patients by 25% to 30%. However, not until 1986 did more than half of all reviews recommend the use of these drugs (Antman et al., 1992; Lau et al., 1992).

- By 1981, cumulative evidence showed that intravenous nitrates reduced mortality by 10% to 20%. However, authors of review articles did not consistently recommend their use until 1988 (Antman et al., 1992; Lau et al., 1992).

In addition, the AMI PORT decision modeling team has demonstrated that thrombolytic therapy is a beneficial and cost-effective treatment for suspected AMI in very elderly patients (75 and over) under a wide variety of clinical circumstances (Krumholz et al., 1992).

Prostate Disease PORT

Uncertainty about the natural history of benign prostatic hyperplasia (BPH) and localized prostate cancer, plus the availability of alternative treatments, has led to wide variations in practice. Approximately 400,000 prostatectomies are performed in the United States every year. Enlargement of the prostate and attendant urinary dysfunction affects 8 of every 10 men by the age of 80.

The BPH PORT, based at Dartmouth University, is assessing numerous surgical and nonsurgical interventions for BPH and localized adenocarcinoma of the prostate (Wennberg, 1990). For BPH, the PORT will study variations in use and outcomes associated with transurethral resection of the prostate (TURP, the most common procedure), open prostatectomy, medical therapy, balloon dilation, transurethral incision of the prostate, microwave diathermy, other emerging treatments, and watchful waiting. Assessments for localized adenocarcinoma of the prostate will include early screening, radiation, radical prostatectomy, and watchful waiting.

A special contribution of the Prostate Disease PORT is its establishment of a cohort of approximately 1,000 men with diagnosed BPH who elect not to undergo surgery. Data will be collected for these "watchful waiters" over a period of 2 to 3 years (depending when they joined the study cohort). This will provide the best source of information to date on the natural history of diagnosed BPH to help answer questions about the appropriate indications for treatment. Members of the Prostate Disease PORT have developed a pioneering interactive video production to explain treatment options and their outcomes to patients. Early findings from experiments using this novel dissemination tool show that most patients with BPH who view the video choose watchful waiting rather than surgery.

Low Back Pain PORT

Investigators, based at the University of Washington, are studying alternative treatments for low back pain, the second leading cause for all physician visits and hospitalizations in the United States (Deyo, Cherkin, & Conrad, 1990). Geographic variations in the management of patients with low back pain have been well documented, but the efficacy and effectiveness of some treatments have not been demonstrated (Deyo, Cherkin, Conrad, & Volinn, 1991).

The Back Pain PORT is assessing alternative types of lumbar spine surgery (fusion, laminectomy, and discectomy), a variety of nonsurgical interventions (traction, physical therapy, spinal manipulation, and various therapeutic injections), and diagnostic tests (including myelography, computed tomography, magnetic resonance imaging, and thermography) that are commonly used, especially for patients with back pain due to spinal stenosis, the diagnosis leading to most back surgery among elderly patients.

The following findings are based on two meta-analyses plus analysis of Medicare claims data carried out by the Back Pain PORT:

- Continuing controversy regarding indications for spinal fusion is evidenced by ninefold variation in its use across large geographic regions of the United States. There have been no randomized controlled trials to compare fusion techniques with alternative procedures. The PORT's analyses reveal that, in comparisons of outcomes for back surgery performed with and without lumbar fusion, short-term outcomes were worse with fusion, long-term outcomes were not improved (especially in terms of reoperation rates), and hospital charges were 50% higher (Turner et al., 1992).

- The quality and quantity of existing studies do not provide convincing evidence for the diagnostic value of thermography, a physiologic test for lumbar radiculopathy. Flaws in the design of published studies tend to exaggerate the accuracy of thermography, and no published studies address the value of thermography above and beyond either physical examination or imaging tests. Meanwhile, thermography is widely used by physicians and chiropractors and is reimbursed by Medicare, private insurance companies, and state workers' compensation boards (Hoffman, Kent, & Deyo, 1991).

The Back Pain PORT is developing a decision model that will incorporate the probabilities for observed outcomes, patient preferences for various health states, and costs. The model will be based on data from national and statewide hospital discharge records, Medicare claims, and surveys of patients and physicians. Findings of the Back Pain PORT will be disseminated via targeted feedback to physicians and hospitals in areas with high surgical rates and by means of an educational interactive video designed to give patients a tailored presentation of the expected outcomes of surgical and nonsurgical treatment options.

Cataract PORT

Cataract extraction is the most common surgical procedure performed on Medicare beneficiaries, with more than 1,350,000 procedures per year. The surgery has proved safe and highly effective in restoring sight; however, there are unanswered questions about the effectiveness and cost effectiveness of the techniques used to treat cataract patients before, during, and after surgery, and there is considerable variation in practice. AHCPR's Cataract PORT, based at Johns Hopkins University, is assessing variations in practice and in short- and long-term outcomes and costs associated with cataract management (Steinberg et al., 1990).

PORT findings will compare the outcomes and costs associated with different types of surgical procedure (intracapsular cataract extraction, standard extracapsular extraction, and phacoemulsification), preoperative ophthalmologic diagnostic procedures (including potential acuity testing and speculomicroscopy), preoperative medical evaluation, and follow-up care, including the use of the Nd: YAG laser for treatment of posterior capsule opacification. A complementary study being carried out in Denmark, Canada, and Spain will permit comparisons of outcomes for cataract patients who choose to delay surgery or who are in a queue.

The Cataract PORT has completed syntheses of the published literature regarding preoperative ophthalmologic tests and complications of surgery, as well as preliminary analysis of utilization and outcomes based on national Medicare claims data. Interviews of patients operated on for cataract in cities with low, medium, and high rates of cataract surgery, plus chart reviews, will provide detailed clinical information, as well as information about patients' reports of their experience, preferences, and satisfaction with outcomes. Surveys of clinicians involved in the care of cataract patients (ophthalmologists, optometrists, anesthesiologists, and internists) will help explain the observed variations in practice and will help identify factual or attitudinal information needed for the design and implementation of effective clinical guidelines. A decision model will be developed to project the clinical and economic impact of alternative strategies for management of cataracts over the next 25 years.

The Cataract PORT has demonstrated how analysis of Medicare data, despite its lack of clinical detail, can lead to identification of rare but important events.

- Annually, about 200,000 Americans undergo Nd: YAG laser capsulotomy, an office procedure used to treat opacification of the lens capsule that is left in place following cataract surgery. Analyses performed by the Cataract PORT suggest that laser capsulotomy, while generally safe and effective, may quadruple the risk of sight-threatening retinal complications following surgery (Javitt, et al., 1992).

- Similarly, analysis of 1984 Medicare data suggests that intracapsular cataract extraction, which has been largely replaced by newer procedures, is associated with a higher risk of retinal detachment and serious ocular infection than extracapsular cataract extraction with a lens implant (Javitt et al., 1991a; 1991b).

**TABLE 15.2   Topics Addressed by AHCPR Clinical Practice
Guidelines**

Published
Pressure Ulcers in Adults: Prediction and Prevention
Urinary Incontinence in Adults
Cataract in Adults
Acute Pain Management
Depression in Primary Care
Sickle Cell Disease

Forthcoming
Diagnosis and Treatment of Benign Prostatic Hyperplasia
Management of Cancer-Related Pain
Evaluation and Management of Early HIV Infection
Low Back Problems
Quality Determinants of Mammography
Screening for Alzheimer's and Related Dementias
Diagnosis and Treatment of Anxiety and Panic Disorder in the Primary Care
    Setting
Pressure Ulcers in Adults: Treatment
Heart Failure
Post Stroke Rehabilitation
Cardiac Rehabilitation
Diagnosis and Management of Unstable Angina
Smoking Prevention and Cessation
Otitis Media in Children

Based on formal literature syntheses regarding tests of potential
visual acuity, glare and contrast sensitivity, and specular micros-
copy, tests often included in evaluation of a patient's need for cataract surgery and their personal risk, the PORT concludes that the
clinical benefits of these tests remain to be proved.

CLINICAL PRACTICE GUIDELINES

Another approach for increasing rationality in health care is the
development of clinical practice guidelines. AHCPR is active in
this movement, along with a large number of other public and private groups, including the American Medical Association's Practice Parameters Forum, specialty colleges, the Joint Commission
on the Accreditation of Healthcare Organizations, and states. At
this writing, AHCPR is supporting expert panels and contractors
to develop guidelines for the topics listed in Table 15.2, many of
which affect principally elderly men and women. For example, completed guidelines focus on urinary incontinence (Urinary Inconti-

nence, 1992), prevention of pressure ulcers (Pressure Ulcers, 1992), and management of cataract (Cataract, 1993). Ongoing guideline development addresses the following geriatric conditions: benign prostatic hyperplasia, Alzheimer's and related dementias, heart failure and other cardiac conditions, post-stroke rehabilitation, and treatment of pressure ulcers.

Significantly, AHCPR's mandate requires that the guidelines developed under its auspices will be subject to periodic review and revision to assure that they remain consistent with advances in science (including AHCPR-sponsored effectiveness research). Another important distinguishing feature of AHCPR-sponsored guidelines emerges from AHCPR's emphasis on active dissemination to all audiences. For each completed guideline, separate versions will be prepared, tailored to meet the different informational needs of clinicians, academicians, and patients.

CONCLUSION

This chapter has emphasized the potential and progress of medical effectiveness research, and to a lesser extent clinical practice guidelines, to increase rationality in health care decisions. The federal government's effectiveness program will add—in fact, it already has added—new clinical findings and relevant new perspectives to the clinical decision arena. The positive effects of this work will be felt in geriatric clinical practice and research, as well as in related government and institutional policies.

For geriatric practice, the relevance of AHCPR's medical effectiveness program is guaranteed by the agency's legislative requirement to emphasize conditions and procedures that are common and significant in the Medicare population. Early findings illustrate the capacity of MEDTEP to produce results that are pertinent to virtually any area of geriatric practice, from cardiology to ophthalmology. It has also been shown that this research has the capacity to accelerate the identification and dissemination of clinical findings, through such techniques as meta-analysis.

As with any clinical research, relevance to an area of practice and publication of findings do not assure adoption, especially if adoption necessitates behavior change. However, characteristics of geriatric medicine as a specialty, the involvement of geriatric patients, and the current interest in health care reform all support the view that the influence of MEDTEP activities within geriatric practice is potentially great.

First, geriatricians know that their youthful specialty is undeveloped, that many clinical issues have been unstudied or unresolved. This, combined with the recent entry of many physicians to geriatric medicine, means that practice patterns may be relatively less entrenched and that individual practitioners should be particularly receptive to pertinent new information. The fact that few geriatricians personally perform any of the specific procedures described above highlights the critical role of geriatricians as sources of information and referral for their patients.

Second, MEDTEP's mixing of disciplinary perspectives in identifying issues, framing questions, and designing and carrying out research is consistent with the importance that geriatrics attaches to comprehensive assessments, functional status, and quality of life. This common culture should help to make the results of many effectiveness studies particularly interesting and acceptable to geriatricians.

Significantly, the keen interest and large constituency of organized "aging" groups will give elderly health care consumers rapid access to MEDTEP findings and is expected to exert powerful influence on patient expectations and decision making. Already, the American Association of Retired Persons has been involved in disseminating information to its membership about AHCPR-sponsored clinical guidelines.

Other circumstances favoring the adoption of effectiveness findings in geriatrics are their relevance to and ready ear among Medicare and other insurers, as well as other health-policy-making forums eager to contain costs and improve the quality of care. Conditions currently addressed by AHCPR's PORTs account for roughly one-third of all hospital charges. To the extent that MEDTEP work identifies ineffective treatments and practices, adoption of this information by health insurers will simultaneously reduce costs and improve cost-effectiveness. MEDTEP information regarding the outcomes of alternative strategies and the reasons physicians and patients make the choices they do will also inform policy decisions, made at all levels of government and by health care institutions, regarding quality assurance, patient selection, technology, training, and possibly liability.

The impact of effectiveness work on geriatric research will be of several types. First is its potential to identify some of the most critical and most promising areas for research. Already it has shown that observed relationships between specific clinical interventions and patient outcomes, discernible through analysis of very large data sets, can throw light on previously unasked clinical questions that warrant further study. Other research needs have been identified through comprehensive, critical reviews of the clinical literature that have exposed some weak spots and gaps in the science base underlying current practice. In addition, the involvement of new participants and the certain advances in research methods will be beneficial for geriatric and other clinical research.

This chapter has stressed the dependence of rational health care decisions on the availability of good information. In concluding, it is necessary to stress that even complete and perfect information does not assure a rational decision if the decision making process is flawed. The process must accommodate the inherently different perspectives of physicians, patients, and payors and the myriad variations within each of these constituencies regarding what outcomes are acceptable or desirable.

The decision making processes used by effectiveness researchers include sophisticated statistics, meta-analysis, and decision modeling. They assign relative weights, probabilities, and utilities to the numerous variables and points of view that need to be considered. These synthetic approaches permit us to draw "rational" conclusions about the interaction of clinical data, economic data, and patient preferences, for hypothetical cases and statistical samples. Decisions made during the real-world, real-time interactions of physicians and patients will be assisted by these research findings, but the rationality of these decisions ultimately depends on the communication and mutual trust of those who possess the clinical expertise and those who seek their help.

ACKNOWLEDGMENTS

This chapter was produced in the federal domain under the auspices of the Agency for Health Care Policy and Research, Department of Health and Human Services. The views expressed are my own. No official endorsement by the Agency for Health Care Policy and Research is intended or should be inferred. I wish to acknowledge the helpful comments of Richard Greene, MD, PhD, Director of the Center for Medical Effectiveness Research, and Ira E.

Raskin, PhD, Deputy Director, as well as the PORT investigators whose work is described.

References

Acute Pain Management Guideline Panel. *Acute pain management: Operative or medical procedures and trauma.* (AHCPR Pub. Nos. 92-0019, 92-0021, and 92-0032). Rockville, MD: Agency for Health Care Policy and Research, Public Health Service, U.S. Department of Health and Human Services. 1992.

Agency for Health Care Policy and Research. *Medical treatment effectiveness research.* Program Note, Rockville, MD: Public Health Service, U.S. Department of Health and Human Services. 1990.

Antman, E. M., Lau, J., & Kupelnick, B., et al. A comparison of results of meta-analyses of randomized control trials and recommendations of clinical experts: treatments for myocardial infarction. *JAMA, 268*: 2: 240–248. 1992.

Ayanian, J. Z., & Epstein, A. M. Differences in the use of procedures between men and women hospitalized for coronary artery disease. *New Engl J Med, 325*(4): 221–225. 1991.

Cataract Guideline Panel. *Cataract in adults: Management of functional impairment.* (AHCPR Pub. Nos. 93-0542, 93-0543 and 93-0544). Rockville, MD: Agency for Health Care Policy and Research, Public Health Service, Department of Health and Human Services. 1993.

Chassin, M. R., Brook, R. H., & Park, R. E., et al. Variations in the use of medical and surgical services by the Medicare population. *N Engl J Med, 314* (5): 285–290. 1986.

Clinton, J.J. From the Agency for Health Care Policy and Research: Outcomes research—a way to improve medical practice. *JAMA, 266*: 15: 2057. 1991.

Depression Guideline Panel. *Depression in primary care: 1. detection and diagnosis. 2. treatment of major depression.* (AHCPR Pub. Nos. 93-0550, 93-0551, 93-0552, and 93-0553). Rockville, MD: Agency for Health Care Policy and Research, Public Health Service, U.S. Department of Health and Human Services. 1993.

Deyo, R. A., Cherkin, D., & Conrad D. The back pain outcome assessment team. *Health Services Res, 25*: 5: 733–737. 1990.

Deyo, R. A., Cherkin, D., Conrad, D., & Volinn, E. Cost, controversy, crisis: Low back pain in the health of the public. *Ann Rev Public Health, 12*: 141–156. 1991.

Eddy, D.M., & Billings, J. The quality of medical evidence: Implications for quality of care. *Health Affairs, 7,*1: 19–32. 1988.

Hoffman, R. M., Kent, D. L., & Deyo, R. A. Diagnostic accuracy and clinical utility of thermography for lumbar radiculopathy: A meta-analysis. *Spine, 16*: 623–628. 1991.

Javitt, J. C., Tielsch, J. M., Canner, J.K., Kolb, M. M., Sommer, A., & Steinberg, E. P. National outcomes of cataract extraction: Increased risk of retinal complications associated with Nd: YAG laser capsulotomy. *Ophthalmology, 99*: 1487–1498. 1992.

Javitt, J. C., Vitale, S., & McBean, A. M., et al. National outcomes of cataract extraction: Retinal detachment after inpatient surgery. *Ophthalmology, 98*: 896–902. 1991a.

Javitt, J. C., Vitale, S., & Krakauer, H. D., et al. Outcomes of inpatient cataract extraction: Endophthalmitis following inpatient surgery. *Arch Ophthalmology, 109*: 1085–1089. 1991b.

Krumholz, H. M., Pasternak, R. C., & Weinstein, M. C., et al. Cost effectiveness of thrombolytic therapy with Streptokinase in elderly patients with suspected acute myocardial infarction. *N Engl J Med, 327*: 7–13. 1992.

Lau, J., Antman, E. M., & Jimenez-Silva, J., et al. Cumulative meta-analysis of therapeutic trials for myocardial infarction. *N Engl J Med, 327*: 248–254. 1992.

Pashos, C. L., & McNeil, B. J. Consequences of variation in treatment for acute myocardial infarction. *Health Services Res, 25*: 5: 717–722. 1990.

Pressure Ulcers Guideline Panel. *Pressure ulcers in adults: Prediction and prevention; clinical practice guideline.* (AHCPR Pub. Nos. 92–0047, 0048, and 0050). Rockville, MD: Agency for Health Care Policy and Research, Public Health Service, U.S. Department of Health and Human Services. 1992.

Raskin, I. E., & Maklan, C. W. Medical treatment effectiveness research: A view from inside the Agency for Health Care Policy and Research. *Evaluation and the Health Professions*, June: 161–186. 1991.

Relman, A. S. Assessment and accountability: The third revolution in medical care. *N Engl J Med, 319*, 18: 1220–1222. 1988.

Roper, W. L., Winkenwerder, W., Hackbarth, G. M., & Krakauer, H. Effectiveness in health care: An initiative to evaluate and improve medical practice. *N Engl J Med, 319*, 18: 1197–1202. 1988.

Sickle Cell Disease Guideline Panel. *Sickle cell disease: Screening, diagnosis, management, and counseling in newborns and infants.* (AHCPR Pub. Nos. 93–0562, 93-0563 and 93-0564.) Rockville, MD: Agency for Health Care Policy and Research, Public Health Service, U.S. Department of Health and Human Services, 1993.

Steinberg, E. P., Bergner, M., & Sommer, A., et al. Variations in cataract management: Patient and economic outcomes. *Health Services Res, 25*(5): 727–731. 1990.

Turner, J. A., Ersek, M., Herron, L., Haselkorn, J. K., Kent, D. L., Ciol, M. A., & Deyo, R. A. Patient outcomes after lumbar spinal fusion: A comprehensive literature synthesis. *JAMA, 268*: 907–911. 1992.

Udvarhelyi, I. S., Gatsonis, C. G., & Pashos, C. L., et al. *Treatment and outcome of elderly patients with acute myocardial infarction.* Presentation at the annual meeting of the Society of General Internal Medicine, Seattle, WA, May 1991.

Urinary Incontinence Guideline Panel. *Urinary incontinence in adults*: Clinical practice guideline. (AHCPR Pub Nos. 92–0038, 0040, and 0041). Rockville, MD: Agency for Health Care Policy and Research, Public Health Service, U.S. Department of Health and Human Services. 1992.

Wennberg, J. E. On the status of the prostate disease assessment team. *Health Services Res, 25*(5): 709–716. 1990.

Wennberg, J. E. The paradox of appropriate care. *JAMA, 258*(18): 19–20. 1987.

Wennberg J. E., Freeman, J. L., & Culp, W. J. Are hospital services rationed in New Haven or over-utilized in Boston? *Lancet,* 8543: 1185–1189. 1987.

Wennberg, J. E., & Gittelsohn, A. Health care delivery in Maine: I. Patterns of use of common surgical procedures. *J Maine Med Assoc, 66*: 123–130, 149. 1975.

Index

Activities of daily living (ADLs),
  5
Acute myocardial infarction
  (AMI), 258–259
Advance directives, 76, 81, 84
Advanced cancer treatment
  aging and, 241–243
  approaches to, 244–248
  global organ function, 239–
    241
  outcome, 243–244
  toxicity and, 242–243
  types of, 237–239
Agency for Health Care Policy
    and Research (AHCPR)
  effectiveness research, 253,
    255, 257, 263–264
  topics addressed by, 263
Age-related changes tests, 20
Albumin
  levels of, 16
  screening tests, 33
Alcohol abuse, 13
Alpha coma, 155
Alzheimer's disease, 153–154
American Joint Committee on
    Cancer (AJCC), 215–216

Amyotrophic lateral sclerosis
    (ALS), 160
ANA test, 20
Androgen therapy, 229–231
Anemia, 13, 15, 29, 32
Angina, 120, 174
Angiodysplasia/arteriovenous
    malformations (AVM), 176
Angiography, 124, 162
Angioplasty, 124, 137
Ankle replacement, 198
Antiandrogens, 230
Antibiotic treatment, 59, 61
Anticoagulation, 176
Antiinflammatory medication,
    188
Aortic valve regurgitation (AR),
    138
Aortic valve stenosis (AS),
    137–138
Appliance feedings
  benefits and burdens of, 99
  defined, 96
  discomfort of, 100–101
  goal of, 97
  trial, 108
Arrhythmia, 118–120, 125

Arterial blood gases, 19, 27
Arthritis, treatment of, 187–188;
    see also specific types of
    arthritis
Aspiration, 97–98
Aspiration pneumonia
  feeding disability and, 98
  recurrent, 61–62
Assessment, see Geriatric patient
    assessment
Atherosclerosis
  coronary, 57
  dialysis and, 175
Aterosclerotic coronary artery
    disease (CAD), 135
Autoimmune system, 19–20
Automation, impact of, 20–23

B

Beck Depression Inventory, 6
Beneficence-autonomy conflict,
    79, 82–84, 99, 102
Benign prostatic hyperplasia
    (BPH), 159–160
Bilirubin, 18
Binswanger's disease, 152
Biochemical individuality, 25
Biopsy, 245
Biphosphonates, 51
Blood loss, 21
Bone density, measurement of,
    49–50
Bone loss, pathophysiology of, 49
Brain, aging of, 147–149
Brain lesions, 151, 155, 161
Breast cancer, 51–52

C

Calcitonin, 53
Calcitriol (1–25 dihydroxy
    vitamin D_3), 52
Calcium supplements, 52

Cancer, see also specific types of
    cancer
  advanced, treatment for, see
    Advanced cancer
    treatment
  anemia and, 13
  incidence of, 236
  systemic treatments, 238
Cardioplegia, 133
Cardiovascular disease, advanced
    diagnostic technology
  cardiac catheterization, 121,
    123–125
  cardiac magnetic resonance
    imaging, 120–121
  diagnostic imaging modalities
    comparison, 126
  echocardiography, 113–117
  Holter monitoring, 119–120
  intracardiac electrophysiologic
    studies, 125–126
  nuclear cardiac imaging,
    117–119
  stress testing, 112–113
Cardiovascular surgery
  cardiopulmonary bypass, 133
  coronary artery bypass
    long-term results, 136
    perioperative morbidity,
      135–136
    perioperative mortality, 135
  internal mammary artery,
    136–137
  myocardial protection,
    133–134
  percutaneous transluminal
    coronary angioplasty, 137
  percutaneous valvuloplasty,
    141
  risk factors, 134–135
  valvular surgery
    results of, 139–140
    types of, 137–139
Carotid endarterectomy, 58

Carotid studies, noninvasive, 161
Carpal tunnel syndrome, 180
Cataract PORT, 261–263
Catheterization, cardiac, 121, 123–125
Central pontine myelinolysis, 152
Cerebral angiography, 161–162
Computed tomography scan (CT), 149–151
Cerebrovascular disease, 150
Cervical spondylosis, 152
Charcot joint, 188
Chemistry tests, 15–19
Chemotherapy, 241–242
Cholesterol screening, 16–17, 29, 32
Chronic obstructive pulmonary disease (COPD), 29, 27–28, 156, 210–211
Chronologic age, 240
Cigarette smoking, 13
Clinical ethics, *see* Ethics
Clinical testing threshholds, 24
Cognitive function, aging process and, 147–148
Colon cancer, screening test, 32
Comorbidity, 111, 113, 246
Conduction system disease, 125
Contusions, 149
Coronary angiography, 127
Coronary artery bypass (CABG), 135–136
Coronary artery surgery registry study (CASS), 135–136
Cranial nerve testing, 148
Creatinine, 17–18, 29, 241–242
Creutzfeldt-Jakob disease, 152

D

Decision-making, by physician, 75–93, 105–106

Decision trees, 25
Defensive medicine
    generally, 70–73
    medical malpractice and, 67–70
Degenerative arthritis, 187–188, 201
Dehydration, 27, 32, 98–99, 102
Dementia
    depression, 155
    evaluation of, 155
    multiinfarct, 151, 156
Depression
    in dementia, 155
    sleep disturbance and, 157
Diabetes mellitus
    development of, 16
    screening for, 31–32
Diagnosis, laboratory testing and, 26. *See also specific conditions*
Dialysis
    end stage renal disease, 169
    expenditures for beneficiaries, 172–174, 183
    indications, 168
    medical complications
        cardiovascular, 174–176
        gastrointestinal, 176–177
        genitourinary, 180
        musculoskeletal, 180
        nutrition, 177–180
    quality of life and, 181–182
    rationing of, 182–183
Digital rectal examination (DRE), 216
Do Not Resuscitate policy, 106
Doppler flow mapping, 114
Doppler ultrasound, 114
Dying patients
    comforting, 78
    dealing with, 77
    treatment of, 76

E

Eastern Cooperative Oncology
    Group, 243
Eaton-lambert myasthenic
    syndrome, 159
Echocardiography, 112–117
Effectiveness research
  clinical practice guidelines,
    263–264
  federally sponsored
    appropriateness, 254–257
    cost-effectiveness, 254
    effectiveness, 254
    efficacy, 253–254
  progress of, 257–263
  rationality in health care,
    251–253
Elbow replacement, 200–201
Electroencephalography (EEG),
    154–156
Electrolytes
  aging process and, 17
  function of, 27, 32
Electromyography, 158–160
Elderly elderly, 33
Encephalopathy, 155
End stage renal disease (ESRD)
  demographics of, 169
  incidence, 169
  survival probabilities, 169–170,
    172
Endometrial cancer, 51
Endoscopic retrograde
    cholangiopancreatography
    (ERCP), 209
Environmental influences,
    significance of, 8
Enzymes, functioning of, 17–18
Epilepsy, 154–155
Erythrocyte sedimentation rate
    (ESR), 15
Estrogen replacement therapy,
    effect of, 50–51

Ethics
  life-sustaining technologies
    generally, 80–82
    guidelines for, 83
    tubal feedings, 105–108
Evoked potentials, 157–158
Exercise
  arthritis and, 188
  stress testing, 112–113

F

Falls, 60–61
Fecal occult blood (FOB),
    screening for, 33
Feeding disability, 96–98
Fluoride, 52–53
Follow-up testing, 26
Frail elderly
  cancer screening, 33
  defined, 12
  diagnosis for, 26
  laboratory testing and, 34–36

G

Gait disturbance, 148–149
Gallstone treatment
  cholecystectomy, 207–208
  common duct stones, 208–209
  options, 206–207
  results, 209
Gastrostomy feedings, 96–98
Geriatric Depression Scale
    (GDS), 6
Geriatric patient assessment
  environment, 8
  function, 5–6
  goals of, 2
  mental status, 6
  multidimensional, 1–4
  physical health, 4–5
  socioeconomic status, 6, 8
  structure of, 2

Gleason grading system, 216
Glucose tolerance test, 15
Gonadotropin releasing hormone
    (GnRH), 229–230

H

Health care, rationality in,
    251–253
Health care delivery, 45
Health care proxies, 76, 81
Heart disease, prevalence of, 132
Hematology tests, 13–15
Heparin, 54–55
Hepatitis, 60
Hernias, laparoscopy and, 210
Hip replacement
    overview, 191–193
    result of, 202
Holter monitoring, 119–120
Home care, 108
Hormones, functioning of, *see*
    specific hormones
Hospice care, 108
Hospital admissions, 47
Hyperlipidemia, 175
Hypertriglyceridemia, 175
Hypertension
    end stage renal disease (ESRD)
        and, 174
    isolated systolic, 55–57
    sleep studies and, 156
Hypoalbuminemia, 13, 15
Hypotension, 175–176
Hypothyroidism, 18, 160

I

Immunizations, 45
Immunoassay techniques, 22
Informed consent, 47–48
Instrumental activities of daily
    living (IADL), 5
Insulin, 16

Intelligence, changes in,
    147–148
Internal mammary artery (IMA),
    136–137
Intracardiac electrophysiologic
    studies, 125–126
Intradialytic parenteral nutrition
    (IDPN), 178

J

Joint Commission of
    Accreditation of Health
    Care Organizations
    (JCAHO), 106, 263
Joint replacement
    ankle, 198
    elbow, 200
    hip, 191–193, 202
    history of, 189–191
    knee, 193–198, 203
    shoulder, 200

K

Kevorkian, Dr., 75
Knee replacement
    overview, 193–194, 196, 198
    results of, 203

L

Laboratory tests
    advances in, 10–11
    diagnosis and, 26
    follow-up, 26
    interpretation of, 25
    newer analyzers, accuracy of,
        21–22
    normal values, 11–13
    prognosis and, 26
    purposes and usefulness of, 26
    screening tests, 29–34
    specific tests

Laboratory tests, specific tests
(*continued*)
  types of, 13–20
  usefulness of, 27–29
  specimen size, 21
  steps in, 23–26
Laparoscopic surgery
  development of, 205–206
  as gallstone treatment
    cholecystectomy, 207–208
    common duct stones,
      208–209
    options, 206–207
    results, 209
  significance of, 205–206
  types of, 209–210
Laser hemotology analyzers, 22
Life expectancy
  active, 44
  advanced cancer treatment,
    247
  laboratory testing and, 24–25
  prostatic cancer and, 225–226
  screening tests and, 30
Life-sustaining technologies
  benefits and burdens,
    assessment of, 82–84
  case studies, 87–93
  clinical ethics, 80–82
  decision-making, 80–82
  dilemmas, examples of, 76–77
  physician's role in, 84–87
Litigation, *see* Medical
  malpractice
Liver function, 17
Living Wills, 76, 81
Low back pain PORT, 260–261
Lumbar puncture, 162–163

M

Magnesium levels, significance
  of, 18

Magnetic resonance angiography,
  162
Magnetic resonance imaging
  cardiac, 120–121
  neurological disorders,
    151–152
Malignancy, screening for, 32–33.
  See also Biopsy
Malnutrition, 177–178
Medicaid, 8, 81
Medical history, significance of, 4
Medical jargon, 85–86
Medical malpractice
  elements of, 67–69
  older patients as plaintiffs, 69–70
  risk management, 24
Medical Treatment Effectiveness
  Program (MEDTEP), 253,
  255–257
Medicare, 76, 81, 173–174
Mental status, assessment of, 6
Mitral valve regurgitation, 139
Mitral valve stenosis, 138–139
Motor function, aging process
  and, 148
Motor neuron disease, 160
Movement disorders, 150
Multichannel chemistry
  autoanalyzers, 22
Multidimensional assessment,
  1–4
Multidimensional assessment
  instruments, 3–4
Multiinfarct dementia, 151, 156
Multiple sclerosis, 152
Muscle diseases, 159–160
Myasthenia gravis, 159
Myelography, 153
Myopathies, 159–160

N

Nasogastric feedings, 96–98
Negligence, 68–70

Nerve conduction studies,
158–160
Neurological disorder, diagnostic
tests
cerebral angiography, 161–162
computed tomography scan
(CT), 149–151
electroencephalography (EEG),
154–156
electromyography, 158–160
evoked potentials, 157–158
lumbar puncture, 162–163
magnetic resonance
angiography, 162
magnetic resonance imaging,
151–152
myelography, 153
nerve conduction studies,
158–160
noninvasive carotid studies,
161
positron emission tomography,
153–154
radioscope cisternography,
160–161
single photon emission
computed tomography
(SPECT), 153
sleep studies, 156–157
transcranial Doppler studies,
162
Neuromuscular transmission
disorders, 159
Nocturia, 157
Normal aging
insulin resistance, 16
neurological changes in,
147–149
sleep studies and, 156–157
Normal pressure hydrocephalus
(NPH), 151, 160–161
Nuclear cardiac imaging,
117–119
Nutrition

albumin levels, 29
appliance feeding and, 105
deficiency, *see* Tube feeding
dialysis and, 177, 179
laboratory testing and, 33–34

O

Obesity, 30, 156–157, 187
Ondine's curse, 157
Organ function, 240, 246
Organ Systems Coordinating
Center (OSCC), 216
Osteoarthritis
predisposing factors of, 188
treatment of, 188
Osteoporosis, prevention of,
48–53

P

Parathyroid hormone, 52
Parkinson's disease, 97, 154
Patient autonomy, 80–81, 102
Patient Outcomes Research
Teams (PORTS), 257
Patient Self-Determination Act
(PSDA), 81, 84
Pelvic lympadenectomy, 226
Percutaneous transluminal
coronary angioplasty, 137
Performance status evaluation,
240
Peripheral neuropathy, 159
Persistent vegetative state (PVS),
100–101
Phosphorous, 17
Physical examination, 4–5
Physical health, evaluation of,
4–5
Physician
decision-making, 75–93,
105–106

Physician (*continued*)
litigation, *see* Medical
malpractice
medical training, 78, 85
Physiologic age, 240
Plebotomy, 21
Polymyositis, 160
Positron emission tomography
(PET)
cardiovascular disease, 118
neurological disorders and,
153–154
Postradiation necrosis, 152
Pretest probability, 24
Pretest prognosis, 24
Prevention, types of, 45
Primary prevention, 45, 57
Progesterone, 51
Prognosis, laboratory testing
and, 26; *See also specific
conditions*
Progressive multifocal
leukoencephalopathy
(PML), 152
Prophylactic therapies
aspiration pneumonia,
recurrent, 61–62
falls and associated injuries,
60–61
informed consent, 47–48
isolated systolic hypertension,
55–57
osteoporosis prevention, 48–53
overview, 44–47
pulmonary embolus, 53–55
significant debility, nosology of,
46
stroke prevention, 57–58
thrombophlebitis, 53–55
tuberculosis, 59–60
urinary tract infection, 58–59
Prostate disease PORT, 259–260
Prostate, anatomy of, 214–215
Prostate specific antigene (PSA)

cancer diagnosis and, 218–220,
222–224
screening for, 32–33
Prostatic cancer
incidence of, 214
screening and diagnosis of, 216,
218–220, 222–224
staging, 224–225
treatment
advanced disease, 228–231
organ-confined disease,
225–228
Prostheses
ankle, 198
hip replacement, 191–193
history of, 189–191
knee replacement, 196, 198
MEDLINE search, 202
shoulder replacement, 200
Protein, screening tests and, 33
Prothrombin, 55
Pulmonary embolus, 53–55

Q

Quality control, 10
Quality of life, 136, 181–182

R

Radiation, effect of, 226
Radical prostatectomy, 226–227
Radiculopathies, 158–159
Radionuclide scintigraphy, 112
Radionuclide ventriculography
(RVG), 117
Radioscope cisternography,
160–161
Radiotherapy, 231
Reflexes, aging process and, 148
Renal disease, anemia and, 13;
See also End stage renal
disease (ESRD)
Renal osteodystrophy, 180

Restless leg syndrome, 157
RF test, 20

S

Screening tests, overview, 29–34
Secondary prevention, 45, 57, 59
Senile gait, 148–149
Sensitivity analysis, 25
Sensory examination, 148
Shoulder replacement, 200
Significant debility, nosology of, 46
Silent ischemia, 120
Single photon emission computed tomography (SPECT), 118, 153
Sleep apnea, 156–157
Sleep disturbances, 156–157
Socioeconomic status, significance of, 6, 8
Specimens, size of, 21
Spinal cord, evaluation of, 152
Spoon feeding, 100, 103–104
Staging, 245–246
Steroids, 160
Stress testing, 112–113
Stroke
  blood pressure and, 56
  feeding disability and, 97
  prevention of, 57–58
Subdural hematomas, 151
Successful aging, 44
Surrogacy, 102–104
Swallowing apraxia, 97
Systolic Hypertension in Elderly Program (SHEP), 56–57

T

Tertiary prevention, 45, 57
Test ordering, 23–25
Testosterone, 229–230
Thallium imaging, 118

Thromboembolism, 53
Thyroid dysfunction, 160
Thyroid function, screening test, 18, 32
Thyrotropic hormone (TSH), 18
Tracers
  infarct-avid, 119
  perfusion, 118
Transcranial Doppler ultrasonography (TCD), 162
Transesophageal echocardiography (TEE), 114, 116–117
Transient ischemic attacks, 57
Transrectal ultrasonography (TRUS), 216, 220, 224
Transthoracic echocardiography, 114–115
Trauma, 205, 211
Tricuspid valve regurgitation, 139
Tube feeding
  arguments regarding, 104–105
  autonomy, limitations of, 102
  background of, 96–98
  beneficence, limitations of, 102
  decision-making process, 101–102, 105–108
  ethics, 105–108
  as medical treatment, 98–100
  persistent vegetative state and, 100–101
  risks, 108
  surrogacy limitations, 102–104
Tuberculin sensitivity, 20, 34
Tuberculosis, testing for, 59–60
Tumors, detection of, 151–152

U

Ulcers, rectal, 177
Urinalysis, 33
Urinary tract infection, 58–59

Urine culture, 20
Uterine cancer, 51

V

Valvular surgery
    results of, 139–140
    types of, 137–139

Videofluoroscopy, 97
Vitamin deficiency, 19, 36

Z

Zung Self-Rating Depression
    Scale, 6